Communication Disability in the Dementias

Communication Disability in the Dementias

Edited by

Karen Bryan PhD
University of Surrey

and

Jane Maxim PhD
University College London

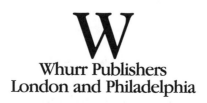

Whurr Publishers
London and Philadelphia

Other Wiley Editorial Offices

John Wiley & Sons Inc., 111 River Street, Hoboken, NJ 07030, USA

Jossey-Bass, 989 Market Street, San Francisco, CA 94103-1741, USA

Wiley-VCH Verlag GmbH, Boschstr. 12, D-69469 Weinheim, Germany

John Wiley & Sons Australia Ltd, 42 McDougall Street, Milton, Queensland 4064, Australia

John Wiley & Sons (Asia) Pte Ltd, 2 Clementi Loop #02-01, Jin Xing Distripark,
Singapore 129809

John Wiley & Sons Canada Ltd, 22 Worcester Road, Etobicoke, Ontario, Canada
M9W 1L1

Wiley also publishes its books in a variety of electronic formats. Some content that
appears in print may not be available in electronic books.

A catalogue record for this book is available from the British Library

ISBN -13   978-1-86156-506-8
ISBN -10   1-86156-506-2

Printed and bound in Great Britain by TJ International Ltd, Padstow, Cornwall

This book is printed on acid-free paper responsibly manufactured from sustainable
forestry in which at least two trees are planted for each one used for paper production.

Contents

Preface

This book was preceded by *Communication Disability and the Psychiatry of Old Age*, published in 1994. When the publisher approached us to consider a second edition it was quickly agreed that this would be inappropriate because the field had advanced substantially in relation to speech and language therapy (SLT) practice, as a result of the growing awareness of the need to treat older people appropriately and substantial advances in the diagnosis and treatment of the dementias. We have therefore approached this volume with a fresh brief and have faced some challenges in terms of the material to include. One challenge is that language and communication are not just the business of SLT, and, quite rightly so, both are considered to be the business of all staff involved with people who have mental health difficulties. We have tried to reflect this issue by including a chapter on team approaches and by urging authors to clarify the exact role of SLTs within older people's mental health services. We hope that these measures will increase the relevance of the book to all members of the multidisciplinary team. A second issue is that of evidence for SLT intervention. When the previous book was published, there was very little evidence, but now there is a more substantial body of research, and given the drive for evidence-based practice, we have encouraged authors to include the relevant research within their chapters. This leads to a possible charge of repetition, but we make no apology for our approach, rather drawing the reader's attention to the consistency of evidence across different parts of the world and across different aspects of the field of older people's mental health.

We have included a chapter on developing new services for older people's mental health and extending existing ones. This represents a challenge for the SLT profession (or indeed any other specialist therapy or rehabilitation services) and requires us to convince commissioners, service managers and colleagues within the multidisciplinary team that a service such as SLT is necessary. However, this is essential if current service inequities are to be resolved. The focus should not be on a service such as SLT itself, but rather on what older people with mental health difficulties require to maintain their independence and to minimize the effects of degenerative disease processes for as long as possible. There is little research which examines the effectiveness of a service such as SLT within the multidisciplinary team. The next major challenge for researchers and research funders is to address this issue.

We are very grateful to all the contributors who have responded to our requests, queries and editorial suggestions with patient goodwill. We owe a great debt to Mrs Enid Tubbs who has assisted us with formatting and tables as well as undertaking the mammoth task of checking all the references. We would also like to thank our colleagues at the University of Surrey and University College London for their support. Our families have, of course, largely ignored our need for time and space to work on the book, as indeed they should!

Karen Bryan and Jane Maxim
April 2005

Contributors

Kate Allan has a background in clinical psychology where she worked in mental health services for adults and older adults for 5 years. She then took up a research post at the Dementia Services Development Centre in the University of Stirling to carry out a study exploring ways for practitioners to consult people with dementia about their views of services. More recent work has investigated the needs of deaf/hard of hearing people with dementia, and how we can communicate with people with very advanced dementia.

Colin Barnes MA, BSc, MRCSLT has worked as a specialist in elderly mental health in Portsmouth for the past 10 years. He also coordinates a regional training organization for dementia care workers, has initiated an activity service for hospital inpatients and runs a dementia carers group. Colin has a particular interest in working with carers and has carried out postgraduate research into the effectiveness of providing specific communication advice for carers of people with dementia. He has also published a presentation/training tool for working with dementia carers on specific communication issues and has participated in a Cochrane review of the literature supporting interventions for dementia carers.

Karen Bryan is a Professor of Clinical Practice at the European Institute of Health and Medical Sciences, University of Surrey. She previously established a specialist NHS speech and language therapy service for older people in Bristol. She continues to practice as a consultant therapist in forensic mental health. Her current research interests include development of the Barnes Language Assessment, care sector training and education and practice development for the healthcare workforce.

Dr **Vari Drennan** is a primary care nurse and senior lecturer in the Primary Care Nursing Research Unit at the Royal Free & University College Medical School. Her clinical work and research interests have focused on the health of older people in primary care since the early 1980s. She is co-author with Dr Steve Iliffe of *Primary Health Care of Older People* (2000), published by Oxford University Press and *Primary Care and Dementia* (2001), published by Jessica Kingsley Publishers.

Helen Griffiths started working as a speech and language therapist in mental health services for older people in 1985 and as part of her post-graduate study undertook training in the neuropsychology of the dementias. She has published in the areas of language disorder in dementia and service delivery.

Mary Heritage is a RCSLT advisor on Older People and has a particular interest in communication and eating/drinking difficulties associated with dementia. She is the manager of the Southern Derbyshire SLT service.

Jennifer Horner PhD JD is an associate professor in the College of Health Professions, Medical University of South Carolina where she serves as Program Director of Communication Sciences and Disorders, and Chair of the Department of Rehabilitation Sciences. She holds a doctorate in speech-language pathology (University of Florida, Gainesville) and a law degree (Boston University). Her past research spans aphasia, neglect, dementia and dysphagia; her current interests include research ethics, clinical ethics, and legal and health policy issues affecting the health professions.

Dr **Steve Iliffe** is a general practitioner in Kilburn, London, and Reader in General Practice at the Royal Free & University College Medical School. His research interests are in health in later life, particularly dementia and depression, and he is on the editorial boards of *Aging & Mental Health*, the *Journal of Dementia Care* and *Geriatric Medicine*.

Jackie Kindell is a specialist speech and language therapist working with people with dementia in Stockport (Pennine Care NHS Trust). She also manages the therapy team within the old age psychiatry department including occupational therapy, physiotherapy and activity services. Jackie is an advisor to the Royal College of Speech and Language Therapists in the area of mental health in older people and has published work previously on dysphagia in dementia.

Jane Maxim is Head of Department and Professor of Language Pathology at the Department of Human Communication Science at University College London. She has a particular interest in language breakdown in different forms of dementia.

David Neary is Professor of Neurology at the Neuroscience Centre, Hope Hospital, Manchester. He is head of the Cerebral Function Unit, which provides a diagnostic service for early onset dementias. His special interests are in the cognitive and behavioural consequences of degenerative brain disease and their neurobiological substrate.

Claire G. Nicholl BSc FRCP DGM is a consultant physician in medicine for the elderly at Addenbrooke's Hospital, Cambridge and an associate lecturer at the University of Cambridge. She developed her special interest in dementia while working with Professor Brice Pitt in the memory clinic at the Hammersmith Hospital.

Victoria Ramsey has worked as a speech and language therapist in Mental Health services in South West London for nearly 10 years. During this time she has managed specialist SLT services to mental health and was project lead for a redefinition of local health and social service provision for older people. She is on the working group for the development of the Barnes Language Assessment and is a visiting lecturer in Mental Health to the SLT course at City University.

Danielle N. Ripich PhD is Dean of the College of Health Professions and Professor of Rehabilitation Sciences and Neurosciences at Medical University of South Carolina. Dr Ripich's FOCUSED program was given the American Society of Aging's Award for Best Clinical Practices. She has edited the *Handbook of Geriatric Communication Disorders* and written numerous articles and chapters on discourse and Alzheimer's disease.

Julie Snowden PhD is a consultant neuropsychologist attached to the Cerebral Function Unit, Greater Manchester Neuroscience Centre, Hope Hospital, which provides a diagnostic service for early-onset dementias. Her special interests are in focal dementia syndromes, particularly those associated with disorders of language.

Susan Stevens is a speech and language therapy manager with wide clinical, teaching and research experience. She established a service for older people across acute and community sectors in Hammersmith, and while managing the service in Hammersmith Hospitals NHS Trust continued clinical and research work in the Memory Clinic at Hammersmith Hospital. Her present commitments include research on the development of the Barnes Language Assessment.

CHAPTER 1

Health, ageing and the context of care

KAREN BRYAN AND JANE MAXIM

Population issues

Across the EU, people over 65 form 17% of the population (ONS 2002a). The UK had a population of 59.2 million at the last census in 2001. For the first time, people over 60 form a larger part of the population (21%) than children under 16 (20%). There has also been a large increase in the number of people over 85: now 1.1 million, which is 2% of the population. In England and Wales there are 336 000 people aged 90 and over, and of these nearly 4000 are providing 50 or more hours of care to another family friend or carer.

Older people receive a large proportion of health and social care spending. In 2000, £28 billion were spent on hospital and community care with nearly two-fifths of this spend on people aged 56 and over (ONS 2001). In England and Wales, 5.2 million people provide informal care, including a million who provide more than 50 hours a week and 1.6 million who are in full-time work.

A major public health issue for the next century is the increase in the number of older people in the UK from ethnic minority groups (OPCS 1993). As of 2000, the largest ethnic group was Indian (984 000 people), then Caribbean and African descent (969 000) and Pakistani and Bangladeshi descent (932 000). Initiatives for these groups have tended to focus on physical health, and this together with the traditional stigma of mental illness in some ethnic groups has led to the relative neglect of older people from ethnic minorities (Rait et al. 1996). The term 'triple jeopardy' has been used to describe the challenges of racism, ageism and in some cases socio-economic deprivation faced by older people from ethnic minority backgrounds (Norman 1985).

Who are older people and where do they live?

Single-pensioner households make up 14.4% of all households, and more than two thirds of these have no access to a car. Many older people live alone: 52.5% of women and 25.7% of men aged 75–84, and 54.5% of women and 36.9% of men aged 85 and over.

The number of places in residential care for older people peaked at 247 000 in 1998, but fell to 237 000 in 2001 due to a levelling off of places available in the private sector and continued reduction in public sector places (ONS 2002b). Around 2 million children or children-in-law provide informal care to older adults living in another household and that figure has remained relatively stable between 1985 and 1995, although there has been a shift from children as the most likely carers to spouses. However there has been a 25% decline in intergenerational care within the same home. This is thought to be associated with trends such as more women working outside the home and the previous rise in institutional care (Pickard 2002).

Attitudes to older people and their health

Greengross et al. (1997) described ageing as a subject that should be top of world agendas. There are more older people living longer with increasingly fewer resources to care for them. Shifts in government policy in developed countries have encouraged preservation of independence. Emphasis is being placed upon providing support to enable people to live with age-related degenerative conditions such as dementia (Benbow and Reynolds 2000). Care of older people is a recognized specialism within medicine and other health professions. Another positive development is that age discrimination is considered a negative factor to be avoided and age is not now a valid criterion to restrict access to services (National Service Framework for Older People, DH 2001). Much has been written about the benefits of preventive care and the need to manage degenerative difficulties rather than accept them as an inevitable consequence of older age. For example, the effects of reduced hearing on communication and psychosocial functioning are recognized (Heine and Browning 2002) and studies have shown that intensive support for older people with hearing difficulty produces significant improvements in social functioning (Sherbourne et al. 2002).

The boundary between cognitive changes associated with normal ageing and those associated with dementia is accepted as unclear (Figure 1.1). The Nun study showed that education may function as a buffer to protect against the effects of dementia on ageing (Snowdon et al. 1996). However, the study also showed that pathological changes associated with Alzheimer's disease are present in the brains of those older sisters who do not show dementia, suggesting that other factors such as environment and lifestyle may mediate in pathological processes (Stern et al. 1994). These findings are helpful in encouraging professionals to take positive attitudes towards the support and care of older people with dementia. In Chapter 3 we look at the contribution of general practice and in Chapter 9 at measures to support carers; Chapter 7 examines whole-system approaches to dementia.

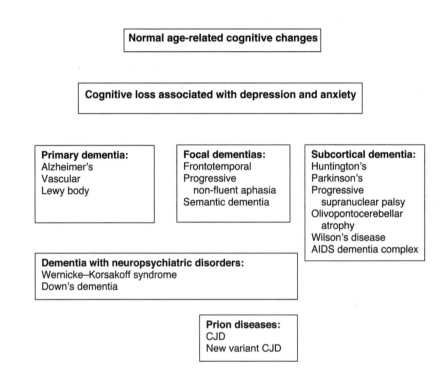

Figure 1.1 Cognitive changes in normal ageing and dementia.

Overview of language and ageing

Age-related reduction in cognitive functioning (including language) has received much attention in recent years (see Nussbaum et al. 1996 for a review of ageing and communication). The traditional view of decline in functioning across the board has long since been shown to be an inaccurate and simplistic view. Losses and gains are now considered, with age-related decline often a function of the exact task. For instance, recognition of pictures and completion of word stems have been convincingly shown to be age-invariant memory tasks (Park 2000). Salthouse (1991) described four mechanisms hypothesized to account for age-related differences in cognitive functioning:

- speed at which information is processed
- working memory function
- inhibitory function (affecting the ability to focus by inhibiting unwanted information)
- sensory function.

These factors need to be distinguished from actual changes in language functioning. The effects of health problems such as cardiac or peripheral vascular disease on cognitive functioning also need to be distinguished from normal ageing (Elwood et al. 2002).

A further important factor is individual variation. Parameters such as education, experience and cognitive style will influence the effects of ageing. Christensen (2001) reported, from an extensive longitudinal study of older people in Australia, that education, good health, genetic factors (such as absence of the APOE epsilon4 allele) and activity were protective of cognitive decline, and that diversity in cognitive ageing suggests that more than one process may be operating to produce cognitive decline. Butler et al. (2004) reviewed the evidence for cognitive decline in normal ageing and concluded that social engagement, intellectual stimulation and physical activity play a key role in maintaining cognitive health and preventing cognitive decline. Factors such as circadian rhythms may also influence processing. Yoon (1997) found that older people's preference for reading the paper and shopping first thing in the morning related to their tendency to be more energetic and mentally alert in the morning.

Age-related changes in cognitive functioning may also result in developmental 'gains' (Dixon 2000):

- Gains despite or independent of constraints provided by losses, e.g. logical, abstract thinking (Sinnott 1996) and the concept of 'wisdom' (Baltes and Staudinger 1993) are thought to emerge post young adulthood.
- Gains as losses of a lesser magnitude, i.e. that some consolation may be taken from cognitive losses that emerge later than expected, at a level less than feared or predicted or at a level that does not impair everyday skills. For example, the Seattle study suggested that 90% of older people in four age groups maintain at least two intellectual abilities (Schaie 1996).
- Gains as a function of losses, i.e. occasioned by losses or that compensate for losses, for example, collaborative experiences during assisted performance (Dixon and Gould 1998).

Attention is a complex area, with no evidence for older people having an automatic decline and assessment findings very much reflecting exact task demands. There is some evidence that older people have difficulty in directing attention, but the exact effects of ageing versus pathology on attention remain uncertain (Perry and Hodges 1999).

Memory is also a complex area of cognition, with considerable interaction between variables such as task demands, familiarity and mode of response (see Stevens et al. 1999). Craik (2000) summarizes what professionals dealing with older people should be aware of in terms of memory functioning, particularly during assessment. It should be expected that older people might be less accurate in recalling recent events, especially if these involve specific details of time and place. Telephone conversations or interviews should avoid complex instructions or questions. Priming effects may have more influence for older people, e.g. providing examples may bias older respondents' choice of answers. Reduced perceptual clarity (visual or auditory) may reduce immediate memory for initial alternatives in a multiple-choice format. The decline in working memory capacity may also bias answers to the most recently presented alternative. Repetition of information may result in that information being viewed more favourably.

Older people may also have sensory losses that affect communication functioning. Age-related decline in hearing (presbycusis) is very common, with 2.5 million people in the UK over the age of 70 thought to have hearing impairment that would benefit from an aid (Hanratty and Lawlor 2000). See Chisholm et al. 2003 for a review of age-related deafness. There are also age-related changes in relation to speech perception. Wingfield (2000) highlighted four important principles relating to adult ageing and spoken language comprehension. The extent to which these broad principles are important to any older individual will depend on their individual profile:

- Older people will use top-down information drawn from linguistic context to supplement an impoverished bottom-up signal (as do younger people under difficult listening conditions). Provision of contextual information will therefore assist comprehension.
- Older people have difficulty in processing speech structures that place a burden on working memory. Therefore long sentences, sentences whose comprehension requires memory for referents that occurred far previously in the passage and sentences with high prepositional density or complex syntax should be avoided.
- Normal prosody (intonation, timing and stress) assists older listeners by aiding the rapid detection of the linguistic structure and the semantic focus of an utterance. Exaggerated prosody (often associated with 'elderspeak') should be avoided (Brown and Draper 2003).
- Pausing at natural processing units (such as sentences and clauses) allows additional time for speech processing and increases comprehension relative to rapid speech.

Age invariance (preservation of a skill despite ageing) has been demonstrated for many aspects of language comprehension and production (Kemper and O'Hanlon 2000). Where age-related changes occur, for example in the comprehension of complex syntax, these reductions are hypothesized to reflect working memory constraints. More recent studies suggest that immediate syntactic processing is age-invariant, although post-interpretive processes required for text integration and discourse comprehension may be vulnerable to age-related working memory reduction (Kemtes and Kemper 1997). Older people tend to adopt strategies of parsing text into smaller units and utilizing background information, resulting in few difficulties in processing narrative prose (Radvansky and Curiel 1998).

For language production, ageing is associated with sensory changes such as dry mouth and muscular changes that result in slowing of motor production. These changes should be regarded as contributing to reductions in efficiency rather than deficits (Xue et al. 2001). Changes in dentition, particularly ill fitting dentures and absent teeth or dentures, can also affect speech production (Roessler 2003).

It is important to exclude other possible reasons for a cognitive impairment before assuming a deficit or a reduction in functioning. For example, older people tend to take more medication than younger people, and are more prone to medication side effects (Swift 2003). Drugs which work on the central nervous system, such as some analgesics and sleeping medications, may depress cognitive functioning and may affect testing.

However, recent research has also shown that older people's daily capabilities often appear not to reflect the age-related 'decline' discussed above (Park and Gutchess 2000). There is considerable evidence that older people function well in most aspects of daily life and work. Two aspects of the ageing cognitive system appear to facilitate functioning:

• Knowledge is maintained across the lifespan and may even increase (Echt et al. 1998), providing an extensive knowledge base for problem-solving and addressing the needs of everyday life.
• Frequent and familiar behaviours become automatized and therefore require little cognitive recourses to perform (Jacoby et al. 1996).

Thus older people can successfully cope with the cognitive demands of complex medication regimes. Park et al. (1999) showed that older people made fewer errors than middle aged people in taking medication for rheumatoid arthritis. Literature is also emerging on positive advantages to older people of working (Park 1994), and on their ability to perform at a high level particularly where they are expert or in a familiar environment and where they continue to train and update their skills (Salthouse et al. 1996).

Recent approaches to older people with dementia

Drug therapies have demonstrated benefits for people with Alzheimer's disease. Studies have assessed benefits of drug therapies in terms of cognitive function, global severity, behaviour, activities of daily living and burden of care. At present the benefits of various drugs are being researched (Birks and Harvey 2003, Areosa Sastre et al. 2004, Loy and Schneider 2004). The NICE appraisal consultation document on donepezil, rivastigmine, galantamine and memantine suggests that the effects are limited and do not assist all patients (NICE 2005). However, there is now renewed interest in demonstrating the benefits of behavioural and psychological interventions (see Clare and Woods 2001 for a review of cognitive rehabilitation).

The concept of treatment has though challenged traditional assumptions that people with dementia cannot be treated. Rehabilitation for older people has been firmly enshrined in the NHS Plan for older people (DH 2000) and researchers are beginning to recognize the relevance of cognitive rehabilitation for people with dementia (Camp and Mattern 1999). Clare and Woods (2001) state that:

> defining rehabilitation as a process of active change aimed at enabling people who are disabled by injury or disease to achieve an optimal level of physical, psychological and social function implies a focus on maximizing functioning across a whole range of areas including physical health, psychological well-being, living skills, and social relationships. Such an approach is just as important for people with dementia and other progressive disorders as it is for people with non-progressive acquired brain injury. (pp. 193–194)

Bayles and Esther (2003) also advocate the value of behavioural interventions to enhance communicative functioning for people with dementia. Alternatives to the medical model of dementia, for example Kitwood's dialectal model (Kitwood 1997; see Chapters 7 and 8 for more information on Kitwood's approach) and Sabat's social constructionist model (Sabat 1994), give a theoretical basis for an approach to dementia that addresses the needs of people with dementia and their carers, taking into account the influence of biology, individual psychology, and social environment. Hagberg (1997) suggests that intervention should aim to enhance coping skills and self-efficacy, combat threats to self esteem and help the person with dementia to make the best possible use of their individual resources. The evidence base for interventions aimed at enhancing language and communication is beginning to emerge.

The evidence base for speech and language therapy intervention in dementia

In the following sections, the evidence for speech and language therapy (SLT) interventions is discussed, considering reduction or mediation of the losses and programmes designed to enhance language for patients with dementia. Interventions designed for carers and the issues involved in working with people with dementia via carers are discussed in Chapter 9.

Mediation of functional losses

In vascular dementia, improvement in language ability and new learning can occur when the disease process is controlled (Swinburn and Maxim 1996) (see Chapter 4). Communication in semantic dementia can be maintained and enhanced by specific interventions such as utilizing the beneficial effects of personally relevant autobiographical memory and retraining concepts within a personally relevant context (Snowden and Griffiths 2000) (see Chapter 5). Communication difficulties in Korsakoff's dementia associated with memory difficulties have been shown to respond to a validation approach to communication management where all behaviour is treated as having meaning and involves responding positively to what a person says (Bryan and Maxim 1998). The possibility of treatment, particularly drug treatments for Alzheimer's disease, has given new impetus to the need for accurate and early assessment and has helped to challenge excessively negative associations about dementia (see Chapter 6).

There are indications that language processing deficits in some dementias may be due to difficulty in accessing information such as vocabulary rather than to complete loss of such information (Bayles et al. 1991, Nebes and Halligan 1996, Arkin et al. 2000). For example, in the semantic (or meaning) system, people with probable Alzheimer's disease may be able to recognize items that they cannot name and may be able to classify them according to semantic categories (e.g. animals versus flowers), therefore indicating preservation of underlying knowledge (Maxim et al. 2000). Priming or cueing by providing relevant information have therefore been established as ways of assisting naming. Recent work also shows that access to the semantic system can be maintained in Alzheimer's disease despite disease progression (Bell et al. 2000, Maxim et al. 2000).

Arkin et al. (2000), in a multiple baseline study, demonstrated significant explicit learning, as well as implicit learning and semantic activation in a group of people with probable Alzheimer's disease, who participated in an eight-session programme. Some were able to name previously unnamed items and all produced new vocabulary items which had not been used in the programme. Arkin (1998), Arkin et al. (2000) and Arkin and Mahendra (2000) have used similar techniques to demonstrate recall and recognition of world and autobiographical events. Mahendra (2001) published a detailed review of interventions for improving the communicative performance of individuals with Alzheimer's disease. Hopper et al. (1998), using a more controversial intervention, found that giving dolls and soft toys to people with probable Alzheimer's disease had an effect on the relevance of their communication. In a case study design, four women produced significantly more relevant information when toys were present.

Other studies have examined the effectiveness of modification of communication to improve communication with people with dementia. Experimental studies have demonstrated that people with probable Alzheimer's disease have difficulty understanding if syntax is complex or sentences have a greater number of words (Kempler et al. 1998); both repetition and rephrasing may be useful techniques in the therapeutic repertoire but require that the person with probable Alzheimer's disease is given time to process and respond. Ripich et al. (1999) found that giving a choice of answers or asking questions requiring only a yes/no response resulted in better conversation with people with probable Alzheimer's disease than open-ended questions. Small et al. (2003), in an empirical assessment of strategies recommended to families of people with probable Alzheimer's disease, found that simplified sentences and yes/no questions produced significantly more effective communication but slow speech did not improve communicative outcome.

Effective communication programmes for patients

Not all communication interventions are necessarily implemented by speech and language therapists and, indeed, given the limited SLT resource, delivering a programme is more likely to fall within the remit of care workers assisting health professionals (see Chapter 7 for a discussion of whole-team approaches to communication in dementia and the interface between these approaches and the specific interventions provided by SLT). Delivering such programmes requires that an appropriate skill mix is available within the multidisciplinary team. Powell (2000) reviews the evidence for the value of communication and discusses efficacy issues, stating that:

> an overall aim of intervention should be to improve 'quality of life' – a notoriously complicated outcome to measure.

Studies of the efficacy of a specific intervention in dementia are seldom carried out to the high standard of randomized controlled trials, but Bourgeois (1991), who conducted an extensive review of the diverse literature relating to the treatment of communication disorders in dementia, concluded that, despite the heterogeneous populations involved, positive outcomes had been reported.

Cochrane reviews are drawing together research that suggests reality orientation and reminiscence are of value (Spector and Orrell 1999, Spector et al. 1999, see also Spector et al. 2003) while the position on validation therapy is not clear (Neal and Briggs 2003) (see Chapter 8 for discussion of these techniques).

However, reviewing evidence that specifically addresses SLT involvement shows that SLT-managed intervention in the dementias may enhance communication. Clark (1995) called for a paradigm shift to move from a focus on skill improvement per se to a broader quality of life orientation, although there is still a need to address the efficacy of such programmes.

Shadden (1995) describes the application of discourse analysis to planning communication interventions in long-term care settings. Orange et al. (1995) describe the application of a communication enhancement model for people with Alzheimer's disease in a single case study. Bourgeois et al. (1997), in a multiple baseline study, trained caregivers to use written cues to reduce repetitive verbal behaviours over a 12 week period and found that carers still maintained use of the cues 6 months after the study. In a single-case study, Brush and Camp (1998) demonstrated that a similar technique was effective in a feeding programme. Burgio et al. (2001) found that care assistants specifically trained to conduct individually tailored communication skill enhancement programmes could improve and maintain communication skills without increasing the amount of time delivering care.

Mahendra and Arkin (2003) showed that a comprehensive cognitive linguistic intervention programme for people with mild to moderate Alzheimer's disease administered by students who were trained and supported by speech and language therapists resulted in maintained or improved performance on multiple discourse outcome measures. Mahendra and Arkin (2003) and Maxim et al. (2001) suggest that speech and language therapists have a valuable role as trainers and supervisors of non-professional rehabilitation partners.

Orange and Ryan (2000) mention the importance of communication between patients with dementia and their physicians, and suggest that speech and language therapists can be effective in enabling other professionals to modify their communication to address the needs of people with dementia. Such evidence suggests that speech and language therapists have a role in assisting other professionals to achieve effective communication with patients who have dementia.

More information on SLT intervention is given in other chapters of the book relating specifically to different forms of dementia (see Chapters 5, 7, 8 and 10). In Chapter 11 the evidence base for SLT intervention is given from an American perspective, reflecting much similarity of approach and an international perspective on the evidence, as would be expected with electronic databases and a willingness to learn from the good practice in other settings.

The evidence base for SLT intervention to enhance communication in dementia is therefore emerging. It is by no means complete, and there is an urgent need for more research into the effects of SLT to be funded. In particular, the evidence for SLT provision within the multidisciplinary team needs to be demonstrated. There is also a need for individual speech and language therapists and departments working with people with dementia to disseminate their work, write up case studies and publicize benefits of SLT such as successful integration of a patient with communication problems into a day care setting, advocacy roles or reduction in carer burden. Such case studies are included in Chapter 8.

At the same time the policy agenda and the views of older people support the drive for increased rehabilitation for older people including those with dementia.

Services for older people

The NHS Plan (DH 2000) and the National Service Frameworks for mental health and for older people (DH 1999, 2001) set the context for services for older people with mental illness. The policy agenda is one of active rehabilitation and access to appropriate specialisms as necessary. However, not all older people with mental health problems have equal access to SLT, given current service disparities across the UK. There is a need to develop more services and enhance those that already exist (see Chapter 10). The recent Royal College of Speech and Language Therapists' Position Paper on Speech and Language Therapy for People with Dementia (RCSLT 2005) provides a comprehensive case for SLT and is written to inform service managers and commissioners.

Empowerment of older people

Older people's views are recognized as important. Easterbrook (1999) showed that older people had definite views about their care and expected to be consulted about this. Older people are active users of resources such as the internet, and are often well informed about health issues. Researchers have shown that even people with advanced dementia can be involved in research studies that evaluate treatment (Vaas et al. 2003). Ethical issues in end-of-life care for people with dementia are actively being debated (Coetzee et al. 2003, De Vries et al. 2003) and the need to involve people with dementia and their carers in care decisions is now widely advocated (Wilkinson and Milne 2003).

The context for examining language difficulties associated with older age mental health conditions and management of the resulting communication problems is therefore one of optimism. Older people are an increasing and ever more powerful sector of the population (through factors such as voting numbers), whose rights to good quality health provision including rehabilitation are strongly advocated.

References

Areosa Sastre A, McShane R, Sherriff F (2004) Memantine for dementia. Cochrane Databases Reviews Issue 4. John Wiley & Sons, Chichester, UK.

Arkin SM (1998) Alzheimer memory training: positive successes replicated. American Journal of Alzheimer's Disease 13: 102–104.

Arkin SM, Mahendra N (2000) Structured information retrieval training yields implicit and explicit learning gains in Alzheimer's patients. Poster presented at the 28th Annual Meeting of the International Neuropsychological Society, Denver.

Arkin SM, Rose C, Hopper T (2000) Implicit and explicit learning gains in Alzheimer's patients: effects of naming and information retrieval training. Aphasiology 14: 723–742.

Baltes PB, Staudinger UM (1993) The search for a psychology of wisdom. Current Directions in Psychological Science 2: 75–80.

Bayles KA, Esther KS (2003) Improving the functioning of individuals with Alzheimer's disease: emergence of behavioural interventions. Journal of Communication Disorders 36: 327–343.

Bayles KA, Tomoeda CK, Kaszniak AW, Trosset MW (1991) Alzheimer's disease effects on semantic memory: loss of structure or function. Journal of Cognitive Neuroscience 3: 166–182.

Bell EE, Chenery HJ, Ingram JCL (2000) Strategy-based semantic priming in Alzheimer's dementia. Aphasiology 14: 949–965.

Benbow SM, Reynolds D (2000) Challenging the stigma of Alzheimer's disease. Hospital Medicine 61: 174–177.

Birks JS, Harvey R (2003) Donepezil for dementia due to Alzheimer's disease. Cochrane Databases Reviews Issue 3. John Wiley & Sons, Chichester, UK.

Bourgeois MS (1991) Communication treatment for adults with dementia. Journal of Speech and Hearing Research 34: 831–844.

Bourgeois MS, Burgio LD, Schulz R, Beach S, Palmer B (1997) Modifying repetitive verbalizations of community dwelling patients with AD. Gerontologist 37: 30–39.

Brown A, Draper P (2003) Accommodative speech and terms of endearment: elements of a language mode often experienced by older adults. Journal of Advanced Nursing 41: 15–21.

Brush JA, Camp CJ (1998) Spaced retrieval during dysphagia therapy: a case study. Clinical Gerontology 19: 96–99.

Bryan K, Maxim J (1998) Enabling care staff to relate to older communication disabled people. International Journal of Language and Communication Disorders 33: 121–126.

Burgio LD, Allen-Burge R, Roth DL et al. (2001) Come talk with me: improving communication between care assistants and nursing home residents during routine care routines. Gerontologist 41: 449–460.

Butler RN, Forette F, Greengross S (2004) Maintaining cognitive health in an ageing society. Journal of the Royal Society for the Promotion of Health 124(3): 119–121.

Camp CJ, Mattern JM (1999) Innovations in managing Alzheimer's disease. In: Biegel DE, Blum A (eds) Innovations in Practice and Service Delivery Across the Lifespan. Oxford University Press, New York.

Chisholm TH, Willott JF, Lister JJ (2003) The aging auditory system: anatomic and physiologic changes and implications for rehabilitation. International Journal of Audiology 42(2): 3–10.

Christensen H (2001) What cognitive changes can be expected with normal ageing. Australian and New Zealand Journal of Psychiatry 35: 768–775.

Clare L, Woods R (2001) Cognitive rehabilitation in dementia. Neuropsychological Rehabilitation (special issue) 11(3): 193–517.

Clark LW (1995) Interventions for persons with Alzheimer's disease: strategies for maintaining and enhancing communicative success. Topics in Language Disorders 15: 47–65.

Coetzee RH, Leask SJ, Jones RG (2003) The attitudes of carers and old age psychiatrists towards the treatment of potentially fatal events in end-stage dementia. International Journal of Geriatric Psychiatry 18: 169–173.

Craik FIM (2000) Age-related changes in human memory. In: Park DC, Schwarz N (eds) Cognitive Aging. Psychology Press, Philadelphia.

De Vries K, Sque M, Bryan K, Abu Saad HH (2003) Variant Creutzfeldt–Jacob disease: need for mental health and palliative care team collaboration. International Journal of Palliative Nursing 9: 512–520.

DH (1999) National Service Framework for Mental Health. Department of Health. HMSO, London.

DH (2000) NHS Plan. Department of Health. HMSO, London.

DH (2001) National Service Framework for Older People. Department of Health. HMSO, London.

Dixon RA (2000) Concepts and mechanisms of gains in cognitive aging. In: Park DC, Schwarz N (eds) Cognitive Aging. Psychology Press, Philadelphia.

Dixon RA, Gould ON (1998) Younger and older adults collaborating on retelling everyday stories. Applied Developmental Science 2: 160–171.

Easterbrook L (1999) When We Are Very Old – Reflections on the Treatment, Care and Support of Older People. King's Fund, London.

Echt KV, Morrell RW, Park DC (1998) Effects of age and training formats on basic computer skill acquisition in older adults. Educational Gerontology 17: 282–293.

Elwood PC, Pickering J, Bayer A, Gallacher JEJ (2002) Vascular disease and cognitive function in older men in the Caerphilly cohort. Age and Ageing 31: 43–48.

Greengross S, Murphy E, Quam L et al. (1997) Aging: a subject that must be at the top of world agendas. BMJ 315(7115): 1029–1030.

Hagberg B (1997) The dementias in a psychodynamic perspective. In: Miesen BML, Jones GMM (eds) Care-giving in Dementia, Research and Applications, Vol. 2. Routledge, London.

Hanratty B, Lawlor DA (2000) Hearing impairment in the older population. Journal of Public Health Medicine 22: 512–517.

Heine C, Browning CJ (2002) Communication and psychosocial consequences of sensory loss in older adults: overview and rehabilitation directions. Disability and Rehabilitation 24: 763–773.

Hopper TL, Bayles KA, Tomoeda CK (1998) Using toys to stimulate communicative function in individuals with Alzheimer's disease. Journal of Medical Speech and Language Pathology 6: 73–80.

Jacoby JJ, Jennings JM, Hay JF (1996) Dissociating automatic and consciously-controlled processes: implications for diagnosis and rehabilitation of memory deficits. In: Hermann DJ et al. (eds) Basic and Applied Memory Research: Theory in Context (vol. 1). Erlbaum, New Jersey.

Kemper S, O'Hanlon L (2000) Semantic processing problems of older adults. In: Best W, Bryan K, Maxim J (eds) Semantic Processing: Theory and Practice. Whurr, London.

Kempler D, Almor A, Tyler LK et al. (1998) Sentence comprehension deficits in AD: a comparison of offline versus online sentence processing. Brain and Language 64: 297–319.

Kemtes KA, Kemper S (1997) Younger and older adults' online processing of syntactically ambiguous sentences. Psychology and Aging 8: 34–43.

Kitwood T (1997) Dementia reconsidered: the person comes first. Open University Press, Buckingham, UK.

Loy C, Schneider L (2004) Galantamine for Alzheimer's diseases. Cochrane Databases Reviews Issue 4. John Wiley & Sons, Chichester, UK.

Mahendra N (2001) Direct interventions for improving the performance of individuals with Alzheimer's disease. Seminars in Speech and Language 22(4): 291–304.

Mahendra N, Arkin SM (2003) Effects of four years of exercise, language and social interventions on Alzheimer discourse. Journal of Communication Disorders 36(5): 395–422.

Maxim J, Bryan K, Zabihi K (2000) Semantic processing in Alzheimer's disease. In: Best W, Bryan K, Maxim J (eds) Semantic Processing: Theory and Practice. Whurr, London.

Maxim J, Bryan K, Axelrod L et al. (2001) Speech and language therapists as trainers: enabling care staff working with older people. International Journal of Language and Communication Disorders 36: 194–199.

Neal M, Briggs M (2003) Validation therapy for dementia. Cochrane Library (Oxford) 2.

Nebes RD, Halligan EM (1996) Sentence context influences the interpretation of word meaning by Alzheimer patients. Brain and Language 54(2): 233–245.

NICE (2005) National Institute for Clinical Excellence Appraisal Consultation Document: Alzheimer's disease – donepezil, rivastigmine, galantamine and memantine (review). *www.nice.org.uk*

Norman A (1985) Triple Jeopardy: Growing Old in a Second Homeland. Centre for Policy on Ageing, London.

Nussbaum JF, Hummert M-L, Williams A, Harwood J (1996) Communication and Older Adults. Sage, Thousand Oaks, CA.

ONS (2001) Hospital and community health service expenditure: by age of recipient 1999–2000. Social Trends 32. Office for National Statistics. HMSO, London.

ONS (2002a) 2001 Census – first results. Population Trends 110 (Winter). Office for National Statistics. HMSO, London.

ONS (2002b) Places available in residential care homes: by sector. Social Trends 33. Office for National Statistics. HMSO, London.

OPCS (1993) Census: ethnic groups and country of births, Vol 1/2. Office of Population Censuses and Surveys. HMSO, London.

Orange JB, Ryan EB (2000) Alzheimer's disease and other dementias: implications for physician communication. Clinics in Geriatric Medicine 16: 153–173.

Orange JB, Ryan JB, Meredith SD, MacLean MJ (1995) Application of the communication enhancement model for long-term care residents with Alzheimer's disease. Topics in Language Disorders 15: 20–35.

Park DC (1994) Aging, cognition and work. Human Performance 7: 181–205.

Park DC (2000) The basic mechanisms accounting for age-related decline in cognitive function. In: Park DC, Schwarz N (eds) Cognitive Aging. Psychology Press, Philadelphia.

Park DC, Gutchess AH (2000) Cognitive aging and everyday life. In: Park DC, Schwarz N (eds) Cognitive Aging. Psychology Press, Philadelphia.

Park DC, Hertzhog C, Leventhal H et al. (1999) Medication adherence in rheumatoid arthritis patients: older is wiser. Journal of the American Geriatrics Society 47: 172–183.

Perry J, Hodges JR (1999) Attention and executive deficits in Alzheimer's disease. Brain 122: 383–404.

Pickard L (2002) The decline of intensive intergenerational care of older people in Great Britain 1885–1995. Population Trends 110. HMSO, London, pp. 31–41.

Powell JA (2000) Communication interventions in dementia. Reviews in Clinical Gerontology 10: 161–168.

Radvansky GA, Curiel JM (1998) Narrative comprehension and aging: the fate of completed goal information. Psychology and Aging 13: 69–79.

Rait R, Burns A, Chew C (1996) Age, ethnicity, and mental illness: a triple whammy. BMJ 313: 1347–1348.

RCSLT (2005) Position Paper on Speech and Language Therapy Provision for People with Dementia. Royal College of Speech and Language Therapists, London.

Ripich D, Ziol E, Fritsch T, Durand EJ (1999) Training Alzheimer's disease caregivers for successful communication. Clinical Gerontologist 21(1): 37–56.

Roessler DM (2003) Complete denture success for patients and dentists. International Dental Journal 53: 340–350.

Sabat SR (1994) Excess disability and malignant social psychology: a case study of Alzheimer's disease. Journal of Community and Applied Social Psychology 4: 157–166.

Salthouse TA (1991) Theoretical Perspectives on Cognitive Aging. Erlbaum, Hillsdale, NJ.

Salthouse TA, Hambrick DZ, Lukas KE, Dell TC (1996) Determinants of adult age differences on synthetic work performance. Journal of Experimental Psychology 71: 432–439.

Schaie KW (1996) Intellectual Development in Adulthood: The Seattle Longitudinal Study. Cambridge University Press, New York.

Shadden BS (1995) The use of discourse analyses and procedures for communication programming in long-term care facilities. Topics in Language Disorder 15: 75–86.

Sherbourne K, White L, Fortnum H (2002) Intensive rehabilitation programmes for deafened men and women: an evaluation study. International Journal of Audiology 41: 195–201.

Sinnott J (1996) The developmental approach: Post formal thought as adaptive intelligence. In: Blanchard-Fields F, Hess TM (eds) Perspectives on Cognitive Change in Adulthood and Aging. McGraw-Hill, New York, pp. 122–162.

Small JA, Gutman G, Makela S, Hillhouse B (2003) Effectiveness of communication strategies used by caregivers of persons with Alzheimer's disease during activities of daily living. Journal of Speech Language Hearing Research 46: 353–367.

Snowden JS, Griffiths H (2000) Semantic dementia: assessment and management. In: Best W, Bryan K, Maxim J (eds) Semantic Processing Theory and Practice. Whurr, London.

Snowdon DA, Kemper SJ, Mortimer JA et al. (1996) Linguistic ability in early life and cognition function and Alzheimer's disease in later life: findings from the nun study. JAMA 275: 528–532.

Spector A, Orrell M (1999) Reality orientation for dementia: a review of the evidence of effectiveness. Cochrane Library (Oxford) 1.

Spector A, Orrell M, Davies S, Woods RT (1999) Reminiscence therapy for dementia. Cochrane Library (Oxford) 2.

Spector A, Thorgrimsen L, Woods B et al. (2003) Efficacy of an evidence-based cognitive stimulation therapy programme for people with dementia. British Journal of Psychiatry 183(3): 248–254.

Stern Y, Gurland B, Tatemichi TK et al. (1994) Influence of education and occupation on the incidence of Alzheimer's disease. JAMA 271: 1004–1010.

Stevens FCJ, Kaplan CD, Ponds RWKM, Diedericks JPM, Jolles J (1999) How ageing and social factors affect memory. Age and Ageing 28: 379–384.

Swift CG (2003) The clinical pharmacology of ageing. British Journal of Clinical Pharmacology 56: 249–253.

Swinburn K Maxim J (1996) Multi-infarct dementia: a special case for treatment? In: Bryan K, Maxim J (eds) Communication Disability and the Psychiatry of Old Age. Whurr, London.

Vaas AA, Minardi HA, Ward R et al. (2003) Research into communication patterns and consequences for effective care of people with Alzheimer's and their carers. Dementia 2: 21–48.

Wilkinson H, Milne AJ (2003) Sharing a diagnosis of dementia: learning from the patient's perspective. Aging and Mental Health 7: 300.

Wingfield A (2000) Speech perception and the comprehension of spoken language. In: Park DC, Schwarz N (eds) Cognitive Aging. Psychology Press, Philadelphia.

Xue SA, Neeley R, Hagstrom F, Hao JP (2001) Speaking F-O characteristics of elderly Euro-American and African-American speakers: building a clinical comparative platform. Clinical Linguistics and Phonetics 15: 245–252.

Yoon C (1997) Age differences in consumers' processing strategies: an investigation of moderating influences. Journal of Consumer Research 24: 329–342.

Chapter 2

Mental health in older age

Claire Nicholl

This chapter is written from the perspective of a physician dealing with medical illness in frail older people in a teaching hospital. If there is concern about a patient with mental health problems in the hospital or community, advice should always be sought from the old age psychiatry team. In hospital, a specialist liaison nurse can be particularly helpful.

Mental health problems are common in old age, particularly the '3 Ds' – dementia, delirium and depression. They interact with physical problems and are often the most distressing aspect of the person's condition for the family, carers and health and social care staff. This chapter outlines the range of psychiatric illness in older people and gives a brief description of common conditions. It concludes with some general principles about the legal implications of mental health problems.

Background

Normal ageing

Normal age-related changes in cognition have been outlined in Chapter 1. It is important to understand that, in comparison with younger people, the population of older people show much more individual variation in function. However well older people function in their normal setting, they have much less 'reserve' if they are physiologically stressed, for example by illness (delirium is common with infections), a change in environment (a patient with mild dementia can become very disorientated when moved between wards) or extremes of climate (for example the rapid increase in death rate of older people in Paris in the summer of 2003).

Interaction with physical health and social circumstances

Multiple pathology is present in a few unfortunate younger people (usually due to premature vascular disease), but in those over 75, and particularly over 80 years, multiple pathology is usual. As the population is ageing, chronic disease management is increasingly recognized as a challenge with initiatives being designed to address these diseases (e.g. Evercare schemes in the US and community matrons in the UK). Evercare is a health-care improvement programme developed in the US to improve the quality of care for vulnerable older people. It involves the use of specially-trained nurses to identify and monitor at-risk older people so that treatment can be given before a visit to hospital is necessary (DH 2004).

General fitness, the social support around an individual and physical illness all interact with any psychiatric problems (Figure 2.1).

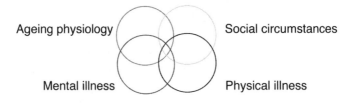

Figure 2.1 Interactions in multiple pathology.

If a patient with dementia falls, the likelihood of hip fracture will depend on previous fitness (she may put out an arm to save herself and break her wrist rather than her hip; if well nourished she may bruise but not fracture); the outcome is influenced by social support (those living alone will suffer a longer lie) as well as co-existing medical problems (heart failure and renal impairment make surgery more risky), and chronic conditions (such as arthritis or age-related macular degeneration) will make rehabilitation more difficult.

Prescribing in old age

As older people have multiple pathology, they are the major consumers of prescription and over-the-counter drugs. The oldest 15% of the population receive 40% of all prescriptions. Few drug trials recruit many participants in their 80s, so evidence for efficacy and safety of drugs is often lacking in this group. However, denying older people drugs that are beneficial to those a decade younger may not be justified. Older people are likely to be more sensitive to the effect of drugs for a variety of reasons. Standard drug dosages are developed for the 'standard 70 kg man'. In paediatrics, careful account is taken of body weight, but this may be overlooked in adult medicine, so that a 40 kg woman may receive a relatively large dose per kilogram of body mass. Pharmacokinetics (what the body does to a drug) and pharmacodynamics (what the drug does to the body) are both affected by ageing. The ratio of fat to lean muscle tissue increases with age, so the same dose of a hydrophilic drug (e.g. alcohol) will result in a higher plasma concentration in an older person. Most drugs are excreted by the kidney, but renal function declines with age, so plasma drug levels tend to be higher and dose and frequency of administration may need to be reduced to prevent toxicity. In the UK, The British National Formulary (BNF) has an excellent section on drug dosage in renal impairment (Appendix 3). For a given plasma concentration of some drugs, such as benzodiazepines, older people seem to be more sensitive; this is thought to be because of changes at and beyond the drug receptors.

Drugs that cross the blood–brain barrier, which includes all drugs for psychiatric problems, have the potential to cause drowsiness and confusion. Side effects (effects caused by a drug other than the intended therapeutic effect) are common in older people, and neuropsychiatric side effects are more common if brain function is already compromised, as it is in dementia. In younger patients, the dose of dopaminergic drugs for Parkinson's disease is usually limited by the development of unwanted abnormal movements (dyskinesias) but in older patients, neuropsychiatric complications such as confusion and hallucinations often limit the dose that can be given.

If a side effect occurs, it often has more serious consequences in a frail older person. For example, long-acting hypnotics, tricyclic antidepressants and antipsychotics are all associated with hip fracture because they may exacerbate drowsiness, confusion and postural hypotension. Other biological and social factors make a risky situation more likely to arise; an older person is more likely to get up at night to urinate (decreased renal concentrating ability, prostate enlargement in men, etc.) and is more likely to have poor vision (70% of new visual impairment occurs in the over 70s). Cardiovascular reflexes become less efficient with ageing and may be impaired by concomitant drugs (e.g. diuretics), so on getting up from a warm bed to a cold room, the patient is more likely to experience postural hypotension (impaired homeostatic mechanisms) and fall, sustaining a hip fracture (because of osteoporosis). If the patient is then left lying on the floor for a period this in itself can have its own sequelae (incontinence, pressure sores, hypothermia and rhabdomyolysis, i.e. kidney damage from muscle tissue breakdown).

When a person is taking many drugs (polypharmacy), there is more scope for muddle, poor concordance (the terms 'compliance' or 'adherence' are thought to sound too authoritarian as the doctor and patient are meant to agree on a plan of drug management), drug reactions and drug interactions (BNF Appendix 1). Most drugs used in psychiatry interact with each other and with alcohol. For example, selective serotonin reuptake inhibitor (SSRI) antidepressants have potentially hazardous interactions with other antidepressants, antipsychotics, anxiolytics, hypnotics and lithium, drugs for neurological conditions e.g. antiepileptics, dopaminergics and a variety of seemingly unrelated drugs, usually by altering their metabolism e.g. some beta blockers and warfarin.

Adverse drug reactions (ADRs) are noxious unintended responses to drugs given in normal doses and may be classified into five groups:

- **Anticipated effects:** These are common, predictable from the pharmacology, usually dose related and often arise because of altered pharmacokinetics. Many side effects fall into this group, e.g. anticholinesterase inhibitors commonly cause nausea because of their cholinergic effects on the gut.
- **Bizarre effects:** These are much less common, unrelated to pharmacology and dose and unpredictable. The commoner ones may still be listed as 'side effects', e.g. liver problems with lofepramine, agranulocytosis (lack of white blood cells) with mirtazapine, urticaria ('nettle rash') with SSRIs. Serious effects often take the form of anaphylaxis where there is an extreme allergic reaction associated with hypersensitivity following earlier exposure.
- **Chronic effects,** e.g. parkinsonian symptoms with antipsychotic drugs.
- **Delayed effects** occurring years after treatment
- **End of treatment effects** when drugs are withdrawn suddenly. This is relatively common with psychoactive drugs such as benzodiazepines, antipsychotics and antidepressants.

Managing drugs in older people

The 'whole person' must be considered when prescribing. Patients should not be denied drugs that are likely to be beneficial because of their age alone. A good plan with any new drug is to 'start low, go slow' and only change one drug at a time. However, the dose should be increased to a therapeutic level for an appropriate period before, for example, deciding that the patient 'does not respond' to an antidepressant.

Regimens should be kept as simple as possible (once-daily medication is preferable at any age). There needs to be an appropriate balance between drugs for symptom relief, prevention and the patient's overall condition. Dementia increases the chance of accidental overdose or underdose, and prescribing may need to be modified. For example, paroxysmal atrial fibrillation increases stroke risk, as when the heart flips between atrial fibrillation and sinus rhythm any clots which have formed in the dyskinetic left atrium may be thrown off to cause emboli in the cerebral arteries. Anticoagulation with warfarin reduces this risk. However, if the patient also has dementia and falls, the likely risk/benefit ratio of treatment with warfarin changes. The blood may become too thin if the patient cannot be relied on to take the correct dose and to have their clotting checked regularly. In such a patient, it may be better to pre-scribe low-dose aspirin which is less effective but also less hazardous. Depression increases the risk of deliberate overdose, so extra care must be taken with all prescription drugs.

Most patients appreciate clear written instructions about their drugs and need a list with both generic and trade names (e.g. donepezil/ Aricept). People need to understand which drugs are for symptom relief and can be stopped if the symptom settles (e.g. analgesics), which drugs must be continued for a course (e.g. antibiotics) and which drugs should be continued long-term until further discussion with the clinician (e.g. antihypertensives and antidepressants). In some instances, patients bene-fit from a detailed explanation as to why a drug is needed. Prejudice about mental health problems is still widespread amongst older people who equate depression with mental 'weakness'. An explanation that depres-sion is a 'real' illness at a biochemical level and an outline of the neurotransmitter theory of depression may improve willingness to con-sider medication. Concordance may be improved if the patient understands that initial side effects usually decrease over time and that benefit will not be apparent for 4–6 weeks.

Medication may be a small component of the overall management plan; for example, in depression support from a community specialist (in the UK often a community mental health nurse) and day hospital attendance may be crucial both in ensuring concordance with the drug regimen and as part of the therapeutic strategy. An exercise pro-gramme may also help, but must be appropriate for the person's physical abilities.

Patients are at particular risk from confusion over drug regimens on discharge home from hospital, as they may restart drugs they were taking before admission. Drugs may be dispensed in 'Dosette' boxes, but some patients require direct supervision. In principle, covert medication (e.g. putting drugs in tea) should be avoided, but if there seems no alternative, there must be multidisciplinary discussion which includes the patient's family or advocate, clear documentation and regular review.

Service provision

Many people develop mental illness for the first time in old age partly because of changes in the brain associated with dementia and partly because of the increasing burden of other problems including bereave-ment and infirmity. Just as 'geriatric' medicine grew from the observation that many people were kept unnecessarily in long-stay institutions, old age psychiatry grew from recognition that older patients in long-stay psy-chiatric hospitals needed a specialist approach. Specialist status for old age psychiatry was obtained in the UK in 1989, and doctors undertake general psychiatry training before specializing, though they often work more closely with their colleagues in old age medicine than general psychiatry. In the UK, old age psychiatry has developed as a multidisciplinary community-orientated service and a similar pattern is seen in Australia. (See Chapter 3 for discussion of the role of primary care in managing dementia and Chapter 10 for further discussion of service provision in old age mental health.)

In much of continental Europe, people with dementia (which accounts for up to two thirds of all referrals to old age psychiatry services in the UK) are managed by neurologists. In the US, services for older people have lagged behind those for younger people because of the limitations of the reimbursement system (see Chapter 11 for further information on services in the USA). Services in many third world and transition countries have been almost non-existent, but in India for example the number of older people in the population is increasing very rapidly and the traditional model of family-based care is under strain as western patterns of work are adopted. There will be an urgent need to improve service provision.

A comprehensive old age psychiatry service would include:

• psychiatrists
• doctors in training: middle grade; aspiring old age psychiatrists, junior grades and those preparing for related careers e.g. general psychiatry, general (family) practice
• mental health nurses, including some specializing e.g. in dementia or hospital liaison psychiatry
• social workers, psychologists, occupational therapists (OTs), physiotherapists (PTs), speech and language therapists (SLTs), chiropodist, dietitian, pharmacist.

A typical service would provide:

• community and hospital clinics
• home assessments
• day unit places
• acute assessment and treatment beds
• ongoing care and respite beds (ongoing care is increasingly carried out in the private sector in residential homes or nursing homes according to need). If a patient has severe behavioural problems or wanders, a place in a specialist elderly mentally infirm (EMI) facility may be sought.
• liaison services (working with patients with mental health problems in general hospitals)
• educational activities (including work with the private and voluntary sector and providing programmes for carers).

One group of patients with particular problems is people with a life-long mental health problem who become old. Historically, people in this group were institutionalized for most of their adult life and faced problems with resettlement at a time when increasing physical frailty was combined with chronic mental health problems and institutionalization. Nowadays, these patients, who are termed 'graduates', are more likely to have lived in the community. However, perhaps because of lack of resources, these patients can fall between general adult and old age psychiatry services.

Links with the voluntary sector

One of the strongest aspects of old age psychiatry is that it usually has excellent links with the voluntary sector. Societies for dementia are well developed in the UK, although organizations such as the Alzheimer's Society and Age Concern are increasingly becoming worldwide organizations. The Alzheimer's Society includes 'related disorders' in its remit, so that anyone concerned about a dementia can be referred. The Alzheimer's Society provides superb educational literature, practical support for patients and carers and in some areas care provision, as well as fulfilling a campaigning and fundraising role. (Websites for such information are given at the end of this chapter.)

Importance of carers

Life for the carer of a patient with a mental health problem is tough at any age, but perhaps particularly difficult when faced with the combination of physical frailty and mental decline that is seen in old age. A caring spouse may well be older and may have their own health problems. Carers need consideration, education and emotional and practical support. They are entitled to a social services assessment in their own right. (See Chapter 9 for further information on supporting family carers.)

Elder abuse

Poor mental health is a major risk factor for elder abuse. This takes many forms and includes physical abuse, neglect, psychological abuse, financial exploitation and sexual abuse. Abuse occurs in all settings from the teaching hospital to the home of the person with a dementia living alone, and the perpetrators may be informal carers or employed staff. Standards of what is acceptable to society change with time and over the years there have been a number of scandals involving institutional abuse. Age Concern produce brochures for practitioners and students on what to do if abuse is suspected (see Action on Elder Abuse website, listed at the end of this chapter). Practitioners should alert the multidisciplinary team and be aware that a carer may be unable to cope. In extreme circumstances the police should be alerted.

Evaluation of the older patient

History

The history is taken from the patient but it is often necessary to get information from other informants, such as family, carer or GP. The presentation must be considered in the context of the patient's cultural background.

Use of standardized instruments

Standardized instruments are available for several diagnoses, particularly depression and dementia. They do not replace a clinical assessment for diagnosis but can be used to identify those who need a full assessment, in the research setting and to monitor change. For example a low Abbreviated Mental Test (AMT) (Yesavage et al. 1983) score may be due to dementia, delirium caused by acute infection, not speaking the language used to administer the test, deafness, depression, dysphasia or refusal to cooperate, but it raises awareness that the patient's mental state needs closer scrutiny.

The mental state examination

This examination includes an assessment of appearance and behaviour, speech, thought form and content, perceptions, mood and cognition.

Table 2.1 The mental state examination

Areas of examination	Example of signs
Appearance	Hair, clothing and personal cleanliness speak volumes about cognitive impairment. Flowers and fruit on the bedside locker suggest someone cares
Behaviour	Poor eye contact in depression, restlessness in mania, oro-facial dyskinesia suggests previous antipsychotic medication
Speech	Language breakdown and perseveration in dementia, reduced spontaneous speech in depression, pressure of speech in mania, neologisms in schizophrenia
Thought form	Flight of thought in mania, lack of logical sequencing in schizophrenia (sometimes called knight's move thinking)
Thought content	In schizophrenia, obsessions (persistent thoughts that enter the patient's consciousness unbidden but are recognized as his own), delusions (beliefs that persist despite evidence to the contrary that are out of context for that individual's background), and thought alienation (can take the form of thought insertion, withdrawal or broadcasting). Obsessions are also a hallmark of obsessive compulsive disorder

Table 2.1 continued

Areas of examination	Example of signs
Perception	Illusions (misperceptions) and hallucinations (perceptions in the absence of a stimulus) can occur in schizophrenia, psychotic depression and some dementias (e.g. Lewy body)
Mood	Abnormally low in depression and elevated in mania
Cognition	Impaired in dementia and delirium and to some extent in depression

Classification of psychiatric illnesses

Diagnosis in psychiatry continues to be a matter of some debate. Two major classifications are current: the *Diagnostic and Statistical Manual of Mental Disorders*, 4th edition, Test Revision (DSM-IV-TR) (APA 2000) and the Tenth Revision of the *International Classification of Diseases and Related Health Problems* (ICD-10) (WHO 1992). Differences in classification have important consequences. For example, the prevalence of depression in a community study depends on the definition of a 'case' (one explanation of the wide range of estimates in different studies) and the results of a drug trial in dementia should only be extrapolated to a patient with a similar type and severity of dementia. In this text, the detail of the two classification systems is not pursued. However, it should be remembered that a diagnostic label, or its lack, has consequences for an individual and the carers. Families struggling with a relative whose behaviour is becoming increasing difficult can be relieved by the diagnosis of a dementia, which opens doors to a range of services.

The psychiatric disorders described here are depression and mania, anxiety disorders including obsessive-compulsive disorder (OCD), delirium, dementia, late onset psychosis, substance abuse, sleep disorders and the Diogenes syndrome.

Prevalence of psychiatric illness in older people

The figures for the prevalence of psychiatric disorders given in recent publications encompass such wide ranges that it is difficult to give accurate figures. There is great variation depending on the type of population, age structure and diagnostic criteria etc. The key message for clinicians is that patients with the disorders represented by the '3 Ds' (depression, delirium and dementia) are common in the community and overrepresented in hospitals. Depression is a common accompaniment of chronic physical disease, dementia makes a person more vulnerable and delirium often reflects physical illness (such as a chest infection) in a vulnerable patient. Perhaps as hospitals are known to generate anxiety, a degree of anxiety may be regarded as 'normal', so that formal diagnosis of anxiety disorders does not seem much higher in hospitals than in the community.

Table 2.2 Prevalence of psychiatric disorders in older people

Category	Community residents (%)	Medical/surgical inpatients (%)	Notes
Depression			Wide range
symptoms	10	40	depending on
disorder	3	25	diagnostic criteria
Dementia	5	30	Very age dependent
Delirium	3	15	Often missed and overlaps dementia
Anxiety disorders	5	5	
Alcohol abuse	1	5	Often overlooked
Late-onset psychosis	< 0.5	< 0.5	Relatively rare

Specific disorders

Mood disorders

Most people have ups and downs in their mood, but, if they are extreme, the person may be suffering from a mood or affective disorder. Mood disorders can be unipolar, in which there are only downswings in mood (depression), or bipolar, in which episodes of low mood are interspersed with periods of elevated mood and overactivity (mania).

Depression

Depression is the most common mental health problem of older people, but can be difficult to diagnose. Depressive symptoms are often recognized, but may be attributed to life events or a reaction to physical disability and depressive illness may be overlooked. Bereavement is frequent in this age group and the normal grief reaction which follows has many features in common with depression. It can be hard to identify the cases where grief does not resolve but develops into depression. Diagnosis is important because a combination of support (e.g. through CRUSE), counselling and drugs may be needed.

There is no universally accepted way of classifying the range of clinically significant depressive illness seen in older people. The ICD-10 diagnostic criteria include mild, moderate and severe classifications.

Studies using various diagnostic criteria report a 5–25% prevalence of depressive disorders in the community, the range reflecting different diagnostic criteria as well as differences in population.

In older age, depression can present as it does in younger people. However, there may be more interaction with physical symptoms. Patients with physical illness may have symptoms that might suggest 'depression' in a younger age group; for example poor appetite, feeling of lassitude and poor sleep could all occur with heart failure or rheumatoid arthritis. The stigma of mental illness may be more prevalent in the older generation, who may be reluctant to seek help for depression. Some older people present with a very physical-sounding illness, but all investigations to find the 'occult cancer' are persistently normal and after a battery of unpleasant and costly tests, it may be recognized that depression is the cause.

The presentation of depression may be complicated by a dementia. In the early stages of a dementing illness, many patients become depressed – either because it is a rational response for someone to feel down when they realize they are beginning to lose their grip, or because the brain pathologies that underlie dementia predispose to depression. Once dementia is established, a patient who also has depression may lack the language to convey her misery and despair, so the diagnosis has to rely on observation of behaviour rather than history. In severe depression, slowness, poor concentration and apathy may lead to the presentation with some similarities to that of the dementias, and when treatments for depression were limited this was sufficiently common for a special term, 'pseudodementia', to be used. Older patients with depression usually present with a mixture of psychological and biological symptoms and may be agitated or retarded. Because of the interaction with physical symptoms described above, a particularly useful symptom strongly suggesting depression in older people is anhedonia (loss of pleasure in activities that the individual would normally enjoy). Depression may also present as a psychosis with delusional convictions of disease or guilt, alcohol dependence occurring for the first time in old age, an anxiety state or deliberate self-harm.

Diagnosis of depression
In settings where depression is likely to be common, but where specialist diagnosis is limited, screening tests may be useful to identify those who need a clinical opinion. The 15 point Geriatric Depression Scale (GDS) (Yesavage et al. 1983) and the Brief Assessment Schedule Depression Cards (BASDEC) (Adshead et al. 1992) are two examples. In the clinical setting, the following information may be needed to assist diagnosis:

- detailed history, from the patient and an informant
- the person's underlying personality traits, as results of treatment may be less obvious in a dysthymic (chronically gloomy) patient
- examination of the mental state, including an assessment of cognition

- drug history: this provides a practical prompt for co-morbidity, and a number of drugs are associated with mood change; most commonly steroids and beta-blockers
- physical examination, because of the overlap with major illness
- a number of blood tests, to exclude physical disease that can present with low mood:
  - full blood count, as low haemoglobin with large red cells (macrocytic anaemia) may suggest vitamin B_{12} deficiency or alcoholism
  - bone profile to check for high calcium (most often due to hyper-parathyroidism, but metastatic cancer is not rare)
  - thyroid function (high thyroid stimulating hormone in hypothyroidism)
  - blood glucose
  - renal and liver function tests, to rule out major pathology and prior to drug treatment
- ECG may be needed before treatment, and chest X ray if there is a suspicion of cancer
- CT brain scan if there is concomitant dementia or neurological findings.

Management of depression
This is usually multifactorial and includes talking (ranging from education and counselling to cognitive behavioural therapy), ongoing social and therapeutic support (CPN, day unit or the voluntary sector), drugs and electroconvulsive therapy (ECT). Although the results of ECT were often excellent for patients with severe depression unrelieved by drug therapy (particularly in patients refusing to eat or who are suicidal) the adverse publicity has meant that, except in areas where the local psychiatrists are keen proponents, ECT is now rarely used.

Drug treatment for depression
The range of drugs used is similar to that in younger people. Table 2.3 below lists some of the common drugs. For the full range of drugs and details see the British National Formulary. In general, benzodiazepines (e.g. Valium) are best avoided.

Table 2.3 Drug treatment for depression

Name	Mechanism of action	Common side effects	Indications	Points to watch
Citalopram	Selective serotonin reuptake inhibitor (SSRI)	Nausea, agitation	General use	Hyponatraemia, caution in epilepsy, risk of bleeding from the gut
Mirtazapine	Presynaptic alpha2 antagonist	Weight gain, sedation	Agitation and anorexia	Patients must report sore throat – risk of marrow suppression

Table 2.3 continued

Name	Mechanism of action	Common side effects	Indications	Points to watch
Trazodone	Tricyclic-related	Sedation, dry mouth	Impaired day/night rhythm	
Lofepramine	Tricyclic-related		Try in those with nausea on SSRIs who do not need sedation	Check liver function tests if patient feels unwell
Venlafaxine	Serotonin and noradrenaline reuptake inhibitor (SNRI)		Resistant or severe cases	

The most severe form of depression, psychotic depression, in which there are symptoms such as hallucinations and delusions, may require antipsychotic drugs such as haloperidol or risperidone. Modest doses are often sufficient, and the maintenance dose is often lower than the initial dose needed to control symptoms and lower than that needed in younger people. In recurrent episodic depression, mood stabilizers, particularly lithium, may be useful, but this and another group of antidepressants, the monoamine oxidase inhibitors, are usually only prescribed by psychiatrists.

Suicide

This is one of the saddest consequences of depression, and its effects cascade through the generations. One in five suicides in the US is in patients older than 65 years, and unlike parasuicide (apparent attempt at suicide but with no actual intention to kill oneself) in young people about two thirds of older people attempting suicide have an underlying psychiatric disorder. In the acute medical setting doctors often assume that the unconscious old lady must have had a stroke and overlook the fact she may have taken an overdose. White older men are the group most at risk, and are more likely to choose a lethal method. When judging risk of suicide, consider the person's occupation or previous occupation; for example farmers and gamekeepers have ready access to guns (see Chapter 10).

Mania

Manic episodes are divided into hypomania ('mild' mania) and mania with or without psychotic symptoms. Surprisingly, the number of first admissions with mania increases with age. However, the prevalence of those with mania in the community does not seem to grow steadily, possibly because of the high death rate of those with bipolar disorder and perhaps because some cases 'burn out'. The usual range of symptoms is seen: decreased sleep, physical hyperactivity, flight of ideas, overspending, grandiose delusions, irritability, thought disorder and hypersexuality.

Mania can be associated with steroids, psychoactive medication, thyrotoxicosis, brain tumours or brain damage, but usually it is part of the spectrum of mood disorders occurring as a cyclical condition with periods of depression or a mixed syndrome of manic and depressive symptoms. Depression may precede mania by 25 years in a quarter of patients, so the eventual manic phase will take everyone by surprise. In severe brain damage, disinhibition syndromes (involving difficulties in controlling urges and impulses to speak, act or show emotions) may have some features of a manic condition.

The mainstay of treatment for mania is lithium, although there is little trial data to support this. Lithium toxicity can be a particular problem in older people, and regular checks of the level and renal function are needed. Thyroid function should also be monitored and drug interactions, e.g. with thiazides, ACE inhibitors and NSAIDS, can be significant. Sodium valproate and carbamazepine can also be used for their mood stabilizing effect.

Anxiety disorders

Anxiety is a relatively common symptom and is often made worse by concern about physical infirmity. The experience of a frightening event such as a heart attack (in the patient or spouse) or a mugging may predispose to anxiety. Anxiety is a side effect of a number of drugs, e.g. overprescription of thyroxine, salbutamol (particularly via a nebulizer as the dose is higher), aminophylline (a drug related to caffeine used for severe chronic obstructive pulmonary disease) and fluoxetine. If a patient becomes extremely anxious a day or two after hospital admission, think 'drugs and alcohol' or, in this case, their absence. Is the patient beginning to experience alcohol withdrawal (some older women drink a surprising amount of sherry each day without realizing that they have an alcohol problem), or has their longstanding benzodiazepine night sedation been omitted from the prescription card?

Most older people with anxiety of sufficient severity for it to be classified as a generalized anxiety disorder have suffered for years. Anxiety often coexists with depression. Phobic disorders, where severe anxiety occurs in a specific situation, can be longstanding or late onset; the latter often take the form of agoraphobia. Longstanding phobias may be more difficult for the individual to cope with in old age – for example, a needle phobic will have problems on insulin therapy. It can also be difficult to judge what is a reasonable level of fear of a situation – an elderly woman on diuretics may refuse to go out because of the fear of incontinence, but this may be a realistic scenario. Panic disorders in older people are probably more often seen by cardiologists or neurologists than psychiatrists. The patient may focus so much on the physical sequelae of their anxiety that the underlying cause may be overlooked.

Obsessive-compulsive disorders

Patients with obsessive-compulsive disorders (OCD) are disabled by recurrent intrusive thoughts (obsessions), which often lead to an irresistible urge to perform repetitive voluntary actions (compulsions). OCD tends to start early in life and has a chronic fluctuating course. The infirmities of old age may challenge the ability of an affected individual to keep coping with their symptoms. For example, it is difficult to keep up washing routines as an inpatient and nurses may need persuasion to allow the wearing of rubber gloves on the ward. Preoccupation with routine may also occur in early dementia.

Delirium or acute confusional state

Delirium, or an 'acute confusional state', is characterized by changes in consciousness, attention, cognition and perception. (The word is derived from the Latin *lira*, a ploughed furrow, so delirium means 'to go out of one's furrow'.) Delirium can occur at any age but is commonest in the old and in young children, who may also become delirious with a high fever. When an older person presents with sudden onset or worsening of confusion in the community, a full work-up is essential as there are many diagnostic possibilities, which cannot be elucidated without investigation. Emergency placement in a residential home is not an appropriate way to manage this situation. The facilities of a general hospital may be needed for diagnosis, but such patients often do poorly in a busy ward. Once there is a diagnosis and management plan, if adequate care can be provided at home this is preferable; otherwise an intermediate care setting may be suitable.

Delirium is very common in older patients in hospital (around 15%), especially in those with pre-existing cognitive impairment. The most common settings are the admissions unit or after surgery, especially orthopaedic wards after surgery for fractured neck of femur. Patients present with disorientation, agitation (which may include shouting or physical aggression) or apathy and may cooperate poorly with treatment. They may have visual hallucinations and delusions and, particularly in substance withdrawal, marked autonomic features such as tachycardia, unstable blood pressure and tremor. 'Clouding of consciousness' is a classic sign but it is not very helpful in practice to distinguish delirium from dementia as it fluctuates, mild degrees of impairment (failure to maintain attention and distractibility) are hard to detect and people with dementia can be drowsy for many reasons, including sedation. Patients with dementia and delirium tend to be worse in the evenings and at night (sundowning).

The mechanism underlying the clinical presentation is not understood, but the final pathway may involve central cholinergic and dopaminergic neurones that mediate attention and arousal. Different causes of delirium may bring about these effects in different ways, e.g. by hypoxia in chest

infection or following myocardial infarction or the presence of an endogenous benzodiazepine-like substance in hepatic encephalopathy. Delirium
can be hard to distinguish from dementia when there is no information
about time course. Agitated or retarded (slowed activity) depression and
stroke with fluent dysphasia may also be mislabelled as delirium.

The patient's appearance may give clues to previous function, but history must be sought from other informants (pre-existing dementia,
information about the acute deterioration and past history; for example,
breast cancer years previously may present with confusion due to high
calcium from bone secondaries). A drug and alcohol history is important.
Drug and alcohol withdrawal is usually seen the day after admission, but
if the person became too ill to drink before admission, they may present
with confusion. Could the patient have had a hypoglycaemic attack or an
epileptic fit? Physical examination will include:

- vital signs including oximetry (measurement of oxygen saturation in
  the blood)
- full systems examination looking particularly for infection (chest,
  urine, cellulites (check under any bandages) and meningitis, although
  this is rare), and signs of cerebrovascular disease
- vision and hearing should be checked as sensory deprivation predis-
  poses to confusion and may be treatable
- check that the patient has not got an unrecognized fracture
- exclude simple but commonly overlooked conditions such as consti-
  pation and retention of urine.

Investigations include:

- full blood count
- urea and electrolytes
- liver and bone profile
- blood glucose
- thyroid function
- B_{12} and folate
- troponin
- C-reactive protein
- arterial blood gases
- blood cultures
- urinalysis
- chest X ray
- ECG
- CT brain scan may be needed if there has been a fall (subdural
  haematoma) or stroke or metastatic disease is possible.

Management should be in a calm, well-lit environment with familiar
staff (almost impossible in a modern hospital: try for a side room and
persuade any relatives to stay with the patient). The priority is to diagnose

and treat the underlying medical problems. Approaching the patient formally, with a clear introduction and an offer to shake hands, may gain cooperation. The team should use opportunities to re-orientate the patient with reminders as to where she is, why and how she came to be there, as confused people will not remember the trip in the ambulance. A clock, 'Get Well Soon' card and family photo on the bedside locker may help. A low bed is safer than a normal bed with cot sides, as confused but mobile patients will try to climb over, so the 'safety measure' increases the chance of hip fracture. A very agitated patient may need one-to-one care, for their own safety and that of their neighbours, preferably from a nurse with mental health training. In extreme cases, urgent referral to a psychiatrist may be needed, but the Mental Health Act is rarely used in this situation. Even if the patient is initially compliant, good nursing is essential to ensure that the patient eats, drinks and remains mobile and continent, but doesn't fall on the ward.

Unnecessary drugs, particularly anticholinergics (e.g. amitriptyline), should be avoided, but it can be difficult to decide what to do about regular medication such as nitrazepam (a benzodiazepine prescribed for sleeping difficulty or anxiety) which is undesirable but where withdrawal may cause problems. Antiparkinsonian medication should not be stopped abruptly; if the patient cannot swallow, a nasogastric tube will probably be needed. Common sense is helpful in providing pragmatic treatment the patient will accept rather than ideal treatment that the patient refuses. For example, antibiotic syrups and regular cups of tea will be more use even in severe infection than an intravenous regimen if the drip is always pulled out. Staff should try to maintain a day/night routine, but sedation may be needed. Conventional neuroleptics (e.g. haloperidol 0.5 mg orally) or atypical neuroleptics (e.g. risperidone 0.5–1 mg or olanzapine 2.5–5.0 mg) can be used although lorazepam (0.5–1 mg orally or by intramuscular injection) is used more often now.

The dementias

The dementias, of which Alzheimer's disease (AD) is the commonest cause, are a public health problem of enormous magnitude. The dementias are acquired syndromes marked by chronic, global (*not* just *memory or* just *language problems*) impairments of higher brain function, occurring in alert patients (*not drowsy*), which interfere with the ability to cope with daily living.

The following mnemonic has been suggested by Brice Pitt (Emeritus Professor of Old Age Psychiatry at St Mary's) as a way of helping students to think about possible identification of a patient where a dementia could be a possible diagnosis:

- my (memory)
- old (orientation)

- grandmother (grasp)
- converses (communication)
- pretty (personality change)
- badly (behaviour disorder).

Dementia contrasts with delirium, an acute confusional state with impaired consciousness. An acute confusional state resolves as the underlying illness gets better. Since delirium is particularly common with a background of dementia, the confusion will improve, but to a limited extent.

Causes of the dementias

The *primary dementias*, where the disease mainly affects the neurons in the brain, include AD, dementia with Lewy bodies (DLB), other frontotemporal lobar atrophies including Pick's disease, semantic dementia and frontotemporal dementia and Creutzfeldt–Jakob disease (see Chapter 5 for details of managing semantic dementia).

The commonest *secondary dementia*, in which the neuronal damage is secondary to pathology in other tissues, is vascular dementia (VaD) (sometimes called multi-infarct dementia), which includes multiple small infarcts and white matter ischaemia. Other important causes are listed as a mnemonic below:

- drugs and alcohol
- eyes and ears
- metabolic (thyroid dysfunction, recurrent or severe hypoglycaemia)
- emotional (really, psychiatric problems)
- nutritional (B$_{12}$ deficiency)
- trauma and tumour
- infections (syphilis is very rare now in the UK; HIV is also very rare in old age)
- atheroma – VaD

Dementia is rare below 55 years of age, but its prevalence increases dramatically with age to about 3% in the over 65s, rising to about 20% in the over 80s, and there is a slight female preponderance. In elderly people, AD probably accounts for half to two thirds of all cases of dementia. About 700 000 people in England and Wales have dementia.

The onset of dementia is insidious, with gradual changes in memory and concentration, thinking processes, language use, personality, behaviour and orientation, although the rate of deterioration varies in individuals and preservation of certain functions may occur. Short-term memory is impaired early – long-term recall is often much better. Thinking becomes rigid and concrete. The condition progresses to obvious problems with short-term memory and managing basic activities of daily living, increasing disorientation and sometimes difficult or distressing behaviour such as night-time wandering, aggression or apathy. A tendency to lose things easily leads to suspicion and paranoia. Eventually, the patient is completely disorientated, no longer recognizes close family, ceases to communicate and becomes doubly incontinent, bed-bound and totally dependent.

The presentation of dementia depends on the level of cognitive function and the demands of the environment and this can lead to conflicting opinions. An old woman in a residential home can get by with a good social front and moderate dementia, because of the undemanding routine and care by staff who know her well. Care staff may therefore insist 'she is not confused' and there may be concern when her mental function appears to deteriorate rapidly on admission to hospital. Careful questioning can usually reveal the actual extent of previous functioning. (See Chapter 4 for more information on the presenting symptoms of the dementias.)

Why does dementia matter?

Dementia is devastating for the patient and the family and has major economic consequences. Demographic changes are resulting in marked increases in the oldest old, 1 in 5 of whom may have dementia, a major cause of dependency and institutional care. Politicians and society are beginning to grapple with the cost and difficult of providing adequate health and social care. The direct costs of AD in the UK have been estimated at between £7 billion and £15 billion (2001), greater than the costs of stroke, heart disease and cancer. In addition to the considerable morbidity, it is estimated that AD is the fourth leading cause of death in developed countries although it is often not cited on the death certificate.

How is a diagnosis of dementia made?

The GP is usually the first port of call, but a survey performed by the Alzheimer's Disease Society suggests that it is often difficult to obtain a diagnosis. Many old people are slightly forgetful and it can be difficult to distinguish ageing changes from early dementia. The term 'age-associated memory impairment' is applied to a subjective complaint of forgetfulness in those over 50, with a performance on memory testing one standard deviation below the normal for a young adult. Almost 20% of people over 50 meet these criteria, and the significance is uncertain.

GPs may be reluctant to diagnose an 'untreatable' condition. If the patient lives alone there may be no one to give a history and unless a simple test of cognition is performed, it is easy to be misled by 'a good social front'. Quick screening tests include the AMT Score (Hodkinson 1972). As a general rule, if family members are concerned there is usually a problem, whereas if only the patient is complaining the diagnosis is often anxiety, depression or 'worried well'. Although dementia may have been developing for months, the patient often presents acutely because of a social crisis (e.g. death of caring spouse) or physical crisis (any illness, which worsens the confusion). Having identified possible dementia, the GP may manage the patient or refer to a geriatrician, an old age psychiatrist, a neurologist, or in some areas, a specialist memory clinic. (See Chapter 3 for discussion of the role of general practice in the management of dementia.)

What are the aims of a clinical assessment?

- Is it dementia? A full history, with more detailed cognitive function testing, including assessment of language, visuo-spatial skills and reasoning (e.g. the Mini-Mental State Examination (Folstein et al. 1975)), usually answers this question. At this stage, other conditions must be ruled out. The differential diagnosis includes acute confusional state, depression, communication difficulties due to deafness, poor vision, or language deficits, Parkinson's disease, schizophrenia and mania.
- What type of dementia is it? The next step is to identify the cause. The dementia may be reversible (e.g. hypothyroidism), treatment may slow disease progression (e.g. treating hypertension in VaD), specific treatment may be available (e.g. AD), genetic counselling may be required (e.g. familial AD) or it may be important to avoid certain medication (e.g. neuroleptics in DLB).

There is no diagnostic test for most of the primary dementias until a post-mortem examination, so the *likely* cause is determined by the clinical features and the results of investigations. Common conditions such as VaD and AD may co-exist. More detail about the different types of dementia is given in later subsections, but broadly speaking, progressive deterioration is common in AD whereas stepwise deterioration is characteristic of VaD. Neuropsychiatric phenomena and sensitivity to major tranquillizers suggest DLB. Parkinsonian features point to VaD or DLB. Fluctuation can be surprisingly marked in DLB, even affecting conscious level. Weighted scores, such as the Hachinski ischaemia score (Hachinski et al. 1975), may improve diagnostic accuracy and work is in progress to determine whether patterns of change found on neuropsychological and language testing add to diagnosis.

Investigations typically include:

- blood tests to exclude reversible causes or other major pathology (blood count, ESR, glucose, biochemical profile, thyroid function, B_{12} and folate and occasionally syphilis serology)
- chest X ray
- ECG
- CT scan or MRI. In the late stages, CT scan shows cerebral atrophy but many patients with AD have a normal-looking scan initially. The main purpose of the scan is to rule out a space-occupying lesion and identify major vascular disease

- genetic tests, such as determining the apolipoprotein E alleles which predispose to AD, are not routine.

Management of dementia

Management depends on the severity of the dementia and whether the patient lives alone, and it comprises a multidisciplinary, multiagency package of care. The package needs to be well coordinated and to evolve as the needs of the patient and carer change. Options include:

- coping strategies and psychological techniques, reminiscence work and validation therapy
- optimization of hearing, vision and improve general health
- treatment of other conditions which may impair cognition (e.g. anaemia, heart failure)
- treatment of risk factors (e.g. hypertension in VaD)
- treatment of behavioural and psychiatric symptoms of dementia (e.g. night sedation, neuroleptics)
- education and support for carers (Alzheimer's Society, Carers' National Association, Age Concern)
- genetic counselling (only in rare early-onset dementias)
- legal advice (e.g. an Enduring Power of Attorney may obviate the need for the Court of Protection at a later date, advice about driving, advance directives, etc.)
- therapy assessments (OT, SLT for swallowing and communication, PT and dietetics: aim is usually assessment to plan appropriate care and advise carers, rather than treat the patient)
- assessment by social services (financial entitlements, especially Attendance Allowance, provision of services such as home help and access to 'care management', the process by which frail old people are assessed for substantial packages of care at home or residential care)
- use of 'smart' home equipment – technological solutions to prevent and detect problems, e.g. automatic lighting to the toilet triggered when a person gets out of bed, cooker gas cut-off and bath overflow detectors and sensors to detect falls or wandering behaviour
- regular district nurse/community mental health nurse support
- sitting services (Crossroads), day hospitals, respite care
- proper provision of long-term care.

This list demonstrates just how much can be done in dementia, but until recently no specific treatment was available. Drug management focused on the effects of the disease. In the UK, no drug is specifically licensed for the treatment of the behavioural and psychiatric symptoms of dementia; the choice is often between typical and atypical antipsychotics. Typical antipsychotics are more likely to cause extrapyramidal side effects such as tardive dyskinesia, and their anticholinergic effects may worsen cognition. Low-dose thioridazine was popular as it caused less parkinsonism, but was found to increase the risk of ventricular arrhythmias so it has been withdrawn (apart from specialist prescribing in schizophrenia). This left haloperidol as the major drug used in this group, but in recent years the atypical neuroleptics (risperidone and olanzapine) had become the drugs of choice because they appeared to cause fewer side effects, particularly less parkinsonism. However, in 2004, a caution was issued about these drugs because they were found to increase the rate of cerebrovascular events, including stroke, around threefold. However, the risks and benefits of continuing, stopping or changing treatment must be considered for each individual.

Advances in our understanding of the pathological processes in AD have led to the development of drugs to ameliorate the underlying biochemical changes.

Alzheimer's disease

Alzheimer's disease (AD) is divided into early onset familial AD (EOFAD) and the usually sporadic late-onset form (LOAD). The pathology of both is identical, with characteristic amyloid containing extracellular plaques and the abnormal material which develops inside the neurons, the neurofibrillary tangles. In the late 1980s it was proposed that the neuronal degeneration in AD may be caused by deposition of amyloid beta-peptide (Aβ) in plaques in brain tissue. According to the amyloid hypothesis, accumulation of Aβ in the brain is the primary influence driving AD pathogenesis. The rest of the disease process, including formation of neurofibrillary tangles containing tau protein, is proposed to result from an imbalance between Aβ production and Aβ clearance. Three genes have been linked with EOFAD and all probably increase brain levels of amyloid precursor protein:

- the β amyloid gene (*APP*) on chromosome 21
- presenilin 1 (*PSEN1*) on chromosome 14q (the commonest gene defect in EOFAD)
- presenilin 2 (*PSEN2*) on chromosome 1q.

In addition:

- Apolipoprotein E (*APOE*) on chromosome 19q is polymorphic; e2, e3 and e4 are the common isoforms.
- e4 is associated with atherosclerosis, coronary heart disease, VaD, and early and late onset AD.
- Numerous other loci have been postulated to have linkage with AD.

Risk factors for Alzheimer's disease

- Down's syndrome: Essentially all people with trisomy 21 develop the neuropathological hallmarks of AD after age 40 years. More than half such individuals also show clinical evidence of cognitive decline. The

presumed reason is the lifelong overexpression of the amyloid precursor protein and resultant overproduction of Aβ amyloid
- Increasing age
- Female sex
- Apolipoprotein e4 genotype
- Head injury
- Elevated homocysteine levels (an aminoacid that is a marker of certain disease processes in older people)

Protective factors for Alzheimer's disease

- Education (partly a threshold effect, but possible confounding with social class, e.g. diet high in antioxidants)
- Continued brain activity (keep reading!)
- Tobacco (may be the nicotinic effect on cholinergic transmission, but not worth it)
- Wine and coffee (so it's not all bad)
- Exercise
- Diet rich in foods containing vitamin E, but not vitamin E supplements
- Possibly non steroidal anti-inflammatory drugs (but trials of rofecoxib and naproxen are negative in AD patients) and aspirin
- Possibly hormone replacement therapy. Observational data suggested benefit, but HRT users tend to be fitter and to date, prevention trials with combined progesterone and oestrogen and oestrogen only have been negative (Women's Health Initiative, DH 2002)
- Possibly statins (via reduction in vascular damage, but to date prevention trials with simvastatin and pravastatin are negative)

Trials are in progress with vitamins B_6, B_{12} and folic acid, oestrogens, simvastatin, selenium, ginkgo and a number of drugs including glutamate modulators (N-methyl-D-aspartate (NMDA) antagonists and AMPA agonists) will report by 2008. Various strategies to modulate amyloid plaque formation have been tried. Vaccination with Aβ was successful in a mouse model of AD, but early human studies were stopped when some of the subjects developed encephalitis. Other options include beta- and gamma-secretase inhibitors and gene vectors carrying neprilysin, which reduces plaque growth. Defects in astrocyte cell clearance of Aβ may contribute to the formation of AD plaques. Trials of adeno-associated virus-delivered nerve growth factor continue.

The specific treatments for AD which are currently in use are based on historical work showing that the neurons which bear the brunt of the damage are those which use acetylcholine to transmit messages (Figure 2.2).

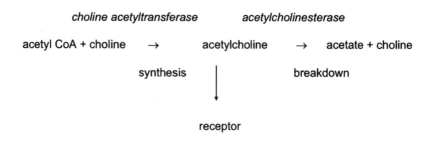

Figure 2.2 The metabolism of acetylcholine.

Cholinergic transmission can be enhanced by increasing the availability of precursor, direct stimulation of the receptors or preventing the breakdown of endogenous acetylcholine. Three drugs which inhibit acetylcholinesterase are available:

- donepezil has been available for longest and has the advantage of once daily dosing at night
- rivastigmine, which also acts on butyryl cholinesterase, which may be more important as the AD advances require twice daily dosing
- galantamine, which also has a direct effect on the nicotinic receptor enhancing acetylcholine release.

Both rivastigmine and galantamine require twice daily dosing. All the drugs tend to cause nausea and bowel upset at first, so it is important to start at a low dose and work up to the maximum tolerated dose. Acetylcholinesterase inhibitors should be prescribed according to NICE guidelines:

- diagnosis of AD made in specialist clinic
- MMSE = 12 or more
- carer's views considered and feasible to expect compliance
- drug continued if cognitive or behavioural benefit (stable MMSE indicates benefit as decline is expected)
- 6-monthly review and drug stopped if benefit no longer apparent or MMSE falls below 12.

Although the licensed indication is AD, trials have shown benefit in DLB and VaD, so the lack of diagnostic precision is not a danger. However, the results of the AD2000 study of donepezil (Courtney et al. 2004) have led to further controversy as, although the study confirms modest benefits on certain tests, the authors challenge claims that the drug is cost-effective. The other drug licensed for AD, memantine, a glutamate inhibitor which blocks NMDA receptors, has few side effects, but there is less clinical data on efficacy. A recent NICE consultation document (2005) suggests that the criteria for prescription of these drugs may be tightened (see Chapter 8).

Dementia with Lewy bodies

Dementia with Lewy bodies (DLB) is probably the second commonest primary dementia and is characterized by dementia, parkinsonism and psychiatric features. In comparison with AD of similar severity, in DLB attention and visual perception are affected more than delayed recall. There may be marked day-to-day fluctuation in cognitive function, particularly attention, to the extent that the patient may become unrousable for periods. There are often well-formed visual hallucinations, but delusions and hallucinations in other modalities are less frequent. The patient develops parkinsonism, particularly rigidity and bradykinesia, and falls are common. There is some pathological overlap with AD with plaques but relatively few tangles. Lewy bodies, intracytoplasmic inclusion bodies containing alpha synuclein, which are restricted to the basal ganglia in Parkinson's disease, are spread through the cortex. Patients can be very sensitive to the effects of neuroleptic medication, so care must be taken with prescribing if DLB is a possible diagnosis.

Progressive supranuclear palsy

The main features of progressive supranuclear palsy (PSP) are early downward gaze palsy, which with the development of instability tends to result in falls especially on stairs, symmetrical parkinsonism and dementia. The pathology shows tangles but these are distinct from those in AD, and gliosis without plaques. The presence of visual hallucinations would suggest a diagnosis of DLB.

Frontotemporal dementia

Frontotemporal dementia (FTD) is characterized by gradual changes in personality, social behaviour, and language ability. Symptoms depend on whether the damage has primarily affected the right (behavioural problems) or left side (language deficits) of the frontal and anterior temporal lobes which control executive functioning. FTD usually develops between the ages of 35 and 75, so although it is rare (about 3% of dementia cases), it may present at an age when patients are labelled AD. Orientation and memory are better preserved than in AD. Pathologically, it is characterized by neurofibrillary tangles. These are known to be abnormally processed microtubule proteins. The microtubule-associated protein tau promotes tubulin polymerization and has a role in stabilizing the microtubules which are responsible for neuronal architecture and transport. A mutation in the tau gene causes a form of FTD called frontotemporal dementia with parkinsonism linked to chromosome 17 (FTDP-17). Mutations in the tau gene impair the binding of tau protein to the microtubule, so FTD is one of the 'tauopathies'.

Vascular dementia

There are several subtypes of VaD. Cognition may remain impaired after a single stroke in a critical area, e.g. the thalamus, recurrent small strokes may produce multi infarct dementia, classically with a stepwise decline, or there may be progressive small vessel disease (Binswanger's disease), characterized by cerebrovascular lesions in the deep white matter of the brain visible on brain CT scan. Risk factors for stroke and VaD appear similar (hypertension, smoking, etc.) but the interesting question is why atheroma (arterial disease) has different consequences in different people. There is a rare familial form of VaD, cerebral autosomal dominant arteriopathy with subcortical infarcts and leukoencephalopathy (CADASIL), characterized by a history of migraine, adult onset (30s–60s) of cerebrovascular disease progressing to dementia and diffuse white matter lesions and subcortical infarcts on neuroimaging. The pathological hallmark of CADASIL is electron-dense granules in the media of arterioles. Another familial condition, congophilic amyloid angiopathy, presents initially with recurrent brain haemorrhage and eventually dementia supervenes.

Normal pressure hydrocephalus

The triad of cognitive impairment, early urinary incontinence and gait disturbance (often apraxic) suggests normal pressure hydrocephalus (NPH). Brain scan shows enlarged ventricles with relatively normal sulci but CSF pressure, as the name implies, appears normal. NPH can be idiopathic or secondary, e.g. to haemorrhage which leads to impaired CSF reabsorption. The pathogenesis is debated but it is assumed that during development of the condition the pressure is higher, perhaps at night. The results of shunting are controversial.

Transient global amnesia

This curious episodic disorder predominantly affects older people. It is of unknown cause and is not predictive of stroke or dementia. There is sudden-onset amnesia – retrograde for recent events and anterograde preventing new memories being laid down – and perplexity, but preservation of alertness, verbal fluency and motor activity. An episode lasts a few hours, although complete recovery may take a few days and there is a low recurrence rate.

Late-onset psychosis

The classification of the psychotic states of late life remains confused (Howard et al. 2000). Psychotic features can be present in depression and dementia, but in this group of conditions they are the major psychiatric phenomenon. On the one hand some believe that this is just a form of schizophrenia seen in older age. Others believe that it is a different disorder, as both the aetiology (schizophrenia in younger people is thought to have a neurodevelopmental basis) and the symptomatology are different. The term 'paraphrenia' is often used in British texts; 'very late onset schizophrenia-like psychosis' is used in the US. The prevalence varies in different studies according to the diagnostic criteria used.

Many factors have been associated with late-onset psychosis including being female, hearing and visual impairment, social isolation and cortical damage on brain scan. The most common symptoms include persecutory delusions and auditory hallucinations. In comparison with young-onset schizophrenia, thought disorder, catatonic symptoms and negative symptoms (including lack of speech inflection and reduced output) are quite unusual.

Management will depend on how the patient presents – the patient rarely seeks help and it is often the family or social services that seek a medical opinion. It is generally helpful to try to establish rapport and to rule out cognitive decline and a mood disorder as the major problem. A stance of 'respectful disagreement' has been recommended towards the patient's delusions. Assessment often has to be made in the home setting and compulsory admission may be required. Multidisciplinary management is usual. Atypical antipsychotics are generally used (e.g. risperidone, olanzapine and quetiapine) in much smaller doses than in younger subjects, but there is little trial data. It was hoped that these drugs would have far fewer side effects than their predecessors such as chlorpromazine, but whilst parkinsonian side effects may be less evident other problems such as weight gain, diabetes, and an increased incidence of stroke are beginning to be recognized.

Substance abuse

Drug and alcohol abuse may be a significant problem in older people. Use may be long term or become a problem in old age, perhaps because of major life events or concomitant physical illness. Drug abuse is most often iatrogenic, benzodiazepine use being the most common. Opiate addiction is seen much more rarely and in the context of chronic pain, not terminal care. An amount of alcohol that would not have caused problems when younger may do so in old age, because of several factors: increased body fat results in higher blood alcohol levels, concomitant physical and cerebral frailty and more scope for interaction with other drugs. Some older people have a poor grasp of units of alcohol and home-poured measures may become more and more generous. If the person is very frail it is helpful to establish who is colluding by supplying the alcohol.

The first step in management is to consider the diagnosis, particularly where alcoholism is associated with self-neglect or falls. Most hospitals have a protocol for managing alcohol withdrawal, usually a reducing course of chlordiazepoxide over 3 days, but for frail old people the regular dose should be reduced by around a half (with the rest prescribed 'if needed'), to avoid oversedation. Patients should not be left in an agitated state as self-discharge is difficult to manage in this group. If the diagnosis is not apparent, agitation and disturbed behaviour may appear a day or so after hospital admission. Even then, the diagnosis of alcohol or benzodiazepine withdrawal will be overlooked unless it is actively considered. Many body systems are damaged by alcohol so that sequelae include neurological damage (fits, Wernicke's encephalopathy – triad of ophthalmopelgia, ataxia and delirium caused by acute thiamine (B_1) deficiency; Korsakoff's psychosis – apathy, poor short-term memory, loss of insight and confabulation; dementia, cerebellar degeneration, peripheral neuropathy), liver damage with cirrhosis and portal hypertension, gastrointestinal bleeding from varices or gastritis, cardiovascular disease including cardiomyopathy, hypertension and haemorrhagic stroke, bone marrow depression and increased incidence of some cancers.

Management follows similar lines to that in a younger group but once alcohol has caused significant brain damage, this is difficult. Other assessments, e.g. by therapists (apart from for immediate treatment) should not be performed until the patient has stabilized after the withdrawal phase. Vitamin B and dietary supplementation should be routine as older people with alcoholism may be particularly at risk of (low income) and vulnerable to (co-existing morbidity) poor nutrition. The management of benzodiazepine withdrawal is well described in the BNF. Success will be much higher if the patient agrees and understands the plan. The dose of the benzodiazepine being taken is converted to the equivalent amount of diazepam and this is very gradually withdrawn. Many psychotropic and neurological agents can cause a withdrawal syndrome if stopped suddenly, and the safest thing is always to wean such medication down. Parkinsonian medication should never be stopped suddenly. If the patient is unexpectedly agitated after changing environments, always compare the previous and current drug regimens.

The immediate management of drug and alcohol abuse is relatively easy, but helping the patient to maintain abstinent behaviour is much harder and usually needs a multidisciplinary approach and involvement of the family or carers. Support from the voluntary sector, education and increased social engagement can contribute. Most social workers with a special interest in substance abuse work mainly with younger clients where the approach is to hand responsibility to the client. This may not be appropriate for the older client with significant brain damage who requires more directive support, and this can cause a culture clash. The management of alcoholism may not have a satisfactory outcome; I have seen ongoing alcohol abuse in a frail brain-damaged man lead to eviction from his residential home.

Sleep problems

Sleep becomes more fragmented with ageing. It can take longer to go to sleep, sleep is less deep and awakening more common, so coupled with the fact that many older people go to bed earlier, complaints of insomnia are common. Aspects of ageing physiology such as reduced urine concentrating ability, most mental illnesses and many physical problems and drugs impair sleep further. A proper history is essential – a patient in her 70s referred for extreme daytime somnolence admitted to staying up every day until around 5 a.m. watching films! The suggestions for better sleep hygiene are the same at any age.

If poor sleep is due to depression, trazodone may be helpful; if due to pain, provide appropriate analgesia. Night sedation (e.g. temazepam, zopiclone) must be used with great caution because of the greater propensity for accidents if the person has to get up in the night, the risk of hangover effects the next day and, at all ages, dependence. Where poor sleep is part of the loss of diurnal rhythm in dementia, increasing daytime activity may help, but regular disturbed nights can be the final straw for a carer; night sedation with its attendant risks may enable a carer to keep coping and may prevent the patient from being institutionalized.

Diogenes (senile squalor) syndrome

Diogenes was a Greek philosopher in the fourth century BC who lived in a barrel. He believed that happiness could only be achieved by self-contemplation, without reliance on other people. In this rather oddly named syndrome, an older person without a major psychiatric diagnosis lives in increasing and often extreme squalor. The person rarely complains but usually attracts hostility from the neighbours who demand that 'something must be done'. It is generally regarded as a personality disorder. A visit to the person's home can be a shocking experience. Typically the rooms will be stacked high with useless things, leaving a narrow track between bed, kitchen, toilet and perhaps a chair. The state may vary from merely dirty to filthy with excrement and infestations of vermin, but the occupant who does not have major dementia or depression will be puzzled by the concern. A long battle with the housing department or the council often intervenes. The prognosis tends to be poor but it is rarely appropriate to apply mental health legislation, as the person usually does not have an identifiable mental illness. Recourse to public health law may be necessary (in the UK Section 47 of the Public Health Act).

Legal aspects

Ethical principles

Many aspects of psychiatry are fraught with ethical issues. In old age it is often dementia that causes additional difficulty. The four basic principles of ethics are:

- beneficence; doing good
- non-maleficence; avoiding harm
- autonomy; allowing self-rule
- justice; distributing goods fairly.

One of the key tensions in old age psychiatry is the conflict between beneficence and autonomy. Should an alcoholic with dementia be allowed to continue drinking? How should the consequences for the individual, his neighbours and his family be judged?

Driving

Suppose a patient with dementia still drives? All four ethics principles and the issue of confidentiality arise. In the UK, everyone is obliged to surrender their driving licence at the age of 70. A new licence is issued which can be renewed every 3 years on completion of a declaration of good health. Certain conditions are considered to render the driver unfit to drive, e.g. poorly controlled epilepsy, but the situation is more difficult where there is concern about driving. Patients should be informed that they must contact the Driver and Vehicle Licensing Authority (DVLA) and their insurance company if there is any change in health status, e.g. developing dementia. A medical or driving assessment may be arranged.

Capacity

In order to make decisions about their care and the future, a person must have mental capacity. People are assumed to have capacity unless the reverse is demonstrated. The assessment of capacity is specific to the task in hand. Contrary to popular belief, a score in a cognitive function test is not the way forward. For whatever task is proposed (e.g. consenting to treatment, drawing up an advance directive, making an Enduring Power of Attorney, making a will) the person must be able to understand, believe and retain the relevant background information, weigh up the risks and benefits and then arrive at a decision (although the choice made may seem eccentric to others).

Enduring Power of Attorney

An Enduring Power of Attorney (EPA) is a document in which an individual, the 'donor', appoints another person or persons to be his or her 'attorney'. This power, which has to be arranged when the donor has capacity, endures or remains in force in the event the donor becomes mentally incapacitated but only if it is registered with the Court of Protection. An EPA authorizes an attorney to make decisions about the property and financial affairs of the donor. This is a simple step to take and should be recommended to the family in which a member has early dementia, but it should be noted that financial abuse has been estimated to occur in 10–15% of such arrangements. It should be noted that different rules may apply in different countries; indeed, within the UK, regulations are different in Scotland.

Court of Protection

The Court of Protection is an office of the supreme court of England and Wales. Where a patient has a mental disorder and is incapable of managing her affairs, and has not previously made arrangements for an EPA, an application can be made to the court. The court appoints a receiver (usually a relative) to manage the patient's financial affairs on a day-to-day basis. The receiver is obliged to present an annual account to the Court, so although the system is more cumbersome than taking out an EPA, it offers more security. The legal frameworks in Scotland and Ireland are different and a specialist text should be consulted.

Mental Health Act

The current legislative framework in England and Wales is the Mental Health Act 1983. The legislation is under revision and the latest version is the draft Mental Health Bill 2004. The Bill provides for both the compulsory treatment of people with mental health problems, in the interests of their own health and safety, as well as the safety of others. A revised Mental Capacity Bill is also to be introduced.

End-of-life decisions and advance directives (living wills)

These allow people to make decisions about what treatments they would wish to accept or refuse in the event of personal loss of competence occurring. For example, in the event of developing dementia, the individual would not want cardiopulmonary resuscitation to be attempted. The principle is sensible, but people are very prone to changing their minds when the situation changes. A number of patients now have a living will but they are often rather vaguely worded and so do not help with clinical management decisions. However, as advance directives become more commonplace, some of the initial problems may be resolved.

References

Adshead F, Cody D, Pitt B (1992) BASDEC: a novel screening instrument for depression in elderly in-patients. BMJ 305: 397.

APA (2000) Diagnostic and Statistical Manual of Mental Disorders, 4th edn, Text Revision. American Psychiatric Association, Washington, DC.

Courtney C, Farrell D, Gray R et al. (2004) Long term donepezil treatment in 565 patients with Alzheimer's disease (AD2000): randomised double-blind trial. Lancet 363(9427): 2105–2115.

DH (2002) Risks and Benefits of HRT: results of the US Women's Health Initiative and implications for long-term use of combination HRT. Department of Health, London.

DH (2004) New Health Programme Trial to Improve Older People's Care. Department of Health, London.

Folstein MF, Folstein SE, McHugh PR (1975) 'Mini-mental state' – a practical method for grading the cognitive state of patients for the clinician. Journal of Psychiatric Research 12: 189–198.

Hachinski VC, Illiff LD, Zilkha E et al. (1975) Cerebral blood flow in dementia. Archives of Neurology 32(9): 632–637.

Hodkinson M (1972) Evaluation of a mental test score for assessments of mental impairment in the elderly. Age and Ageing 1: 233–238.

Howard R, Rabins PV, Seeman MV, Jeste DV and the International late-onset schizophrenia group (2000) Late-onset schizophrenia and very-late-onset schizophrenia-like psychosis: an international consensus. American Journal of Psychiatry 157: 172–178.

NICE (2005) National Institute for Clinical Excellence Appraisal Consultation Document: Alzheimer's disease – donepezil, rivastigmine, galantamine and memantine (review). *www.nice.org.uk/*

WHO (1992) *International Classification of Diseases and Related Health Problems* (ICD-10). World Health Organization, Geneva.

Yesavage JA, Brink TL, Rose TL et al. (1983) Development and validation of a geriatric screening depression scale: a preliminary report. Journal of Psychiatric Research 17(1): 37–49.

Useful websites

Action on Elder Abuse (*www.elderabuse.org.uk*): Elder abuse information including a practitioner booklet.

Alzheimer Research Forum (*www.alzforum.org/home.asp*): One of the best research sites about Alzheimer's disease.

British National Formulary (*www.bnf.org*): up-to-date drug information, site requires (free) registration.

National Institute of Neurological Disorders and Stroke (NINDS) (*www.ninds.nih.gov/disorders/disorder_index.htm*): information on neurological diseases including dementia.

OMNI, the UK gateway for psychiatry and psychology (*http://omni.ac.uk/browse/subject-listing/WM100.html*): a fantastic up-to-date selection of scientific, service and user-focused sites right across the topic range.

Royal College of Psychiatry London (*www.rcpsych.ac.uk*): has excellent leaflets for patients on depression in the elderly, manic depression, schizophrenia, anxiety disorders, etc.

CHAPTER 3

Managing dementias in primary care

VARI DRENNAN AND STEVE ILIFFE

The dementias are one of the most pressing problems facing health and social care and are also the fourth commonest cause of death in people aged 75 and over (Gray and Fenn 1993). Approximately 5% of those over 65 years and 20% of those 85 years old have some kind of dementia, prevalence rates that appear similar across Europe (Hoffman et al. 1991). In 1998 it was estimated that there were nearly half a million people with dementia in the UK, and this figure was predicted to rise to 650 000 by 2021 (Bosanquet et al. 1998). The estimated annual cost of dementia in the United Kingdom is £5.5 billion, of which three fifths are borne by patients, carers and social security funds, one fifth by social services and one fifth by the National Health Service (Bosanquet et al. 1998).

The National Service Framework for Older People (DH 2001) emphasizes the need for early detection and diagnosis of dementia in primary care (delivered through GPs and other community-based health services), to allow access to treatment and planning of future care, and to help individuals and their families come to terms with the prognosis. Similarly, the Audit Commission report 'Forget Me Not 2002' recommends that GPs make increased efforts to diagnose dementias early (Audit Commission 2002). This report points out that the cost of failing to diagnose early is often a crisis situation for the person with dementia and his or her family, with specialist services being called in at too late a stage to establish supportive care packages.

A GP with a list of 2000 patients and an average age distribution will see one or two new cases per year and have up to 14 patients with a dementia at different stages of the disease process at any one time. A practice serving a young population (for example, in the inner city areas) may not notice much change as out-migration of retired people changes the population profile further, but in retirement areas GPs may already have 20 or so people with dementia registered with them, and this will rise to nearer 25. In such a locality, a group practice of 5 full-time equivalent GPs may be managing a caseload of 100 individuals with dementia, and should anticipate adding another 25 in the next few years. Most of these people will be referred to specialist, social care and rehabilitation services, with an increase in early referrals if current plans are implemented. A district nursing team with a caseload of 80 patients will typically have between 5 and 15 individuals with dementia amongst them. Many of these individuals will be cared for by family members or neighbours whose own health may suffer from the prolonged and difficult work of caring. Given the increased awareness of the public about dementia, and an increasingly consumerist attitude amongst younger generations towards the care of their parents, primary care services should prepare for an expanding workload, without necessarily being able to enlarge the workforce proportionately.

Dementia is a progressive disease process with a community-wide impact (Gallo et al. 1991), and its usually unremitting course challenges the diagnostic, management and support skills of primary care workers, and the capacity of specialist services to support people with dementia and to contain and ameliorate the disease process. This chapter offers a brief framework for community-based practitioners to aid their diagnostic, management and support activities; a fuller exploration of the themes in this chapter can be found in Iliffe and Drennan (2001). We do not underestimate how difficult this condition is for everyone concerned and suggest that this framework is but a starting point in a situation of great complexity with no easy solutions.

The features of the dementias

The dementias are much misunderstood, and their diagnosis and management are a challenge. At the beginning memory deficits and other changes in cognition, behaviour or mood (including some features of depression) may be attributed to old age. The personality may begin to change, with emotional lability, disinhibition and sometimes verbal or even physical aggression emerging. Functional losses can appear before evident memory loss, so that individuals cannot remember which medicines to take, or how to make a telephone call. As the dementia process proceeds, awareness of memory or other problems with cognition diminishes, so the patient becomes a less reliable witness. As a consequence, relatives' complaints about the memory of a family member are suggestive of dementia, whereas complaints of memory loss made by the patient suggest depression rather than dementia. However, there is no classic presentation, since one in three patients with dementia will also have features of either a depressive disorder, or symptoms attributable to bereavement, or generalized anxiety, or an alcohol problem.

Later in the disease process higher mental functions are seemingly lost, so that the affected individuals experience disorientation and loss of comprehension, lose the ability to calculate, and lack learning capacity, language and judgement. In the last phases of dementia the individual loses almost all functional capacity. However, an individual's pathway through dementia is unique and influenced by their previous life experience and their social and family relationships, so that dementia emerges through the personality, which remains visible and active as the disease process progresses.

Recognition of dementia

People with early dementia may not be recognized as having a problem for a considerable period; the time between first noted symptoms by patient or carer and medical evaluation for dementia is on average 30 months (Haley et al. 1992). The reasons for this are complex:

• Individuals with cognitive impairment and their carers may attribute symptoms such as memory loss and other cognitive changes, functional loss or emotional lability to ageing (Pollitt 1996).
• Feelings of shame, guilt and incompetence in the affected individual or their family may impede seeking help.
• Carers may not tackle the issue out of respect for their spouse or parent (Antonelli Incalzi et al. 1992).

Seeking help is affected by many factors: those from higher socioeconomic groups are more likely to seek medical attention earlier (Pollitt 1996), and cultural background may influence the timing of presentation to GPs (Rait and Burns 1998). Lack of awareness or insight and denial may account for some late presentation of dementia (Verhey et al. 1995); in one study nearly half of all patients were unaware that they had a problem at first contact (Newens et al. 1994). Nevertheless, informant histories are crucial to investigating the suspicion of dementia, and carers may be the first to reach the diagnosis (O'Connor et al. 1988), even if they do not voice it or act upon it.

The triggers that start the process of recognition of dementia for both lay people and professionals are commonly:

• important functional changes, e.g. not taking prescribed medication regularly
• behavioural disturbances, e.g. wandering or acting in a disinhibited way
• major loss of memory, e.g. losing the way home from the shops
• other cognitive and mood changes, e.g. the expression of paranoid ideas
• crises – e.g. when the spouse, who has compensated so long for the failing ability of their partner with dementia, has to be admitted to hospital.

Moving from suspicion to greater certainty can be a lengthy process, but it has a logical path. Distinguishing dementia from other changes in thinking and behaviour that can occur at different stages of life is not a simple task, especially in the early stages of the process. The two processes that can be mistaken for dementia are acute confusion and depression. Table 3.1 gives a brief guide to the differences between them. Acute confusion is the easier to distinguish from dementia because it begins suddenly, whereas dementias do not, but it may also reveal an underlying dementia process that has been masked by the compensations made by others. Loss of abilities or memories in one person can be replaced by increased effort from another, who becomes, in effect, the memory for the affected individual. Depression is more common than dementia (up to 20% of the population over 65 may report significant depressive symptoms) but can co-exist with dementia in up to 40% of individuals with cognitive impairment, especially in the early stages of the process. Treatment of the depression seems to be effective in terms of restoring some function and reducing psychological distress, in up to 85% of those with both disorders. The important message for community-based practitioners is to think twice about the causes of changed behaviour in their older patients, for the seemingly obvious symptoms of one condition may conceal another process, and diagnoses can be labels that stick even when wrong. The solution to this dilemma is to seek other opinions, from those who know the person (their family and friends), and from those who know dementia well (old age psychiatrists and community mental health nurses).

Table 3.1 A brief guide to the differential diagnosis of dementia, acute confusion and depression

	Dementia	**Acute confusional state**	**Depression**
Onset	Insidious	Acute	Gradual
Duration	Months/years	Hours/days/weeks sometimes	Weeks/months
Course	Stable and progressive	Fluctuates: worse at night, lucid periods	Usually worse in mornings, improves as day goes on
Alertness	Vascular dementia: usually stepwise	Fluctuates	Normal
Orientation	Usually normal	Always impaired: time/place/person	Usually normal
Memory	May be normal but usually impaired for time/place	Recent impaired	Recent may be impaired, remote, intact

Table 3.1 continued

	Dementia	Acute confusional state	Depression
Thoughts	Slowed Reduced interests Perseveration	Often paranoid and grandiose, sometimes with bizarre ideas and topics	Usually slowed, preoccupied by sad and hopeless thoughts
Perception	Normal Hallucinations in 30–40% (often visual)	Visual and auditory hallucinations common	Mood congruent Auditory hallucinations in 20%
Emotions	Shallow, apathetic, labile, irritable, careless	Irritable, aggressive, fearful	Flat, unresponsive or sad and fearful May be irritable
Sleep	Often disturbed nocturnal wandering common	Nocturnal confusion	Early morning wakening
Other features	Nocturnal confusion	Other physical disease may not be obvious	May have past history of mood disorder?

Reproduced with permission from: *Dementia tutorial: diagnosis and management in primary care: a primary care based education/research project*, Stirling University and RFUCLMS.

Diagnoses in general practice are made through pattern recognition over time, with particular symptoms or problems described by the patient or carer triggering an iterative process of hypothesis testing (De Lepeleire and Heyrman 1999). The overall ability of GPs to recognize dementia is moderately good, with positive predictive values for GP diagnoses against gold standards (e.g. CAMDEX) ranging from 32% to 79% in seven studies reviewed by van Hout (1999). Clearly there is considerable scope for improvement but, unless primary care professionals are aware of the early signs of dementia, they are unlikely to begin the diagnostic process (Lagaay et al. 1992).

Early identification of dementia can be important for planning care, for education of patients, families and professional teams, and for mobilization of resources. Also, recent therapeutic advances have renewed calls to improve detection and management of people with dementia because of some evidence of therapeutic benefit from selective use of the newer anti-dementia drugs. Early diagnosis is also important because it allows for individuals and carers to be informed, and to be introduced to appropriate agencies and support networks that can relieve the disabling psychological distress that carers may experience (Levin et al. 1989), even without the support being called upon (Briggs 1993). One of the commonest criticisms of GPs, and to a lesser extent of specialist services, is that they provide too little information about dementia and its consequences, with too little practical content that is helpful to patients and families.

There is no consensus on the optimal methods for recognizing dementia in the community (Toner 1992, Audit Commission 2002). The majority of GPs in the UK (Ireichen 1994) and a large minority of family physicians in the USA (Fortinsky and Wasson 1997) report no use of cognitive function tests in helping to reach a diagnosis of dementia. GPs may be embarrassed or anxious about carrying out cognitive function tests (van Hout 1999), and do not benefit from using standard diagnostic criteria presented as clinical guidelines (Downs et al. 2000). Practitioners who have most difficulty in making the diagnosis of dementia also have more problems in disclosing the diagnosis, particularly to the person with dementia (Cody et al. 2002). Primary care physicians may be especially concerned about making 'false positive' diagnoses in a climate which increasingly encourages early disclosure, and when a wrong diagnosis may have significant impact on doctor–patient relationships (Eefsting et al. 1996). The Alzheimer's Society (2003) have produced a CD-ROM on the diagnosis and management of dementia in primary care, to assist GPs in diagnosing and supporting people with dementia and their carers. Practitioners may be sceptical about the benefits of anti-dementia drug treatment, inhibited in making early diagnoses by the limited availability of local resources to support the person with dementia (Olafsdottir et al. 2001), uncertain about the clinical management of people with dementia (Freyne 2001), or have difficult relationships with patients and carers (Fortinsky 2001). A willingness to accept a family's reluctance to disclose the diagnosis may clash with a desire to communicate honestly and directly with a patient (Gordon and Goldstein 2001), creating dilemmas for long-term relationships. Practitioners are being encouraged to undertake activities that they find particularly difficult, but that are urgently needed (Marriott 2003), such as providing education, offering psychological support for carers and mobilizing carer social support (Cohen et al. 2001).

Disclosing the diagnosis

Sharing the diagnosis is the task that everyone finds most difficult, but it is essential to families, carers and friends that their anxieties about dementia are dealt with directly. Knowing the diagnosis may dispel the patient's belief that she is 'going mad', but the recognition of dementia by patient and family may result in social withdrawal, and a tendency to maximize deficits and minimize strengths and successes. Every disclosure must therefore lead on to follow-up, and to what Kitwood (1997) called 'positive person work' that counters the impact of neuronal losses in a realistic, accepting way. The progressive nature of the dementias needs to be acknowledged, but not as a cruel fate against which all effort is futile. False hopes about cures or even short-term improvements are equally unhelpful. There is evidence from other clinical domains that presenting bad news in an unhurried, honest, balanced and empathic fashion leads to greater satisfaction with disclosure. Prior knowledge of individuals and families can be of enormous importance here, but is not available to old age psychiatrists or community psychiatric nurses coming to an individual with dementia for the first time at some point in the disease process. Whatever the benefits of specialist appraisal, the GP or community nurse with background knowledge of people, families and communities has a great deal to contribute.

Early interventions

There are some interventions with medication or psychosocial techniques (Brodaty et al. 2003) that appear to be beneficial in dementia. In summary they are:

- The medications donepezil and galantamine improve cognitive function and global clinical state in some people with mild to moderate Alzheimer's disease, for up to one year, although this has been challenged recently (Courtney et al. 2004).
- Ginkgo biloba, oestrogen (but only in women) and the medicine selegiline seem to improve cognitive function in Alzheimer's disease, as does reality orientation in all dementia types but not all stages of severity (Spector et al. 2005).
- The medication rivastigmine seems to improve cognitive function in Alzheimer's disease and Lewy body dementia, but adverse effects are common and unpleasant.
- Widely discussed therapies of uncertain effectiveness include vitamins, reminiscence therapy (but see Woods et al. 2005) and non-steroidal medication (such as aspirin or ibuprofen)

More therapies for dementia are being evaluated rigorously, and new medications are being developed, so the potential for modifying the disease process will increase over the coming years. Therapies able to stop or reverse the dementia process are not on the horizon.

Gateways to support, information and services

The message from all the literature is that the person with dementia and their family need to be in touch from the earliest point with those people who can best provide the network of support, information and services. There is significant variation in statutory and voluntary provision in the four countries of the UK. However at a minimum, the GP should ensure that the person with dementia and their family have gateways to people, information and services that can:

- confirm the diagnosis of a dementia
- help them with their psychological distress
- help them access services
- help them deal with financial and legal issues
- provide a care management framework to help detect and address changes in their needs.

So at a minimum the aim from general practice is to:

- refer to specialist secondary care services for confirmation of diagnosis (in some instances) or to seek further diagnostic help when the dementia type is uncertain and to enable access to information about the range of specialist support for people with dementia
- refer to the local social care and/or health personnel who can undertake detailed assessment, care planning and provision of support and services within a care management process
- provide sources of information on dementia
- provide details of the national Alzheimer's Society and its local branches.

Early referral to specialist services, such as memory clinics, can be helpful to all concerned, in confirming the diagnosis, helping mobilize resources, and initiating as appropriate the new drug treatments for mild to moderate levels of dementia.

The broad goals of support from primary health care are to:

- maintain cognition and daily living skills
- reduce excess disability and distress
- maintain the quality of life of patient and carers
- sustain living in the community.

Local sources of expertise to support these broad goals may vary considerably and it is here that the local knowledge of primary care practitioners is invaluable.

Joint working and people with a dementia

The GP working with the patient and the family may be the first to share the diagnosis with them and it may be obvious that they meet the eligibility criteria of the local authority for a full comprehensive assessment under the Community Care Act to prevent a breakdown in their present arrangements for care and support. In this situation, immediate referral to the relevant social work team is required. In other situations, it may be very early in the progress of the dementia and it is more appropriate to establish a baseline of abilities with a mechanism for monitoring and review as well as provide a source of information and support. There are different local arrangements for the provision of this second source of help. In some areas it can be provided by health visitors for older people, in others by community psychiatric nurses for older people. Some areas have specialist dementia nursing services (the Admiral Nursing Service) to provide specialized care management functions, information and support to carers. A baseline assessment of the person with dementia would include information on:

- the person's view of any difficulties or problems at the present
- the network of people in the daily life of the person with dementia
- household composition
- interests/social activities and pattern of a typical day
- other significant recent events, e.g. bereavements
- emotional and other mental health issues, e.g. loneliness
- the medication being taken – on prescription, bought over the counter or borrowed from helpful friends and neighbours
- ability to communicate – speech, hearing, writing, reading, using a telephone
- ability to undertake domestic and household tasks
- mobility inside and outside the home
- sleep patterns
- diet, ability to get meals and changes in appetite
- orientation inside and outside the home
- ability to undertake personal care, e.g. dressing, washing, going to the toilet
- financial/benefit issues
- balance of risks.

Not all of this information can or necessarily should be collected in one discussion and some of it (e.g. financial affairs and incontinence) has to be discussed with additional sensitivity. Here a prior relationship with the person and their family may be more helpful than a systematic interview, and GPs may contribute knowledge to that gained by nurses or social workers. The introduction of the single assessment process (DH 2001) as part of the National Service Framework for Older People, combined with the development of electronic records, has the potential to improve the continuity between agencies and ensure timely offers of services, support and information.

The GP has an ongoing responsibility to provide medical services to patients. The primary health-care team, while addressing specific needs associated with dementia, also has a responsibility to continue to promote healthy, active living which includes those tenets of a balanced diet, sufficient fluid intake, frequent exercise, adequate sleep and minimal alcohol. Health maintenance activities such as dental check ups, eyesight testing and influenza vaccination should not be lost through a focus on dementia-related issues.

There are two other legal issues that need broaching at this point:

- **Driving:** A patient diagnosed as having dementia has a legal duty to inform the DVLA. They may be given a Group 1 licence, if there is no significant deterioration in time and space orientation, and retention of insight and judgement, but an annual medical review is needed for renewal. The GP should inform the DVLA if the patient cannot understand this advice.
- **Financial affairs:** Family carers should be encouraged to seek advice and background information from the Alzheimer's Society on Enduring Power of Attorney, the Court of Protection and Public Office Trust and Guardianship.

Informal carers of people with dementia

In the UK, informal carers (i.e. people who provide unpaid care to others) are:

- more likely to be women than men
- more likely to be aged 45–64 than any other age group
- more likely to be a relative than not
- more likely to be looking after someone aged over 75
- more likely to be a spouse (equal numbers of men and women) than not if the dependent person is elderly and married (ONS 1998).

There are two further salient issues for primary care professionals in supporting informal carers of people with dementia:

- There are often others (usually family members) besides the primary caregiver who form a network of relationships and who may be profoundly affected by the progress of the dementia.
- The carers' roles shift and change with the progress of the dementia. The carer role continues, even if the person with dementia is living in an institutional setting.

The notions of carer and transition are very helpful in understanding changes in roles and relationships. All informal carers start off in one role, such as husband or daughter, with a history and way of being in their personal relationships with this other adult. As the dementia progresses, parts of this original role recede and the caregiver assumes some or all of the following roles:

- **decision-maker:** with and then on behalf of the person
- **protector:** preserving the self image of the person as well as physically protecting them from harm
- **advocate:** promoting the interests of the person with dementia
- **supervisor:** ensuring the person with dementia is able to undertake activities appropriately

- **monitor:** observing changes in the individual as well as the quality of care provided by others
- **instrumental carer:** the provider of the activities of daily living, including the physical, emotional and social tasks the person with dementia can no longer perform
- **preserver:** repository of knowledge about the person who can no longer communicate for themselves their history, their personality or their preferences.

Separating the roles out in this way helps elucidate how others in the caregiving network can contribute, even when they are not providing direct physical care. However, this is not to underestimate the degree to which some kinship networks can generate conflict as well as concordance in caring. It is also important to point out that there are positive aspects to being a carer if only because health and social care professionals rarely think about the positive aspects (Grant and Nolan 1993). Carers of people with dementia have described satisfaction in caring stemming from

- a feeling of satisfaction
- a way of expressing ongoing affection and love
- continued reciprocity
- companionship
- the fulfilment of a sense of duty (Murray et al. 1999).

There is also a significant body of knowledge which demonstrates how the caring role may have negative effects on carers' lives, particularly primary carers, in four interacting domains – economic, social, mental and physical. The economic impact on carers includes:

- the costs incurred while caring
- reduction of income through giving up paid work for some carers
- reduction of future financial security and pension for some carers (Caring Costs Alliance 1996).

Primary health-care professionals should ensure that information is available to carers on the levels of state financial support for carers:

- Disability Living Allowance care component (under 65)
- Attendance Allowance (65 and over)
- Invalid Care Allowance for carers
- reduction in or exemption from Council Tax.

Other benefits and grants are available to those on low incomes. A number of studies have demonstrated the effectiveness of providing information on welfare benefits through primary care (Toeg et al. 2003).

The link between being able to maintain a social life and emotional well-being is very important for carers of people with dementia. Feelings of loneliness and of having no time for leisure activities are implicated in the high levels of poor psychological health reported by carers of people with dementia (Buck et al. 1997). An increased incidence of depression in carers is associated with behavioural problems and with situations where higher levels of care are required by the person with a dementia (Russo and Vitaliano 1995). Although there is a paucity of high-quality research to demonstrate effective interventions on carers' burden (Thompson and Thompson 1998), carers themselves request and praise the following forms of help:

- access to local groups for the provision of support and information
- regular respite services throughout the course of the dementia
- training in carer activities
- multidimensional assessment and support
- financial support for caring.

In England the first government National Strategy for Carers (DH 2000) provides a checklist to help primary care practitioners to improve their attention to carers' needs (see box).

Checklist for GPs and primary care teams to help carers

- Have you identified those of your patients who are carers, and patients who have a carer?
- Do you check carers' physical and emotional health whenever a suitable opportunity arises, and at least once a year?
- Do you routinely tell carers that they can ask social services for an assessment of their own needs?
- Do you always ask patients who have carers whether they are happy for health information about them to be told to their carer?
- Do you know whether there are carers' support groups or carers' centres in your area, and do you tell carers about them?

(DH 2000, p. 57)

Caring for people at home as the dementia progresses

As the dementia progresses, the person with dementia and their carers require greater levels of assistance – either at home or in some form of care setting. Primary health-care professionals have to have knowledge and systems within which to offer their own expertise at the right points while helping the person with dementia and carers access those other services they need. A monitoring and review process agreed by members of the practice team and its attached members, such as the district nurses, is important to ensure that timely support and increased services are offered. Those people who have already been assessed within a community care process will have a named social work care manager and an agreed review process that incorporates the assessments of the GP and other primary care professionals.

The losses experienced at the beginning of dementia may provoke reactions and adjustments as described in the staged model of Cohen et al. (1984), including:

* recognition and concern
* denial
* anger, guilt and sadness: these are the common emotions that emerge after the diagnosis is learned, but they may persist throughout the course of the illness and beyond
* coping: adaptation to the impact of dementia, and the increasing demands of the person with dementia, forces family and other carers to 'get by'
* maturation: an element of acceptance and understanding in individuals with good coping strategies allows both the patient and the carers to do more than 'get by'
* separation from the self.

This last stage, the separation from the self, may be easily misunderstood as the disappearance of the self, but this view may reflect the inability of those around the affected individual to keep up with that person's changing state. Since we do not consist of memory alone but have feelings, imagination, energy, desires and will, the person with dementia can retain and express a sense of uniqueness until death, losing mostly their public or social self (Downs 1997). Professionals may be particularly affected by the loss of the social person, focusing on the illness and its problems, while family members or friends may have a stronger sense of the normality of the person with dementia. Kitwood suggested from his observations that well-supported carers rarely talk about 'personality change' or the 'loss of the person', but rather behave as if dementia represented a loss of resources, and a breakdown of defences in the affected individual (Kitwood 1997). The person who was once overcontrolled emotionally may express rage as their dementia progresses, and the individual who has been sexually inhibited may become embarrassingly disinhibited.

In general practice and community nursing, the knowledge that practitioners acquire about their patients, their families and the local community can help other professionals to understand the changes that are occurring within an individual with dementia. This knowledge can be conveyed to others – to the old age psychiatrist, to social care workers, or to the staff of a nursing home – who do not have the advantage of prior knowledge of the person. And it can be used to tailor support to the patient and their carers.

Through a combination of primary care nursing services, social services, mental health care of older people services and the voluntary sector, a range of services can be provided for the person with dementia and their carers in the home:

- personal care activities
- managing continence problems
- chiropody, dentistry and optometry
- obtaining and taking medicines
- obtaining shopping and meals
- household tasks
- aids to daily living and adaptations to their environment
- social stimulation and activities
- respite from caring
- counselling
- behaviour management.

The levels of provision, eligibility criteria and payment rates for non-NHS services vary according to national and local agreements and thus local knowledge is essential for primary care practitioners.

People with dementia can develop a range of behaviours that can be disturbed and disturbing for all concerned and which need to be investigated carefully to tailor a specific response. Some of the behaviours that can occur in the course of dementia (IPA 2002) are listed below:

- repetitive questioning
- following someone around
- hiding and losing things
- pacing and searching
- repetitive phrases and actions
- fidgeting or restlessness
- continual shouting or wailing
- laughing or crying uncontrollably for no apparent reason
- lack of inhibition
- high levels of suspicion
- hallucinations and delusions
- aggression – verbal and/or physical.

Some behaviours are obviously more problematic than others, although primary health-care professionals should not underestimate the effect of living with someone who continually repeats the same questions or is continually rearranging and then losing possessions. In trying to understand and then address the behaviour it is important to elicit:

- a clear description of the behaviour
- events leading up to the behaviour and contributory factors
- who else was involved and what they were doing
- the environment in which the behaviour happened
- previous occurrences of the event
- any previous interventions or actions that helped.

It can be difficult to understand the origins of behavioural changes in dementia, particularly when they emerge in a crisis on a Sunday evening. A useful mnemonic to help determine the causes of behavioural problems and how best to approach them is 'PAID':

- **Physical** problems can be a cause of behavioural disturbance. For example, the pain from osteoarthritis can make somebody more aggressive than usual.
- **Activity-related** behavioural disturbances may appear when the carer is undertaking a particular activity. For example, helping with intimate tasks such as dressing or bathing may trigger aggressive responses. Such responses may also appear when there is lack of activity, for example pacing up and down may be providing occupation.
- **Intrinsic to dementia:** There are some behaviours intrinsic to dementia, especially, but not exclusively in the later stages of the disorder. For example, people may wander more or repeatedly stroke another person. Unaccountable laughing or crying uncontrollably is often a feature of vascular dementia.
- **Depression and delusions:** People with delusions or hallucinatory experiences can become behaviourally disturbed and have an acute psychosis. The focus for treatment should be the psychosis rather than the behavioural disturbance itself, but caution is required with medication and a specialist in old age psychiatry or medicine for the elderly should be involved if there are any doubts.

Management of behavioural disturbance or psychological symptoms in dementia can be very difficult, partly because the changes may be related to the person's environment, or be very specific to their past experience, or reflect other disease processes – particularly infections or conditions causing pain. Treatment may be complicated by the inability of the individual to give informed consent to it. Antipsychotics are widely used in these situations, but there is little evidence to support the use of these drugs, which may produce profound adverse effects such as increasing confusion and agitation, parkinsonian-type effects, and acute collapse in Lewy body disease (DTB 2003). As a rule, specialist advice should be sought whenever behaviour disturbance becomes unmanageable by non-medical means.

Carers need to be offered ideas and support in coping with the behaviour of the individual, as well as strategies to avoid confrontation: for example, suggestions of simple measures to make wandering safer such as having contact details pinned inside all clothes and on a bracelet. Carers should be directed to the comprehensive information sheets produced by the Alzheimer's Society for strategies across the spectrum of behaviours that the person with dementia might have (Alzheimer's Society 2000).

The following are some suggestions for avoiding confrontation with people with dementia which practitioners and staff in primary care settings should be made aware of:

- Talk in a calm, reassuring tone at normal volume.
- Approach the person in their line of vision before talking.
- Pay attention to your and their body language; try and remain at the same physical level as them.
- Allow enough time to undertake conversations and activities at their pace, not yours; this may often mean not trying to do too many things one after another.
- Find ways of enhancing communication with non-verbal cues.
- Provide reassurance rather than outright denial of their fears or delusions.
- If you start getting irritated or feel angry with the person, take time out, calm down and then come back.
- If the person with dementia starts showing signs of agitation or aggression, cease what you are doing and withdraw, returning later perhaps in the company of someone they know or trust more.

Despite all the best efforts on the part of carers and professionals to find ways to cope and manage the change in behaviour and loss of abilities, it is common to meet refusal or rejection of help from the person with dementia. Refusal to be helped often makes family carers and professionals distressed or worried. The questions to ask out loud are:

- How do the risks balance against the choice of the individual?
- What strategies for coping are available, and which professionals and services should be involved in thinking about risk and risk management?
- When should we review the situation?

Refusal to accept admission to residential care can be the most challenging of all, and should prompt all concerned to think:

- How can risks be limited?
- Is extra community support available?
- Are compulsory procedures appropriate?
- Is there anyone who can be appointed guardian?

The full range of expertise from across the heath and social care agencies may be needed to manage such situations.

Addressing the knowledge and attitudes of primary health-care professionals

Kitwood and Bredin (1992) argued that reliance on a neuropathological framework for understanding the progress of dementia, combined with a history of dehumanizing institutional care traditions, has supported a 'malignant social psychology' in caring for people with dementia. This malignant social psychology in professionals and carers, while not intentionally evil, reduces the person to an object and fails to recognize the importance to them of the psychosocial environment. Primary health-care professionals are not immune from this malignant social psychology, and two strategies are suggested to help counteract its pervasive nature. The first is awareness-raising for all primary care staff in appropriate practical communications skills with people with dementia. Some of these are outlined in the box.

Simple, practical aspects of communicating with a person with dementia

- Reduce the chance of alarming the person by approaching them in their line of vision and conduct your conversation at a similar voice level to theirs
- Ensure the surrounding environment does not provide competing distractions
- Make sure all aids to communication are operational, e.g. glasses in place, hearing aids switched on
- Reinforce your words with non-verbal communication, i.e. try to make and keep eye contact; use a calm, reassuring tone; consider using touch, such as holding hands, if appropriate
- Illustrate your words with pictures or the real thing, e.g. a stethoscope
- Be a good listener and observer of non-verbal clues
- Allow enough time between statements and actions for comprehension and responses
- Use short, jargon-free, simple sentences which deal with one issue at a time
- Avoid complicated linguistic devices such as rhetorical questions and the royal 'we'

Table 3.2 Recognizing signs of well-being and the converse in a person with dementia

Signs of well-being	Signs of ill-being
Being able to assert own will and desires	Distress or despair
Being able to show a range of emotions including pleasure and sadness	Intense anger
Initiating contact with others	Physical discomfort/pain
Having self-respect	Fear/anxiety
Enjoying humour	
Showing pleasure	
Being able to relax	
Being helpful	

Adapted from Kitwood and Bredin (1992).

The second strategy is to pay greater attention to signs of well-being and ill-being in a person with dementia. Again, Kitwood and Bredin (1992) proposed a framework for this within institutional settings. We have adapted this (see Table 3.2) and argue that its use could help primary care professionals move beyond the label of dementia.

Primary health-care and care homes

GPs and nurses are often involved at the point where the decision is made to use a supported care residence as a break for carers in the home or as a permanent move. It is invariably associated with factors such as the person with dementia having increased physical dependence, irritability, nocturnal wandering, incontinence and carer stress (Eccles et al. 1998). This is a major life event for the person with dementia and their relatives, and creates enormous stress and often distress. Primary health-care professionals can offer support, opportunities to express those emotions and reminders or introductions to the wider local support network to share those emotions. While primary health-care professionals are not likely to have in-depth knowledge to assist in the selection of a residence they need to be able to pass on basic information, for example:

- Social work care managers can supply lists of local residential provision.
- The websites of government bodies responsible for social care inspection in the countries of the UK list care homes and provide copies of all inspection reports.
- Helpful publications on how to choose a care home are available from voluntary organizations such as Age Concern.
- The provision of care homes registered for the residence/care of people who have dementia is largely in the independent sector although the financial support may come in full or part from public funds. National policy and local interpretation determines issues such as to what extent the public purse supports long term care of older people, eligibility criteria, and local financial ceilings on the amount for the care of an individual. Up-to-date knowledge of the local system is important for primary care professionals.

Medical care continues to be provided by GPs for all residents of care homes. This care may be organized in different ways so that some GPs are contracted to provide medical care for all the residents in a care home, while in other homes residents register with a local GP in the usual way. Access to primary health-care services is important for people with dementia in residential and nursing homes, not just for immediate health care but also as a gateway to other specialist services.

Unfortunately, there is evidence that residents in care homes do not have the same access to primary care as people in their own homes (Glendinning et al. 2002). It is also important that relatives are able to access the GP of the person with dementia, particularly if the GP has changed on entry to a care home. Discussions on emotive issues such as the level of medical intervention appropriate when a person with dementia becomes seriously ill (for example with pneumonia) are made marginally easier by having prior knowledge of each other and of any views the person with dementia may have made at an earlier time. Whatever decision is made, in each situation based on prior wishes and quality of life, the most important aspect for most relatives is that the person with dementia should not experience pain or discomfort and should be able to look to the GP and nursing staff to use all their palliative care knowledge and skills.

Abuse of older people is not new although now more widely recognized in all its forms: physical, psychological, financial, sexual and neglect. In domestic settings perpetrators can be relatives, friends, volunteers, paid workers or professionals (McCreadie and Tinker 1993). In institutional settings it can be the act of one person or a reflection of a wider culture where poor standards and poor leadership result in systematic abusive as well as criminal acts (House of Commons Health Committee 2004). A national survey of relatives' experiences of care in residential and nursing homes makes salutary reading (Alzheimer's Society 1997). People with dementia are very vulnerable to abusive situations. Most areas have agreed multi-agency guidelines for action on elder abuse. Every area in England has guidance agreed between health and social care organizations on the detection and action to be taken in the event of suspected abuse to adults (DH&HO, undated, c2000). It is important that all practitioners in primary care are aware of the range of indicators suggestive of abuse and neglect as well as the local joint agency guidance, specific general practice and employer policies. Key principles on action if abuse of a vulnerable adult is suspected include:

- Accurate, contemporaneous records of assessments and evidence suggestive of abuse or neglect.
- Assessment of urgency for action, i.e. whether the person is in immediate danger, and/or in need of immediate medical assistance and/or a crime has recently been committed.
- Referral to the appropriate agency to investigate and coordinate a multi-agency protection and action plan. This may be the social services, the police, or the employing organization dependent on both the situation of the vulnerable adult, the nature of the perpetrator and local guidance. If the concern arises in a registered care service the regulatory body, e.g. the National Care Standards Commission (NCSC) in England, should be informed.

Outlining a framework for practice in primary health care

In conclusion, we suggest there is a framework of good practice in primary care that can guide clinical care for individual patients. It can also be used as part of a clinical audit or in a critical incident study and, if used as a template for data capture, can generate the knowledge needed to commission care for a whole population. When a confirmed diagnosis of dementia has been made, then the GP and primary care team should check that they have also achieved the following components of this framework:

- Assessed, documented and shared with relevant others the physical, mental, behavioural and social problems of the person with dementia.
- Identified the strengths and remaining skills of the person with dementia and discussed them with the individual, their family and carers.
- Identified what the carer and person with dementia consider to be the main problems.
- Identified and treated any treatable complications of co-existing pathology in the person with dementia.
- Identified the carer's unmet needs and identified the appropriate services to meet these.
- Reviewed the need of the patient and carer at regular intervals in order to solve new problems as early as possible.
- Ensured that there is good liaison with any other professionals involved.
- Arranged to see the carer regularly once the patient dies or is admitted to long-term care because the caring role does not end with the move to a nursing home, or even with death.
- Recorded and collated information on the needs of people with dementia and their carers.

All primary care trusts in England should have had 'shared care' protocols for dementia in place by 1 April 2004, as a milestone in the implementation of the National Service Framework for Older People (DH 2001, p. 107). 'Shared care' can mean systematic, carefully planned and sustainable collaboration between GPs and hospital in the medical management of specific conditions, based on rules (protocols) for monitoring the condition. However, shared care can also be seen as a flexible working arrangement that is more patient-focused rather than driven by rigid rules. In this sense it offers:

- continuity to the person with dementia, and to their family, which creates a sense of security, confidence and familiarity
- opportunities for mutual learning between GPs, other primary care staff and specialists
- a sense that 'something can be done' about dementia, by constructing a sequence of steps that professionals and carers can take

- an example of the benefits of collaborative working, which may spread to work with other patient groups and other medical problems.

Shared care of patients with dementia already exists where long-standing relationships between specialists and GPs have allowed frequent and easy communication (Iliffe et al. 2004a). Such relationships have allowed speedy agreements to be reached about joint funding and management of the new generation of 'anti-Alzheimer' medicines. A recent study of evolving shared care arrangements for people with dementia identified that many primary care practitioners welcomed and benefited from the joint educational opportunities across agencies (Iliffe et al. 2004b).

We have summarized the process of dementia care in the community here, but to implement this practitioners from all disciplines will need to acquire new knowledge. This knowledge is not going to be acquired passively by listening to lectures from experts in old age psychiatry, neurology or community nursing. Dementia is so complex that learning about it occurs through the experience of solving its problems, including the problem of diagnosis itself, and those organizing professional education on the theme of dementia need to understand how knowledge acquisition occurs (Iliffe et al. 2000). GPs and district nurses have much to offer from their experience (and from the evidence growing in their electronic and written records) that can assist in the process of allocating resources to services, stimulating innovation and improvement in care. This is particularly true for the delivery of services to people with dementia and their carers, because the numbers for any one practice are relatively small, the illness lasts a long time, involves so many agencies, and the individual stories are so powerful as lessons, accolades and warnings.

References

Alzheimer's Society (1997) Experiences of Care in Residential and Nursing Homes: a survey. Alzheimer's Society UK, London.

Alzheimer's Society (2000) Advice Sheets for Carers: Unusual Behaviours. London. Alzheimer's Society UK, London.

Alzheimer's Society (2003) Dementia: diagnosis and management in primary care. Available on CD-ROM and at *www.alzheimers.org.uk/working_with_people_with_dementia/primary_care/diagnosiscd.htm*. Alzheimer's Society UK, London.

Antonelli Incalzi R, Marra C, Gemma A et al. (1992) Unrecognised dementia; sociodemographic correlates. Aging (Milano) 4(4): 327–332.

Audit Commission (2002) Forget Me Not 2002: developing mental health services for older people in England. Audit Commission, London.

Bosanquet N, May J, Johnson N (1998) Alzheimer's disease in the UK: burden of disease and future care. Health Policy Review Paper no. 12. Imperial College of Science, Technology and Medicine, London.

Briggs R (1993) Comment: Alzheimer's disease – your views. Geriatric Medicine 23(1): 40–41.

Brodaty H, Green A, Koschera A (2003) Meta-analysis of psychosocial interventions for caregivers of people with dementia. Journal of the American Geriatrics Society 51: 657–664.

Buck D, Gregson BA, Bamford CH (1997) Psychological distress among informal supporters of frail older people at home and in institutions. International Journal of Geriatric Psychiatry 12: 737–744.

Caring Costs Alliance (1996) The True Cost of Caring: a survey of carers' lost income. Caring Costs Alliance, London.

Cody M, Beck C, Shue VM, Pope S (2002) Reported practices of primary care physicians in the diagnosis and management of dementia. Aging and Mental Health 6(1): 72–76.

Cohen CA, Pringle D, LeDuc L (2001) Dementia care giving: the role of the primary care physician. Canadian Journal of Neurological Sciences 28: S72–S76.

Cohen D, Kennedy G, Eisdorfer C (1984) Phases of change in the patient with Alzheimer's dementia: a conceptual dimension for defining health care management. Journal of the American Geriatrics Society 32(1): 11–15.

Courtney C, Farrell D, Gray R et al. (2004) Long term donepezil treatment in 565 patients with Alzheimer's disease (AD2000): randomised double-blind trial. Lancet 363(9427): 2105–2115.

De Lepeleire J, Heyrman J (1999) Diagnosis and management of dementia in primary care at an early stage: the need for a new concept and an adapted structure. Theoretical Medicine and Bioethics 20: 215–228.

DH (2000) National Strategy for Carers. Department of Health, London.

DH (2001) National Service Framework for Older People. Department of Health, London.

DH&HO (undated, c2000) No Secrets: guidance on developing and implementing multi-agency policies and procedures to protect vulnerable adults from abuse. Department of Health and the Home Office, London.

Downs M (1997) The emergence of the person in dementia research. Ageing and Society 17(5): 597–607.

Downs M, Cook I, Rae C, Collins KE (2000) Caring for patients with dementia: the GP perspective. Aging and Mental Health 4: 301–304.

DTB (2003) Drugs for disruptive features in dementia. Drugs and Therapeutic Bulletin 41(1): 1–4.

Eccles M, Clarke J, Livingstone M, Freemantle N, Mason J for the North of England Evidence Based Dementia Guideline Development Group (1998) North of England evidence based guidelines development project: guideline for the primary care management of dementia. BMJ 317: 802–808.

Eefsting JA, Boersma F, Van den Brink W, Van Tilburg W (1996) Differences in prevalence of dementia based on community survey and general practitioner recognition. Psychological Medicine 26(6): 1223–1230.

Fortinsky R, Wasson J (1997) How do physicians diagnose dementia? Evidence from clinical vignette responses. American Journal of Alzheimer's Disease 12: 51–61.

Fortinsky RH (2001) Health care triads and dementia care: integrative framework and future directions. Aging and Mental Health 5: S35–S48.

Freyne A (2001) Screening for dementia in primary care – a viable proposition? Irish Journal of Psychological Medicine 18(2): 75–77.

Gallo J, Franch M, Reichel W (1991) Dementing illness: the patient, caregiver and community. American Family Physician 43(5): 1669–75.

Glendinning C, Jacobs S, Alborz A, Hann M (2002) A survey of access to medical services in nursing and residential homes in England. British Journal of General Practice 52(480): 545–8.

Gordon M, Goldstein D (2001) Alzheimer's disease – to tell or not to tell. Canadian Family Physician 47: 1803–8.

Grant G, Nolan M (1993) Informal carers: sources and concomitants of satisfaction. Health and Social Care 1: 147–159.

Gray A, Fenn P (1993) Alzheimer's disease: the burden of the illness in England. Health Trends 25: 31–7.

Haley W, Clair J, Saulsberry K (1992) Family caregiver satisfaction with the medical care of their demented relatives. Gerontologist 32: 219–226.

Hoffman R, Rocca W, Brayne C et al. (1991) The prevalence of dementia in Europe: a collaborative study of 1980–1990 findings. International Journal of Epidemiology 20(3): 736–748.

House of Commons Health Committee (2004) Elder Abuse: Second Report of Session 2003–04. House of Commons Health Committee, London.

Iliffe S, Walters K, Rait G (2000) Shortcomings in the care of dementia in general practice: towards an educational strategy. Aging and Mental Health 4(4): 286–291.

Iliffe S, Drennan V (2001) Dementia and Primary Care. Jessica Kingsley Publishers, London.

Iliffe S, Wilcock J, Haworth D (2004a) Shared care for people with dementia. Journal of Dementia Care 12(3): 16–18.

Iliffe S, Wilcock J, Haworth D (2004b) A toolbox of skills to share across dementia care. Journal of Dementia Care 12(4): 16–17.

IPA (2002) Behavioral and Psychological Symptoms of Dementia (BPSD). International Psychogeriatric Association Educational Pack. Internet resource available at *www.ipa-online.org/ipaonlinev3/ipaprograms/bpsdrev/toc.asp*.

Ireichen B (1994) Managing demented old people in the community: a review. Family Practice 11: 210–215.

Kitwood T (1997) Dementia Reconsidered. Open University Press, Buckingham, UK.

Kitwood T, Bredin K (1992) Person to Person: a guide to care of those with failing mental powers, 2nd edn. Gale Centre Publications, Loughton, Essex.

Lagaay A, Van der Meij J, Hijmans W (1992) Validation of medical history taking as part of a population based survey in subjects aged 85 and over. BMJ 304(6834): 1091–1092.

Levin E, Sinclair I, Gorbach P (1989) Families, Confusions and Old Age. Gower, Aldershot.

Marriott A (2003) Helping families cope with dementia. In: Adams T, Manthorpe J (eds) Dementia Care. Arnold, London, pp. 187–201.

McCreadie C, Tinker A (1993) Review: abuse of elderly people in the domestic setting: a UK perspective. Age and Ageing 22(1): 65–9.

Murray J, Schneider J, Banerjee S, Mann A (1999) Eurocare: a cross national study of co-resident spouse carers for people with Alzheimer's disease: a qualitative analysis of the experience of care giving. International Journal of Geriatric Psychiatry 14: 662–667.

Newens AJ, Forster DF, Kay DW (1994) Referral patterns and diagnosis in pre-senile Alzheimer's disease: implications for general practice. British Journal of General Practice 44: 405–407.

O'Connor D, Pollitt P, Hyde J et al. (1988) Do general practitioners Miss dementia in elderly patients? British Medical Journal 297: 1107–1110.

Olafsdottir M, Foldevi M, Marcusson J (2001) Dementia in primary care: why the low detection rate? Scandinavian Journal of Primary Health Care 19(3): 194–198.

ONS (1998) Informal Carers. Office of National Statistics. The Stationery Office, London.

Pollitt P (1996) Dementia in old age: an anthropological perspective. Psychological Medicine 26: 1061–1074.

Rait G, Burns A (1998) Screening for depression and cognitive impairment in older people from ethnic minority backgrounds. Age and Ageing 27: 271–275.

Russo J, Vitaliano PP (1995) Life events as correlates of burden in spouse caregivers of persons with Alzheimer's disease. Experimental Ageing Research 21: 273–294.

Spector A, Orrell M, Davies S, Woods B (2005) Reality orientation for dementia. Cochrane Database of Systematic Reviews, Issue 2.

Thompson C, Thompson G (1998) Support for carers of people with Alzheimer's-type disease. Cochrane Collaboration, Issue 3.

Toeg D, Mercer L, Iliffe S, Lenihan P (2003) Proactive, targeted benefits advice for older people in general practice: a feasibility study. Health and Social Care in the Community 11(2): 124–128.

Toner H (1992) What do we mean by assessment? In: Haxby D (ed.) Dementia: diagnosis and assessment. Dementia Services Development Centre, Stirling.

van Hout H (1999) Diagnosing Dementia: evaluation of the clinical practice of general practitioners and a memory clinic. University of Nijmegen.

Verhey F, Ponds R, Rozendaal N, Jilles J (1995) Depression, insight and personality changes in Alzheimer's disease and vascular dementia. Journal of Geriatric Psychiatry and Neurology 8(1): 23–27.

Woods B, Spector A, Jones C et al. (2005) Reminiscence therapy for dementia. Cochrane Database of Systematic Reviews, Issue 2.

CHAPTER 4

Language, communication and cognition in the dementias

JANE MAXIM AND KAREN BRYAN

This chapter will look at language function, significant cognitive parameters of language, and communication disability in a number of diseases which cause a dementia (except for the special case of semantic dementia which is thoroughly described and discussed in Chapter 5). The dementias are an area of great research activity and some of the work on dementia typology reviewed here is very current.

Why is an accurate diagnosis necessary?

Firstly, there are causes of cognitive and language change which are reversible (e.g. depression) or where the progressive decline may be slowed or halted (e.g. vascular dementia). Secondly, research has now taken us to the stage where we can describe different patterns of impairment and retained abilities which suggest that different dementias and different stages of those dementias require different types of advice to family and formal carers. Such specific intervention, whether palliative or not, is aimed at improving quality of life for the person themselves and for their carers. Whether the carer is in paid employment, a volunteer, or a family member, easing the distressed state and distressing behaviour of someone with a dementia promotes more mutual satisfaction between that person and the carer. Thirdly, to manage communication disability in the dementias, an accurate and specific diagnosis is the foundation from which a care plan, involving family, should evolve. An understanding of which areas of language and cognition are retained, as well as those which show breakdown, is essential.

We have been selective, in this chapter, in the depth of our descriptions of language and cognition in the dementias for three reasons:

- Some diseases are major causes of a dementia (such as Alzheimer's disease) and, as such, require considerable description.

- In some diseases such as Parkinson's disease, a dementia is only present in a small percentage of the clinical population, requiring some description, and the disease is otherwise well documented elsewhere.
- The incidence of some rare types of dementia such as normal pressure hydrocephalus (see Duinkerke et al. 2004) is tiny but, more importantly, for some conditions where a dementia may be present, we have found no or very few studies which describe language functions. An example is multisystem atrophy, a progressive neurodegenerative disorder characterized by extrapyramidal signs and with a high incidence of depression (but see Smith and Bryan 1992).

A further area for consideration is that of mild cognitive impairment (MCI), a deficit which does not meet current criteria for dementia (Burns and Zaudig 2002, Davis and Rockwood 2004). Some people with MCI are at risk of developing a dementia, particularly those who have more signs of amnesia who may eventually be diagnosed with Alzheimer's disease. In a large sample study, Grundman et al. (2004) found that people with MCI had memory impairments with relative sparing of other cognitive domains, fitting in between clinically normal adults and those with Alzheimer's disease. Identification of these pre-dementia states may be vital in intervention and thus prevention of the long-term impact of the dementias.

The dementias typically occur in older people (over 65 years), and the term young-onset dementia (YOD) is used to describe those whose dementia begins earlier than this. Such conditions are often familial and some, such as variant Creutzfeldt–Jakob disease, occur most frequently in young people. While estimates of the number of people with YOD vary, Alzheimer's disease is the commonest single cause of YOD (30%) with an estimated 3000 cases in the UK, followed by vascular dementia (15%), the frontotemporal lobar degenerations (13%) and alcohol-related dementia (12%) (Sampson et al. 2004).

Assessing communication in the dementias

For the speech and language therapist (SLT), Maxim and Bryan (1994) suggest that the following questions on language, cognition and communication and their interactions need to be considered:

- Which language processes are disordered, which are spared and how are they disordered?
- Are language and cognition equally disordered, or is there an imbalance between these two systems?
- What level of severity is present and does this knowledge help to illuminate the current processing deficits, i.e. are these deficits severity-dependent or do they contribute to the severity?

- Is a communication disability present?
- If cognitive deficits are present, what is their contribution to the communication disability?
- What is the relationship between the communication disability and other behaviours?
- If there are behaviours which are distressing to the person themselves or their carer, can a change in communication or communicative environment make any difference?

In order to test specific hypotheses when looking at language and cognitive processing, researchers have had to construct their own tests and use a normal age- and education-matched control group to ensure that their findings are valid. While the use of aphasia tests originally constructed to diagnose aphasia is common practice, such assessments have often not been validated on older people, and best practice demands that tests designed for the purpose of identifying language deficits associated with dementia are used routinely. Examples are the Barnes Language Assessment (Bryan et al. 2001) and ABCD (Bayles and Tomoeda 1993). See Chapter 6 for a detailed discussion of assessment of language in the dementias.

Aphasia and the dementias

Researchers have used the term 'aphasia' extensively to describe the language deficits in the dementias. While this is a useful research term, we see little point in using the term in a clinical situation and much reason not to. Use of some syndrome-based descriptions of types of aphasia is helpful as a quick means of identifying a number of features in the dementias. For example, the language impairment seen in many people with Alzheimer's disease has much in common with transcortical sensory aphasia. Similarly, the term 'progressive aphasia' accurately describes a group of disorders which primarily or only affect language function and in which cognitive parameters are either well retained or deteriorate at a slower rate than language functions. One form of non-fluent progressive aphasia results in language output which is similar to a Broca's aphasia. In the clinical arena, we would prefer to use the term 'language disorder secondary to dementia' to differentiate what happens to language in the dementias from the aphasia secondary to a sudden focal lesion. There are of course difficulties with even this differentiation. In vascular dementia (multi-infarct dementia), it is often difficult to draw a dividing line between that condition and one in which an individual has undergone a number of strokes which have produced an aphasia. However, in clinical terms, management and intervention for sudden-onset focal aphasias and progressive language disorders are very different, in terms of the nature of the intervention, the context in which it takes place and the likely outcome.

Alzheimer's disease

Alzheimer's disease is largely a disease of old age. It is the most common condition causing a dementia in Europe and North America, affecting 10% of the population over the age of 65 and rising to 20% of the population aged over 80, with age being the greatest risk factor for Alzheimer's disease (see Jorm 2000). Of the approximately 400 000 people in the UK with Alzheimer's disease, the UK Alzheimer's Society estimates that about 17 000 are below retirement age. While Alzheimer's disease is by far the most common form of dementia in Europe and North America, in Japan the prevalence of vascular dementia and Alzheimer's disease appears to be much closer (Imai and Hasegawa 2000). Estimates of the familial form of Alzheimer's disease vary from 10% to 50% although only about 10% have autosomal dominant Alzheimer's disease (Godbolt et al. 2004, 2005). From diagnosis, life expectancy is usually 7–10 years.

Alzheimer's disease must be distinguished from other forms of dementia such as vascular dementia and from depression, which is also common among the older population and which may give rise to pseudodementia (Erkinjuntti 2000). The neuropathological findings in Alzheimer's disease include neuronal loss, neurofibrillary tangles, neuritic plaques and amyloid angiopathy, but there are currently no biological markers of Alzheimer's disease that allow presymptomatic detection or definite diagnosis. No positive tests are currently recognized and diagnosis is usually by exclusion criteria and examination of behavioural, cognitive and language data, although imaging is now an established part of diagnosis. One of the most widely used criteria for diagnosis in research is the DSM-IV-TR (APA 2000): the DSM-IV criteria define dementia as a syndrome characterized by the development of multiple cognitive deficits including memory impairment, and at least one of the following cognitive disturbances: aphasia, apraxia, agnosia or a disturbance in executive functioning. The deficits must be sufficiently severe to cause impairment in occupational or social functioning and must represent a decline from a previously higher level of functioning. Alzheimer's disease is defined as a dementia syndrome that has a gradual onset and continuing cognitive decline. Other neurological disorders, systemic diseases or substance abuse sufficient to induce a dementia must be excluded. The deficits must not occur exclusively during delirium and must not be attributable to major psychiatric disorder such as depression. In addition, the diagnosis of Alzheimer's disease is unlikely if the disease is of sudden onset, has focal neurological signs or has seizure or gait disturbance presenting early in the disease. Contributions from neurophysiological investigations and imaging have shown:

- slowed background activity in Alzheimer's disease compared to age-matched controls, using electroencephalography
- asymmetric temporoparietal hypoperfusion, which aids differential diagnosis from vascular and frontotemporal dementias

- an increase in cerebrospinal fluid spaces, with an associated atrophy and corresponding decrease in brain volume (CT/MRI) (see Forstl 2000).

Variation and progression

It is now widely recognized that there is variation within the disease entity of Alzheimer's disease, but why this variation occurs and its relationship to the neuropathology affecting brain structures is only now being defined. Schwartz (1990, p. 143) describes this heterogeneity as follows:

> . . . each patient presents a landscape of eroding cognitive and functional capacities, but the landscape contains peaks and valleys. One patient may be seen with particularly severe visuo-spatial confusion and little language disturbance; another patient may show the reverse. . . . More typically most patients show simultaneous dissolution across several domains.

Although recent genetic studies point to a number of aetiologies that eventually lead to Alzheimer's disease, whether it represents a single pathological entity is uncertain but it does present in different forms (early onset, familial, late onset and in association with Down's syndrome). Inheritance in familial Alzheimer's disease is autosomal dominant and the majority of cases are due to mutations in the presenilin 1 (*PSEN1*) gene on chromosome 14 (Sampson et al. 2004).

Specific symptoms may be associated with faster rates of decline (Chui et al. 1992), but whether these symptoms reflect a different biological basis for the disease is not known. For cognitive impairment, there is some evidence that the rate of decline is slower in the early stages of the disease (Morris et al. 1993) and some individuals may 'plateau' (Maxim et al. 2000). The presence of symptoms such as extrapyramidal and psychotic disorder in Alzheimer's disease is thought not to define different clinical entities but to be manifestations of different stages of disease progression (Mayeux et al. 1992). Different profiles of deficits and preserved abilities between individuals with Alzheimer's disease may be influenced by existing individual differences in brain organization for cognition, and normal age-related changes in this organization (Joanette et al. 1992). In familial Alzheimer's disease, for example, myoclonus tends to be more florid and naming may be spared until later in the course. A comparison of early- versus late-onset types shows the major differences between the types (Table 4.1)

Table 4.1 A comparison of early- and late-onset Alzheimer's disease

	Early onset	**Late onset**
Language deficit	Likely	Less likely
Progression	Faster	Slower
Myoclonus	More likely	Less likely

Language deficits in Alzheimer's disease can be significant in both diagnosis and prognosis. The Nun study (Snowdon et al. 1996) found that low linguistic ability in early life was a strong predictor of poor cognitive function and Alzheimer's disease in late life. Chui et al. (1985) found that prevalence and severity of aphasia correlate with duration of illness and that early-onset Alzheimer's disease predicts the early development of language problems. Boller et al. (1991) suggest that poor performance on naming tests may be a good predictor of rapid decline in Alzheimer's disease at initial diagnosis. Early-onset disease (before age 65) is associated with greater language deficits than late-onset (Seltzer and Sherwin 1983, Faber-Langendoen et al. 1988), although Bayles (1991) did not find greater language impairment in her early-onset group. Alzheimer's disease may present in global, visual or verbal forms, all of which share some semantic deficits but different profiles of deficits and neuropathology (Fisher et al. 1997, Lambon-Ralph et al. 2003).

The prevalent view of language in Alzheimer's disease has been of a homogeneous progressive course of semantic deficit, syntactic deficit and finally phonological deficit. However, people with Alzheimer's disease are almost as likely to be atypical as typical in their presentation and in the course of the disease. Ska et al. (1990), for example, found that only just over half of their Alzheimer's disease group conformed to the standard account of disease progression. In early Alzheimer's disease, Hodges and Patterson (1995) found that, while all their Alzheimer's disease group showed deficits in episodic memory and delayed recall, there was considerable variation on semantic memory tasks. Lambon-Ralph et al. (2003) suggested that nearly 60% of the variance in their Alzheimer's disease group was accounted for by severity-based factors and a homogeneous progression, but their findings also confirmed two main patterns of atypical variation: people with more severe semantic or more severe visuo-spatial deficits. While it is possible to describe general characteristics of the disorder in Alzheimer's disease, the underlying processes and the nature of the disruption to these processes are still not clearly understood, despite the large number of research studies, and individual variation in both deficits and progression should be expected.

Information on language functions linked to stages of the disease, measured on the Global Deterioration Scale (Reisberg et al. 1982) can be found in Bayles et al. (1992), who provides comparisons to normal age- and education-matched controls, and in Kempler (1995), who provides an overview of language in Alzheimer's disease. Maxim and Bryan (1996) presented a checklist of functions showing both language and cognitive deficits and sparing at different stages of the disease which is primarily applicable to late-onset Alzheimer's disease (see Table 4.2). Such lists, however, should be seen as merely a snapshot of the disease process: language may be compromised at any stage of the disease and there is an enormous variation in deficits between individuals.

Table 4.2 An overview of Alzheimer's disease

Language	Cognition	Personality/ mental health
Early stage		
Low-frequency word-finding impairment	Episodic memory impaired	Change of affect
Circumlocution in conversation	Autobiographical memory impaired	Avoidance/denial strategies
Word fluency impaired	Time orientation impaired	Increased anxiety
Composite picture description incomplete	Naming of famous faces impaired	Depression
Poor repetition of low-frequency sentences (BDAE)	Attention impaired	
Utterance completion poor in conversation	Time orientation impaired	
Auditory and written complex sentence comprehension impaired		
Single-word recognition maintained		
Midstage		
Naming deficits on high-frequency items	Working memory impaired	Wandering and exit-seeking behaviour
Semantic paraphasias	Knowledge of current events decreased	Increasing apathy
Reference deficit in pronoun use	Ideational perseveration	Sleep disturbance
Errors in complex sentence production	Time and place orientation impaired	Assistance needed in activities of daily living
Occasional phonemic paraphasias	Calculation deficits	
Decrease in semantic cuing response	Visuo-spatial and perceptual deficits	
Sentence reading aloud poor		
Single regular word reading aloud retained		
Decreased use of gesture		
Poor repetition of high frequency sentences		
Single-word recognition impairment		
Sentence comprehension impairments		
Late stage		
Language initiation decreased or ceases	Time, place and person disorientation	Dependent for activities of daily living
Noun use non-specific/non-existent	Face recognition poor	Poor eye contact
Phonemic paraphasias on repetition		Inappropriate social behaviour
Stereotypical utterances		Poor mobility
Verbal perseverations		Purposeless motor movements
Echolalia possible		Incontinence
No use of gesture		Feeding and swallowing disorder

Maxim and Bryan (1994) suggest that research into language disturbance in Alzheimer's disease has been influenced by four separate research trends:

- group studies of the language characteristics in Alzheimer's disease, which describe symptom clusters and severity
- studies which have compared the language disturbance in dementia with that of aphasia using the syndrome-based classification in the Wernicke–Lictheim tradition
- single case studies which have looked closely at the underlying language deficits, sometimes longitudinally
- small group studies which have looked at patients who present with distinct sub-types of Alzheimer's disease.

There is now a consensus that the language symptomatology in Alzheimer's disease is heterogeneous and that, although it is possible to describe language and cognitive functions at different stages in the disease progression, it is more useful to investigate and compare the deterioration of specific processes. One of the main problems in group studies which use a profile approach is that very little can be said about what the individual patient can and cannot do. Single-case studies have helped to some extent, particularly because they often point to specific deficits and dissociations between deficits which are unlikely to be found in group studies. Unless both group and single-case studies are longitudinal, however, only one moment in the disease process is described. Systematic research into how specific processes deteriorate in Alzheimer's disease is still needed.

Language and cognitive processing

While the main cognitive features in early Alzheimer's disease are deterioration in episodic memory (everyday memory for events) and the ability to learn new information, semantic memory also changes, becoming less accessible (Lambon-Ralph et al. 1997). Episodic memories (i.e. unique, specific in time and space) are impaired and autobiographical memory shows a temporally graded memory loss, with remote memories better preserved than recent ones (Piolino et al. 2003). While there is also a working memory deficit, the involvement of short-term (working) memory decrements in the language processing difficulty is currently an area of debate (Waters and Caplan 2002, Bayles 2003).

Language changes are most apparent at the semantic level in Alzheimer's disease. Vogel et al. (2005) suggest that the semantic system may show changes even in the very early and perhaps pre-diagnostic stages. But what happens to the semantic system and to semantic processing in Alzheimer's disease? A central question in research has been the nature of the deficit: is it due to a problem in accessing semantic information, or is the semantic information lost? This question is not only of interest to research but has very practical implications for people with Alzheimer's disease and their carers. If words and their meanings are difficult to access but are still present, then it should be possible to find strategies which will help access in conversation and pharmacotherapy might be expected to help access to word stores. If, on the other hand, semantic information is lost altogether, then strategies will not help and may even be distressing. The investigation of the reduction in naming ability and in correspondences with understanding names has been the focus of much research. Some research has looked at different levels of breakdown as language deteriorates (Appell et al. 1982, Bayles et al. 1992), giving a valuable overall view of the range of language behaviour and viewing language changes as a reflection of cognitive function in decline. A few single-case and small-group studies have discussed the dissociations of impairment which can be found in Alzheimer's disease and have considered longitudinal aspects of language processing deficits (Chertkow and Bub 1990, Funnell and Hodges 1990, Joanette et al. 1992). Sentence processing and the breakdown of conversation in people with Alzheimer's disease has also been another feature of research, with discourse analysis used to describe changes in conversational interactions (Ripich and Terrell 1988).

Naming and understanding names

Difficulty in finding words that are appropriate and specific to the context in which they are needed is one of the most noticeable features of Alzheimer's disease, but is not always an early feature of the disease process (Bayles and Tomoeda 1983, Huff et al. 1986). Other aspects of lexical semantics, on the other hand, such as word fluency (the ability to generate as many exemplars of a given category in a given time) are often a presenting feature. The exploration of this system entails some of the following range of tests:

- object naming
- picture naming
- word fluency/word generation
- word definitions
- word to picture matching
- picture to picture matching
- superordinate category tasks
- probe questions on semantic features.

The nature of the breakdown at the level of lexical semantics is not a clear picture, but there is now some evidence that, in the early stages of the disease, access to the semantic lexicon is the main problem (Funnell and Hodges 1990, Bayles et al. 1992) but, as the disease progresses, specific items in the lexicon are lost (Funnell and Hodges 1990, Hodges et al. 1992). Despite this loss, the semantic system at a single word level may remain partially intact in Alzheimer's disease up to a relatively late stage in the disease process (Schwartz et al. 1979, Nebes et al. 1986, Bayles et al. 1992). The semantic feature system may be susceptible to breakdown with greater difficulty listing features distinctive to particular concepts, compared to those shared by multiple concepts (Alathari et al. 2004). Whitaker (1976), in an early and exceptionally thorough single-case study, provides evidence that the semantic system in dementia can remain partially intact and accessible under certain conditions. HCEM had no useful social language but could repeat even non-words. Given a noun phrase which contained a sound error (*a gold ling), she would correct the phrase when shown the actual object (a gold ring). The ability to make this type of repair involves, at a minimum, recognizing the object by accessing the semantic system and then accessing the correct phonological form, presumably already partially activated. Although naming and understanding nouns has been the focus of most research, the ability to name and use verbs may also parallel that of nouns (Kim and Thompson 2004).

While there is evidence for access difficulty in Alzheimer's disease, there is now increasingly convincing evidence that specific items from the lexicon may be systematically lost. Chertkow and Bub (1990) and Hodges et al. (1992) used similar methodology of the same target items in all tests. Hodges et al. found a significant relationship between the inability to name specific items and the inability to match the same item in a spoken word to picture matching task. There was evidence of preserved superordinate knowledge on definitions and on category sorting when the categories were grossly different (living versus man-made) but deficits emerged as the distinctions to be made required more semantic processing. The Alzheimer's disease group also showed a significant frequency effect when naming. In moderate to severe Alzheimer's disease, superordinate identification (where a stimulus item has to be matched to an appropriate category) is harder than a spoken word to picture matching task, suggesting loss or inaccessibility of semantic categories (Bayles et al. 1992). The same study suggests that confrontation naming is an easier task than superordinate naming. Sorting objects by category was found to be an easier task than recognizing the function or specific features of an object (Martin et al. 1985). But people with Alzheimer's disease have been widely reported to have difficulty on word fluency tasks and to generate fewer exemplars of a category than controls (Troster et al. 1989, Kontiola et al. 1990). Lambon-Ralph et al. (1997) looked at category naming across time to investigate conceptual knowledge, comparing correctly named items at both time points with items correctly named at the first stage but failed at the second stage, and concluded that correct naming depended on a subset of critical semantic features which vary across different categories of semantic knowledge. Garrard, Lambon-Ralph et al. (2005) suggest that distinctive features of concepts are more vulnerable than shared features and the amount of attribute knowledge about a concept is associated reliably, and in a graded fashion, with the ability to name a picture of that item.

The changing semantic system in Alzheimer's disease produces specific naming behaviour. Bayles and Tomoeda (1983) found that over a quarter of incorrect naming responses were correct contexts or functions. Such behaviour suggests that these patients have some ability to monitor and change their language behaviour. Although naming errors are more likely to be semantically associated with the target, people with Alzheimer's disease produce phonemic paraphasias and even neologisms in the later stages of the disease process, particularly in conversational language. They may also use words, phrases or even short sentences repeatedly in their conversational language, sometimes as perseverations and sometimes as markers when other lexical items are not available. Monitoring of language, a normal process, shows a decrease in Alzheimer's disease but still occurs: McNamara et al. (1992) found that their Alzheimer's disease group repaired 24% of their speech errors compared to 72–92% for a healthy elderly control group. The Alzheimer's disease group used very few single-word repairs but relied on adding new syntactic information. People with Alzheimer's disease also produce intrusions or confabulations where correct information is inaccessible (Dalla Barba and Wong 1992, Dalla Barba et al. 1992), some of which may be using remote autobiographical memory when more recent memories are inaccessible (Tallberg and Almkvist 2001).

Most research on large groups of people with Alzheimer's disease has found that single-word comprehension scores are better than naming scores (Bayles et al. 1992). However, when the same items are used both in naming and comprehension tasks, small-group studies have found item consistency across both tasks and similar patterns of impairment (Schwartz et al. 1981, Chertkow and Bub 1990, Hodges et al. 1992). However, the single-case study of Funnell and Hodges (1990) shows considerable dissociation between input and output tasks, suggesting disease variation. Deficits in the use of the semantic lexicon, then, are one of the most common features of language in Alzheimer's disease. Indeed, severity of object naming and overall dementia are highly correlated (Skelton-Robinson and Jones 1984). These deficits also affect language used in conversation and the semantic relationships between words, although there is evidence that semantic priming and, less effectively, semantic cueing are possible (Herlitz et al. 1991). Although semantic deficits are evident in Alzheimer's disease, there is some evidence that semantic errors may arise from accessing the phonological form of words, suggesting that we need to look more carefully at the nature of single-word processing deficits in Alzheimer's disease (Funnell and Hodges 1990, Maxim et al. 2000). Moreaud et al. (2001) found that, on a visual naming task, the majority of semantic errors were related to a deficit in the retrieval of the phonological form of the word. Unrelated errors were more frequently related to semantic deficits than semantic errors in their population. Grossman et al. (2003) suggest that a deficit in executive processes, which are necessary to rule-based categorization, may degrade semantic knowledge, while Manenti et al. (2004) consider that inhibitory processes may be damaged, leading to interference effects.

Such suggestions highlight the nature of our understanding: although we know something of what happens to the semantic system, what drives these changes is not known. People with Alzheimer's disease appear to begin the process of semantic deterioration with an access problem, but this problem demonstrates some systematicity. At a later stage, there may be both access and loss of semantic representations, followed finally by a late stage where it is not possible to demonstrate either process by conventional testing.

Cueing and priming

Whitaker's (1976) single-case study demonstrated that cueing (in this case a visual cue) can be used successfully: given a noun phrase which contained a sound error (*a gold ling), HCEM would correct the phrase when shown the actual object (a gold ring). Priming is an effect which makes use of rapid, automatic (implicit) processes and can be contrasted with cueing which usually makes use of explicit processes. Cueing taps into the use of metalinguistic or metacognitive skills – that is, the ability to think at a conscious level about the task in hand – while priming functions without this attentional knowledge. People with Alzheimer's disease may be unable to name an object (knife) or suggest a function (eat/cut), but they may show a priming effect. Given a word (knife) preceded by a related prime word (cut), their ability to judge that there is a relationship between these words is facilitated (made faster or more accurate) by the prime. This priming effect demonstrates that there is access to the semantic system, and that a semantic representation is available to be accessed.

Chertkow et al. (1989) used the term 'hyperpriming' to describe their finding that people with Alzheimer's disease appear to benefit more than normal controls from priming. People with Alzheimer's disease show hyperpriming in lexical decision tasks but not in associative priming. Semantic priming effects have been observed in Alzheimer's disease (Camus et al. 2003), but the effectiveness of semantic cueing appears weaker (Nebes et al. 1986, Chertkow and Bub 1990, Chertkow et al. 1989, Herlitz et al. 1991). Indeed, Chertkow and Bub (1990) found that their Alzheimer's disease group showed enhanced priming effects on those items that were semantically degraded compared to those that were not, a finding confirmed by Perri et al. (2003). Semantic cueing is an off-line process whereas semantic priming is an on-line phenomenon; we might hypothesize that people with Alzheimer's disease will be able to respond better to contexts that do not require effortful processing and interventions might be best targeted at on-line processes.

Phonological cueing was found to facilitate picture naming in a longitudinal study by Funnell and Hodges (1990) of a single patient with probable Alzheimer's disease. They suggest that access from semantics to the phonological output lexicon, in which spoken word forms are stored, may be another area of deficit. The patient, Mary, was followed over 2 years and initially spoke fluently although word-finding difficulties and circumlocutions were present. Although single-word comprehension declined over the 2 years, her comprehension scores remained much better than her naming scores. On picture naming tests, her performance declined in line with word frequency and she could not name better when given semantic cues. She could, however, repeat the picture names accurately and read them aloud well but she had difficulty in repeating and reading non-words. This discrepancy between word and non-word repetition suggests that the store of word forms (phonological output lexicon) was intact. Mary showed a word frequency effect for naming and was also consistent in her ability to name or failure to name. She could sometimes name when given a phonemic cue after having failed to name spontaneously, but phonemic cueing became less effective as overall naming scores decreased.

Does context have a cueing effect? People with probable Alzheimer's disease may show naming behaviours which may reflect changes to the semantic system. Several studies describe the use of phrases such as *cutting blade* (knife), *hand bell* and drinking *cup* in naming tasks, giving additional information about an attribute or function of the object. Bayles and Tomoeda (1983), for example, found that over a quarter of incorrect naming responses were correct contexts or functions. Such behaviour suggests that people with Alzheimer's disease are attempting to make use of semantic associations in their use of language.

Visual and auditory perception

Some researchers have argued that anomia in Alzheimer's disease is due in part to an agnosic component; that is, people with Alzheimer's disease have difficulty perceiving the nature of the object they are required to label. People with aphasia due to focal lesions, by contrast, have difficulty finding the label. Stevens (1985) has noted this tendency to misinterpret visual information in picture description tasks. Similarly, Rochford (1971) argues that semantic errors in dementia have an agnosic component and Martin (1987) found that a specific subgroup showed visuo-spatial deficits. When writing to dictation, errors are often misperceptions of the stimulus.

People with Alzheimer's disease may also auditorily misperceive and therefore guess responses. Confirmed visual or auditory agnosia appears to be rare in anything but profound Alzheimer's disease. Usually people with Alzheimer's disease are able to match objects and shapes without error in the earlier stages of the disease. Auditory comprehension is frequently impaired in mild and moderate Alzheimer's disease, and language processing deficits are well documented, but auditory agnosia has not been described as a feature of Alzheimer's disease. The ability to repeat single words and short sentences accurately suggests that auditory agnosia is not a significant component.

Visual processing problems, on the other hand, are often cited as a possible cause of naming difficulty in Alzheimer's disease, but careful analysis of the errors made when naming have concluded that the errors are far more likely to be due to semantic processing deficits (Smith et al. 1989, Hodges et al. 1991). However, people with Alzheimer's disease have far greater difficulty recognizing degraded letters or object pictures than the normal elderly, suggesting that their visual processing can be disrupted more easily or perhaps requires more complete information to facilitate processing (Corkin 1982, Heindel et al. 1990, Grist and Maxim 1992). Dissociations between semantic naming and visual perceptual impairment are now well documented and there is now clear evidence for visual perceptual difficulties in subgroups of people with Alzheimer's disease (Shuttleworth and Huber 1989, Martin 1990, Lambon-Ralph et al. 2003).

Written language skills

Alzheimer described both dyslexia and dysgraphia in his original patients, and recent reports have correlated impairment of writing to the severity of the disease (Bayles et al. 1992). The ability to read regularly spelled single words aloud is particularly well preserved in Alzheimer's disease (Nebes et al. 1984, Bayles et al. 1992). People with Alzheimer's disease are able to use regular spelling rules to assist reading but they are less able to read:

- irregularly spelled words, perhaps because of a loss of or impaired access to word representations from the orthographic lexicon
- non-words, perhaps because of an impairment in the ability to segment and blend (Schwartz et al. 1980, Patterson et al. 1994).

They may use a semantic strategy when asked to spell homophones (plane/plain) and regularize the spelling of irregularly spelled words (Cortese et al. 2003). The ability to read declines as the disease progresses, with more phonetically impossible errors and breakdown of regularization rules (Fromm et al. 1991). Reading sentences aloud, however, is often impaired and may, in part, be due to scanning difficulties (Stevens 1985, Hart et al. 1986). Reading and spelling are, however, all part of language processing and therefore likely to be impaired at some stage in the disease process. The ability to read single words aloud even in severe Alzheimer's disease (without necessarily understanding them) has been used by Nelson and O'Connell (1978) in the National Adult Reading Test which gives a measure of premorbid IQ and which exploits the relationship between reading irregularly spelled words, vocabulary and intelligence. It is useful in mild and moderate Alzheimer's disease and where patients have at least 12 years of education (Stebbins et al. 1990). Reading single words and sentences for comprehension does not show the same sparing, and people with severe Alzheimer's disease may be unable to perform at all on such tasks (Cummings et al. 1986, Bayles et al. 1992).

Using a proficiency score to rate written narrative description, Horner et al. (1988) found a significant correlation between writing ability and dementia severity. In a paper comparing the final book written by Iris Murdoch, a well-known novelist and philosopher, before her diagnosis of Alzheimer's disease, with earlier work, Garrard, Maloney et al. (2005) found few disparities at the levels of overall structure and syntax but lexical diversity varied markedly and consistently. Writing and spelling are both vulnerable in Alzheimer's disease because of language disturbances, but disturbances of praxis and visuo-spatial processes may contribute in the later stages of the disease. Writing in Alzheimer's disease may therefore show spelling and language impairment but may also show difficulties in motor coordination, praxis and visuo-spatial orientation. Writing errors may be incomplete words, missed inflections, substituted letters and incomplete spelling. The ability to copy is better preserved than the ability to write spontaneously or to dictation, but it also shows degradation.

Sentence processing

One of the first dissociations reported in Alzheimer's disease was that of an impaired semantic system in contrast to spared grammatical structure in language output (Appell et al. 1982). While language output in Alzheimer's disease may appear well structured, sentence comprehension and more complex grammatical relations in output may be disturbed (Troster et al. 1989). Another aspect of sentence comprehension and production which requires consideration is that of working memory which does show deficits in Alzheimer's disease (Bayles 2003) but may not explain the difficulty in sentence processing. Waters and Caplan (2002), in a carefully controlled study, found that people with early-stage Alzheimer's disease were not impaired in the ability to assign syntactic structure and to use it to determine aspects of sentence meaning, despite reduced working memories (but see also Rochon et al. 2000). Small et al. (2000) found that, although their Alzheimer's disease group had sentence-repetition performances which were significantly correlated with working memory scores, significant effects were also found for branching direction of phrase structure, canonicity of verb-argument relations, and serial position of errors. Difficulty understanding grammatically complex sentences in Alzheimer's disease may also be related to slowed information processing speed which interferes with processing of the sentence structure and use of canonical sentence structure strategies (Grossman and Rhee 2001).

Kempler et al. (1987) found that people with Alzheimer's disease produced a normal range and frequency of structures, using age-matched normal controls, but they have particular difficulty both in understanding and in constructing complex grammatical structures (Small et al. 1997) and in correction of sentences with semantic anomalies (Whitaker 1976). Kopelman (1986), however, looking at recall of anomalous sentences, found that his early-stage Alzheimer's disease subjects were sometimes able to correct these anomalies. The process of reduction to more simple semantic and grammatical forms is a commonly reported finding although in the early stages complex sentence structure may be retained (Blanken et al. 1987, Illes 1989). In a longitudinal study of language production, Kemper et al. (2001) demonstrated that grammatical complexity and propositional content declined over time, regardless of age.

Frequency of word co-occurrence is an important variable in sentence repetition and construction. Obler (1980) looked at the effect of word frequency on the ability to repeat sentences from the BDAE. Her Alzheimer's disease group could repeat long sentences in which the words were both of high frequency in the general vocabulary and had a high ratio of co-occurrence, but both grammatical and semantic relationships were lost in much shorter sentences where the words were of low frequency and low co-occurrence ('the spy fled to Greece' was repeated as 'the fly fed to geese').

The on-line processing of sentences is dependent on spared aspects of the linguistic system which appear to operate with such variables as word frequency and canonical structures. As the disease progresses, structures become more simple but are also likely to be unfinished. Phonological and syntactic systems are functioning with little backup from the semantic system or cognition (Altmann et al. 2001) and therefore communication is severely curtailed. Utterances tend to become shorter as the degree of dementia becomes very severe and the initiative to use language is lost. Fragments of uncompleted utterances are a feature of fluently produced Alzheimer's disease language and may look like ellipses (Ripich and Terrell 1988, Maxim 1991), but the mechanisms by which these fragments are produced are not clear. Some of the fragments may be the unfinished and abandoned attempts at constructing an utterance, but equally some may be examples of successful and unsuccessful elliptical processes. Bayles (1981) tested the ability to correct auxiliaries and modals in tag questions which require a knowledge that the tag clause is related to the main clause and that part of the process involves ellipsis. She found a hierarchy of difficulty with 'BE' verb tags at the top, but could find no explanation why. The ability to correct some tag question errors does show that relationships between clauses not connected by overt conjunctions may remain partially intact in Alzheimer's disease and suggests that other processes such as the production of elliptical utterances may also be possible at some stages of the disease process.

While the ability to correct sentence errors or anomalies and to match sentences to pictures suggests some processing abilities, deficits in sentence comprehension do occur in Alzheimer's disease. Rochon and Waters (1994) tested people with early-stage Alzheimer's disease on nine different sentence types, using a target picture and a syntactic distractor picture. The vocabulary items were chosen from a pilot test, all sentences were reversible and sentence length was controlled. The Alzheimer's disease subjects showed only a mild syntactic impairment, even on sentences with a complex structure such as passives. Their performance was significantly lower than a control group on all three sentences with two propositions, two of which had an embedded clause. Length was not a significant factor. They suggest that 'a separate match is required for each proposition and thus sentences with two propositions require more post interpretive processing' (p. 346).

Research above the single-word level points to the need to consider how linguistic processes interact and how the disease progression in turn impinges upon these processes.

Discourse, cohesion and repair

The ability to use language appropriately in context becomes more severely impaired as the disease progresses and overall cognitive function deteriorates (Johnson et al. 2003). Yet clinicians working with this population report some meta-awareness of appropriate communication. Ripich and Terrell (1988) found that their group of Alzheimer's disease subjects used more words to discuss a topic but the conversational turns were shorter than the normal elderly. Further research by Ripich et al. (1991) on turn-taking and speech act patterns in Alzheimer's disease subjects showed that they used shorter turns and fewer assertive acts but more requests and increased non-verbal information. Conversational partners also modified their discourse by using shorter turns. They conclude that the basic structure of the discourse is preserved and that the differences observed are compensatory. For example, shorter turns decrease the memory load in conversation, making it more likely that the conversation will continue. They also found that their Alzheimer's disease group used more words to discuss topics than the normal elderly, but cohesion was disrupted twice as often.

Almor et al. (1999) considered how semantic and working-memory deficits contribute to impairments in producing and comprehending referring expressions and found the following:

- The spontaneous speech of 11 people with Alzheimer's disease contained a greater ratio of pronouns to full noun phrases than did the spontaneous speech produced by 9 healthy controls.
- People with Alzheimer's disease were less sensitive than healthy controls to the grammatical information necessary for processing pronouns.
- They were more able to remember referent information in short paragraphs when reference was maintained with full noun phrases rather than pronouns (whereas healthy controls showed the reverse pattern).

Performance was linked to working memory performance but not to word-finding difficulty. Repeated use of specific words, phrases or even short sentences, either in monologues or in conversational language, is characteristic of language use in Alzheimer's disease. Such language use is sometimes perseverative, but sometimes words and phrases may be used as markers when other lexical items are not available. Such intrusions or even confabulations may be produced where correct information appears inaccessible (Dalla Barba and Wong 1992, Dalla Barba et al. 1992).

Cohesion also shows changes which may be of diagnostic significance, with Alzheimer's disease patients having difficulty maintaining simple grammatical agreement across clauses within the same sentence. An early study in this area by Hutchinson and Jensen (1980), comparing normal, institutionalized elderly with an institutionalized dementia group, found that the dementia group initiated topics more frequently than the normal group and also violated topic initiation rules more frequently by not signalling or explaining the change of conversational topic. The dementia group also used twice as many commands, requests and questions as the normal group. Nearly 30% of dementia group utterances were classed as inappropriate to the conversational context in which they were spoken, compared to fewer than 2% in the normal group.

Lahey and Feier (1982) found that lexical cohesion was the most stable form of cohesion in their single-case study of Mrs W, but she reiterated the same words across sentences rather than using related words. In particular, the ability to use pronouns as reference decreased across samples. Absence of a clear referent has been reported as occurring far more frequently in the language of Alzheimer's disease patients than in the normal elderly (Ska and Guenard 1993). Similarly, absence of an appropriate topic is far more frequent in dementia groups than in the normal elderly (Hutchinson and Jensen 1980). The ability to use cohesive devices is likely to be dependent on the functioning of a number of linguistic processes, as well as working and other memory components, and its impairment will reflect the decline of these processes.

Another pointer to the level of meta-awareness of language function is the ability to repair, either to correct errors or to change the emphasis of what is being said. Repair ability is impaired in Alzheimer's disease in comparison to the normal elderly and to other diagnostic groups with dementia (Maxim 1991, McNamara et al. 1992). McNamara et al.'s Alzheimer's disease group used very few single-word repairs but relied on adding new syntactic information, suggesting that metalinguistic awareness in the form of monitoring mechanisms is partially intact in the early to mid stages of Alzheimer's disease.

Movement disorder and the dyspraxias

Although movement disorders are not typical of Alzheimer's disease, myoclonus may be present at some stage in the disease process. People with Alzheimer's disease become less mobile as the disease progresses, and a gait disorder may be present. In the last stages of the disease, primitive reflexes such as the sucking and grasp reflexes may reappear. The presence of other movement disorders may also be due to additional pathologies. Extrapyramidal (parkinsonian) features have been found to correlate with the degree of cognitive and functional impairment, with rigidity and bradykinesia being the most frequent extrapyramidal signs associated with Alzheimer's disease. People who have extrapyramidal signs have greater cognitive and functional impairment than those without clinical evidence of parkinsonism (Clark et al. 1997). Far more common, particularly in the middle stages of Alzheimer's disease, is dyspraxia: the inability to perform certain purposive movements and movement complexes, with the conservation of mobility, sensation and coordination. Ideomotor, ideational and constructional dyspraxia may all appear in Alzheimer's disease and these disorders will affect everyday demands of daily living. Such deficits may be discrete or part of larger decrements (Foster et al. 1986, Miller 1986, Kempler 1988).

Oral and verbal apraxia are both rare in early Alzheimer's disease, unlike Pick's disease and non-fluent progressive aphasia where they may be a presenting feature. Oral and verbal apraxia appears more frequently with lesions of the anterior cortex, as in Pick's disease, whereas other dyspraxias are a more common sequel to diseases of the posterior cortex, as in Alzheimer's disease. Dyspraxia for oral commands and dyspraxia for imitation show different loci of cortical deficit (Foster et al. 1986). Ideational apraxia may be found together with parallel deficits in tests of action tool use, visual and verbal semantic tasks, but is dissociated from tasks tapping action knowledge (Dumont et al. 1995). People with Alzheimer's disease who develop an apraxia have been found to decline more rapidly than those who did not (Yesavage et al. 1993).

People with Alzheimer's disease invariably have constructional difficulties on drawing tasks. Reichman et al. (1991) used a drawing test of increasing complexity to identify visuo-constructive deficits in Alzheimer's disease subjects and found that such deficits were highly correlated with severity of dementia, memory and language deficits. Activities of daily living such as dressing, swallowing and feeding are compromised by the dyspraxias. In particular, the interaction between frontal lobe initiation deficits, other cognitive and language disturbance, motoric function and dyspraxia may require careful assessment and intervention in feeding and swallowing.

Vascular dementia (multi-infarct dementia)

Vascular dementia is a special case amongst the dementias because it is not necessarily progressive, there may be improvement of function during the course of the disease, certain forms of vascular dementia may respond to medical intervention and there is some evidence that specific language impairment may respond to remediation (Swinburn and Maxim 1996).

The disease is caused by multiple small infarcts which leave lacunae (small holes) in the white matter of the brain and the brain stem in about 70% of cases, and is often associated with hypertension. The infarcts are largely from the heart and atheromatous plaques in blood vessels outside the cerebrovascular system. There may also be larger cortical infarcts in about 20% of cases and a mixture of cortical and subcortical lesions in the remaining 30% (Meyer et al. 1988). As with Alzheimer's disease, there is considerable debate as to whether the variation in symptoms and disease progression represents heterogeneity within a single disorder or a number of separate syndromes (Emery et al. 2005). Sampson et al. (2004) suggest three main syndromes:

- infarcts involving the thalamus, basal ganglia, or internal capsule may produce a frontal-subcortical disconnection
- multiple cortical infarcts lead to stepwise erosion of cognitive function with a mixture of cortical and subcortical impairments.
- small vessel disease produces a clinical syndrome of subcortical frontal executive dysfunction, gait 'apraxia', pseudobulbar palsy and urinary incontinence (Binswanger's disease); this form of vascular dementia presents insidiously, often without a history of stroke.

It is the second most common cause of dementia after Alzheimer's disease in North America, Europe and Australia but has a similar prevalence rate in Japan (Imai and Hasegawa 2000). Prevalence estimates vary considerably between 9% and 46% in European and North American surveys, the highest estimate being from an area in the USA with a large black population (Folstein et al. 1985). Results from the Rotterdam study (Ott et al. 1995), a large population-based cross-sectional study, suggest that vascular dementia accounts for 16% of the dementia cases. Unlike Alzheimer's disease, where the increased incidence with age is well documented, the Rotterdam study found only a small increase in vascular dementia with age.

A major issue for health-care professionals is that the differential diagnosis of vascular dementia from multiple strokes is not necessarily easy at a clinical level, although brain imaging is usually definitive. Where the medical diagnosis is made on clinical features alone and without neuroimaging information, misdiagnosis can occur. When a major presenting clinical feature is aphasia, tests of cognitive function which are verbally mediated will show deficits which are due to specific language impairment and which do not reflect cognitive damage. For a discussion of recent attempts to clarify diagnostic categories, see Roman et al. (2004).

Differentiating vascular dementia from Alzheimer's disease

Hachinski's (1974) 13-point ischaemia scale helps to differentiate vascular dementias from primary degenerative dementia and is widely accepted as a useful tool in the diagnosis of the disease. High scores suggest vascular dementia whereas lower scores suggest Alzheimer's disease and other non-ischaemic dementias. Features which score most points and therefore make a diagnosis of vascular dementia more likely are:

- abrupt onset
- fluctuating course
- history of strokes
- focal neurological symptoms and signs.

The fluctuating course of vascular dementia may include at least some recovery after an episode, and the disease is considered to be amenable to a range of treatments (Roman 2000). A complication of medical diagnosis is the high incidence of both vascular dementia and Alzheimer's disease in the same people. Tatemichi (1990) suggests that a dementia can result from cerebrovascular disease because the location of cerebral injury is in a region which can affect many cognitive functions such as the association areas of the posterior cerebrum. The volume of the cerebral injury may reach a point where compensation is no longer possible, or the number of injuries may have an additive or multiplicative effect. There may be an interaction of Alzheimer's disease and stroke, where stroke adds to the effects of early Alzheimer's.

Speech, language and cognitive functions in vascular dementia

Although neuropsychological testing alone may not be adequate to reliably distinguish between vascular dementia and Alzheimer's patients (Traykov et al. 2005) there is some evidence that more specific language testing may be able to do so (Kontiola et al. 1990). A longitudinal study of vascular dementia and Alzheimer patients found that those with vascular dementia had preserved recent memory, more diverse language profiles and less decline in their scores over time than the Alzheimer patients. A study of subcortical vascular dementia (Moretti et al. 2005) found poor general cognitive functions, high insight, depression and apathy as the most salient characteristics, while Graham et al. (2004) found that delayed recall and a silhouette naming task differentiated their Alzheimer's disease and subcortical vascular dementia groups.

Powell et al. (1988) compared the language and speech characteristics of a group of vascular dementia subjects with those of an age- and severity-matched group of Alzheimer subjects. They conclude that vascular dementia is associated with a clinically distinguishable pattern of speech and language disturbances. Motor-speech disturbance was present in nearly all of the vascular dementia subjects but few of the Alzheimer subjects, so that a diagnosis of Alzheimer's disease should be questioned in a patient with melodic or articulatory disturbance. Language abnormalities were not as evident in vascular dementia subjects who had fewer characteristics of fluent aphasia. Instead, they produced fewer, shorter, less syntactically complex utterances than Alzheimer patients. There is simplification of structural aspects of sentence production with retained sentence content, and empty words are used less frequently than in Alzheimer patients (Mendez and Ashla-Mendez 1991, Hier et al. 1985). With increasing severity, sentence length and syntactic complexity are further reduced and sentence fragments become more common.

The patterns of language, cognitive deficits and behavioural changes are determined by the specific arteries affected, the location and extent of infarcted tissue (Mahler and Cummings 1991). Because of the variability in motor speech, language and swallowing deficits, the possibility that control of hypertension may stop deterioration in some patients and even that there may be limited improvement in function with controlled hypertension, careful assessment is necessary.

Vascular dementia patients with lacunae infarcts who show cognitive deficits may also have decreased spontaneity, initiative, response inhibition and mental set shifting deficits (Ishii et al. 1986), whereas those with presumed stroke-related white matter degeneration are more likely to exhibit decreased spontaneity, decreased speed of information processing and elaboration (Gupta et al. 1988, Junque et al. 1990).

Cortical and subcortical forms of vascular dementia have been described, having different pathologies and symptomatologies. Subcortical vascular dementia, as might be expected, is likely to be associated with a dysarthria, emotional lability, gait disturbance, bradykinesia and depression whereas the cortical form is more likely to produce an aphasia, apraxia or agnosia and other focal cortical signs. Binswanger's disease, for example, is a subcortical form of vascular dementia, caused by multiple infarcts of the white matter of the cerebral cortex with lacunar infarcts in the subcortical areas of the basal ganglia and the thalamus but sparing of the cortex and subcortical arcuate fibres. Clinical features of the disease are a history of hypertension, vascular disease and possibly acute strokes. White matter infarcts can be clearly seen on MRI scanning. Neurological symptoms are a prominent motor disturbance, pseudobulbar palsy with associated dysarthria, and behavioural and mood changes including agitation, depression, irritability, euphoria and a memory disorder. Binswanger's disease is essentially progressive but, if high blood pressure is controlled, then patients can have periods of relative stability and may be able to benefit from treatment for speech and language deficits (Cummings and Benson 1992).

Depression is often a specific complicating feature in vascular dementia and may not be amenable to medication (Kramer and Reifler 1992). People with vascular dementia under 85 years may have depressive symptoms due to indirect health related limitations, whereas those over 85 years are more likely to have depression which is directly related to the severity of their disease (Mast et al. 2005).

Despite the high incidence of the disease, there are very few studies of language impairment, perhaps due to the problem of reporting fluctuations in performance which may include partial recovery of function. Language impairment may be similar to specific aphasia syndromes (Benson 1979) but there may be a co-occurring dysarthria. Lesser (1989) described a patient with vascular dementia whose language profile was similar to transcortical sensory aphasia. This man had preserved oral spelling and repetition but severe anomia and poor semantic comprehension. His spelling suggested a dissociation between his semantic system and his store of written word forms (graphemic output lexicon). Canning et al. (2004) suggest that word fluency measures may be helpful in distinguishing vascular dementia from Alzheimer's disease. Their vascular dementia group was significantly better on animal fluency and worse on Letter F fluency than an Alzheimer's disease group.

Hachinski et al. (1974) say that early features of vascular dementia are a dysarthria and dysphagia with associated weakness, slowing, a small-stepped gait and emotional lability. Pseudobulbar dysarthria is the most common form of speech disturbance. Because of the focal nature of the damage, there is no characteristic pattern of behavioural deficits in the earlier stages of the disease but language deficits may be present if there is specific left hemisphere damage and dysprosody has been reported where there is right hemisphere damage (Ross 1981).

Primary progressive aphasias, semantic dementia and frontotemporal dementia (Pick's disease)

Consensus criteria for the three prototypic syndromes – progressive non-fluent aphasia, semantic dementia and frontotemporal dementia (Pick's disease) – were developed by members of an international workshop on frontotemporal lobar degeneration (Neary et al. 1998), and the diagnostic distinctions between these dementias are discussed cogently in Hodges (2000). For the clinician, this group of dementias deserves a special mention because a major symptom is often a specific language deficit without significant or any cognitive impairment. In the case of the progressive non-fluent aphasias and semantic dementia, a language disorder is the main or only presenting symptom and it may be so in people diagnosed with Pick's disease (for a discussion of semantic dementia, see Chapter 5). Because language may be impaired, with little cognitive deficit, and the disease progression is often slow, intervention aimed at the individual's specific problems may be appropriate.

A number of excellent single-case and small-group studies look at these specific dementias. Mesulam (1982) first used the term 'progressive dysphasia' to describe a group of patients with a progressive language disorder while semantic dementia was first described as such by Snowden et al. (1989). Pick's (1892) first patient had a language disorder as a major presenting feature and he described a further three patients with temporal or frontal lobe atrophy (see Hodges 2000). Other studies have described a similar picture of language disorder (Holland et al. 1985, Poeck and Luzzatti 1988), yet the clinical descriptions of Pick's disease usually suggest that early behavioural changes are an important feature of diagnosis. People with frontal lobe atrophy may, then, present with either behavioural or language changes or a combination; the language change is usually of a non-fluent type.

Primary progressive aphasias

There is now a considerable literature on people whose language impairment progresses slowly over a number of years without significant cognitive impairment (Mesulam 1982, Chawluk et al. 1986, Poeck and Luzzatti 1988, Tyrrell et al. 1990). Westbury and Bub (1997), in a review of 112 cases, show that this is a dementia which begins early (mean age at onset 59 years) and is very heterogeneous. Poeck and Luzzatti (1988) concluded that only a few out of over 30 patients described in the literature maintained isolated language impairment. Mesulam and Weintraub (1992) distinguished primary progressive aphasia from Alzheimer type dementia and suggested the following criteria for diagnosis:

• progressive decline in language
• absence of deficits in other domains for at least 2 years
• no disturbance of consciousness
• no signs of a more generalized dementia syndrome
• no systemic disorder or other brain disease that could account for the progressive deficits in language.

Most people with a progressive aphasia have a fluent form of language deficit and have been classified as anomic, transcortical sensory or Wernicke's type aphasia, although Tyrrell et al. (1990) describe one patient whose language impairment was non-fluent with good auditory comprehension and who had a number of apraxias. Weintraub et al. (1990) describe the longitudinal course of four other non-fluent patients. There is usually left hemisphere focal atrophy and PET studies now suggest that, in some patients, there may be little or no functional disturbance in the right hemisphere (Chawluk et al. 1986, Tyrrell et al. 1990).

Poeck and Luzzatti (1988) describe a businesswoman who presented with severe word-finding problems. Medical investigations for hypertension or cerebrovascular disease were negative. Her language was fluent but showed severe word-finding problems, empty phrases and semantic paraphasias. She attempted to repair her output errors but was not always successful. She was, at that time, still able to communicate adequately with little help from her conversational partner. IQ tests showed her to be within the average range for the normal population. Over the next 3 years her language deteriorated to the extent that she had to stop work, but she still had an active social life. Subsequent assessment showed few attempts to self-correct and increased use of stereotypes. Conversation needed support from the examiner. Her IQ was lower but still within the average range.

Current descriptions of people with progressive aphasia suggest that they are younger than the Alzheimer's disease population and often develop signs of language difficulty in their late 50s (Westbury and Bub 1997). The disease progression is slow. Cognitive impairment appears late on in the disease process or is a minor component of the disorder, and cognitive deterioration is slower than language loss. The retained functional language and daily living abilities suggest that this group may benefit from different management and advice from those patients with more general cognitive decline.

Frontotemporal lobar degenerations

The frontotemporal lobar degenerations (FTLD) are a group of disorders characterized by focal degeneration of frontal and temporal lobes of a non-Alzheimer type and which now have consensus diagnostic criteria (Neary et al. 1998). Age at onset is 45–60 and there may be a family history in up to 50% of people with FTLD, with a number of genetic causes. Brain pathology shows three types (Brun et al. 1994):

- microvacuolation or spongiosis (frontal lobe type)
- gliosis with or without ballooned neurons and Pick inclusion bodies (Pick type)
- motor neurone type (MND type).

Behavioural disturbances (including overeating), personality changes and loss of empathy or motivation are common in FTLD as presenting features. As the disease progresses, disinhibition, emotional lability, decreased verbal fluency, impaired ability to abstract and difficulty shifting set have all been noted. There may also be motor and verbal perseveration and stereotypies. Janssen et al. (2005), in a single-case study of familial frontotemporal lobar degeneration, describe progressive speech production difficulties, orofacial dyspraxia, dyscalculia, frontal executive impairment, and limb dyspraxia, with significant cognitive impairment at later stages of the disease.

Kramer et al. (2003), in a group study, found that the FTLD group were not impaired on visual memory tasks and were less impaired on verbal memory tasks and confrontation naming than Alzheimer's disease and semantic dementia groups. The FTLD group performed significantly worse on backward digit span and made significantly more executive errors than the Alzheimer's disease and semantic dementia groups. Orange et al. (1998) showed that the pragmatic performance of people with FTLD and primary progressive aphasia could be distinguished, with well-retained pragmatic skills in FTLD and poor topic maintenance and request response in both fluent and non-fluent progressive aphasia.

Pick's disease

Pick's disease (a frontotemporal dementia) often presents with a specific language impairment and relatively spared cognitive function (Hodges 2000). It may be the cause of some cases of progressive aphasia. There are a number of reports in the literature of people whose language impairment deteriorates only slowly over many years, who are not reported as having gross behavioural changes and who are diagnosed as having Pick's disease on post-mortem (Graff-Radford et al. 1990, Scheltens et al. 1990).

The disease is said to have three stages (Cummings and Benson 1992):

- Initially patients present with personality changes such as lack of spontaneity and inactivity and emotional changes such as inappropriate laughter. Impaired insight and judgement are also a feature, but language abnormalities are among the earliest intellectual deficits.
- As the disease progresses, language impairment increases, often with relative sparing of cognitive functions such as mathematical skills, memory and visuo-spatial skills.
- In the final stage of the disease, patients develop extrapyramidal disorders, intellectual decline in all areas, mutism and incontinence.

The disease process is commonly 7–10 years between diagnosis and death.

Pick's disease begins at an earlier age than Alzheimer's, often in the 50s (Lishman 1987). Diagnostic criteria on post-mortem include the presence of Pick bodies and Pick cells in the brain matter. Cortical atrophy is most likely to be significant in the frontal and temporal lobes where one or both hemispheres may be affected. There are also rare reports of parietal, occipital and subcortical changes (Wechsler et al. 1982, Holland et al. 1985, Munoz-Garcia and Ludwin 1984).

Mutism is often reported, although this is not usually a presenting symptom, tending to appear in the middle stages of the disease process, unlike Alzheimer's disease where it is common only in the final stages of the disease process. Why people with Pick's disease become silent is not clear, but a specific verbal dyspraxia may be present. In Holland et al.'s (1985) single-case study, they report that Mr E was heard to make non-speech sounds for 2 years after he stopped talking. Early on in the disease process, his speech was described as stumbling and he produced what might have been phonemic paraphasias but there is evidence that he might have had dyspraxic difficulties too. For Mr E, his eventual mutism was restricted to speech output. At first, he was able to communicate well by writing and even in the later stages of the disease he could still communicate meaning through single words although he was unable to construct sentences correctly. Mr E's writing showed that he initially retained good access to his semantic lexicon although low-frequency words were sometimes substituted for higher-frequency ones. He was still able to understand most written material until 1 year before he died. The most striking feature of his progressive language disorder is his auditory agnosia. Hearing acuity was good, but he had difficulty understanding spoken language. At first he could understand if the speaker slowed the rate of speech or repeated for him. He understood better, he wrote, if the conversational context was known to him. Approximately 7 years after language changes were first noted, he asked his family to write when they wished to communicate with him. A trial training period of Amerind was begun about 18 months before he died; he learned 50 signs but could not combine or use them despite encouragement from his family. Mr E showed no sign of echolalia but he did have auditory comprehension deficits. Both symptoms are signs of transcortical sensory aphasia, the aphasic syndrome Pick used to describe his patient.

The case of Mr E suggests that communication can be maintained until late on in the disease process because of specific modality sparing. Another patient, EK, however, presented with marked behaviour changes but developed quite marked changes in language and cognition over a 1-year period (Maxim and Bryan 1994). She was a 78-year-old widow who lived alone and was diagnosed as having Pick's disease after referral to a psychogeriatric assessment team. A CT scan demonstrated frontal atrophy. EK had a history of 10 years of deteriorating relations with family and neighbours, and she developed suspicious thoughts about the local butcher. On assessment, she was found to have a moderate dementia, with disorientation in place and a poor knowledge of current events. She was able to identify objects by name and function without difficulty but her auditory comprehension was reduced. Like Mr E, her verbal output and, in particular, her ability to initiate language deteriorated, but she did not demonstrate the same depth of specific modality sparing and her behavioural symptoms were very apparent.

As Pick's disease may progress very slowly, with major language change and less cognitive change, then, as with the progressive aphasias, specific intervention may be appropriate.

Dementia with Lewy bodies

Dementia with Lewy bodies (DLB) is a primary degenerative dementia sharing clinical and pathological characteristics with both Parkinson's disease and Alzheimer's disease and characterized by interneuronal inclusions similar in structure to the Lewy bodies found in Parkinson's disease. These inclusions reflect neuronal loss and are found in the cortex and the subcortical nuclei. It was considered a rare form of dementia, but now is thought to be the second most common form of dementia after Alzheimer's disease, 15–20% of older people with a dementia who reach autopsy having DLB (Burns et al. 1990, Ala et al. 1997, McKeith et al. 2003). DLB may have a faster cognitive decline and accelerated mortality than Alzheimer's disease (Olichney et al. 1998).

The clinical features of DLB are:

- people present with striking fluctuations in cognitive state and transitory episodes of confusion
- cognitive impairment is less than would be expected in Alzheimer's disease in the early stage, with fluctuating impairments in attention, visual recognition and construction
- extrapyramidal deficits of rigidity and tremor (parkinsonism) are present
- visual hallucinations and paranoid delirium are a common finding
- the progress of the disease is variable but all develop dementia and have at least one extrapyramidal deficit
- hypersensitivity to neuroleptic drugs.

Symptoms range from a parkinsonian syndrome with subsequent dementia to dementia with subsequent parkinsonian syndrome, with fluctuations in severity of symptoms from day to day (Byrne et al. 1989). There may be memory deficits, motor disturbances, hyperkinetic dysarthria and aphasia (Galloway 1992, Fearnley et al. 1991), but more studies of speech and language functioning in patients with DLB are needed. Lambon-Ralph et al. (2001) found that people with DLB were impaired across a range of semantic memory tasks, with greater semantic deficits for comprehension of pictures than words, unlike Alzheimer's disease where the impairments are equal. In word fluency tasks, letter and category tasks were equally difficult while in Alzheimer's disease, letter performance was significantly better.

Some overlap with Alzheimer-type pathology has been found, but a strong case is now being made for its distinction as a separate form of dementia: DLB has pathological continuity with Parkinson's disease but can be pathologically differentiated from Alzheimer's disease (Iseki 2004).

Huntington's disease

Huntington's disease is inherited as an autosomal dominant condition, caused by the expansion of a CAG trinucleotide repeat sequence on the short arm of chromosome 4. Because of the familial nature, the diagnosis is not usually difficult: members of families in which it is present are often aware of the possibility that it may develop. This progressive and familial disease, affecting both sexes, usually has a mean age of onset between 30 and 45 years, beginning with either involuntary movement or personality changes, with depression, apathy, aggression, disinhibition, and social disintegration being common (Paulsen et al. 2001). It is associated with cortical and basal ganglia degeneration, with a progressive cognitive and behavioural decline, chorea and other extrapyramidal signs; a subcortical dementia with gaze apraxia typically develops.

A hyperkinetic dysarthria with sparse speech, altered prosody, decreased phrase length and lack of speech initiation is a feature (Podoll et al. 1988). Impairment of comprehension of prosody (Speedie et al. 1990) and language changes including simplified syntax and press of speech (Illes 1989) have been reported. Visual processing impairments may contribute to word-finding difficulties, rather than specific semantic impairment (Bayles and Tomoeda 1983, Hodges et al. 1991). People with Huntington's disease have difficulty on initial letter and semantic category fluency tasks but their performance showed the same pattern as a normal age-matched control group, suggesting that the difficulty is one of initiation and retrieval rather than lexical semantic loss (Rosser and Hodges 1994). People with early Huntington's disease have specific memory disorders associated with difficulty in acquiring new information and reduced verbal fluency, due to difficulty in retrieval from long-term memory, rather than a specific language dysfunction, as naming was intact on other tests. In the later stages there is generalized non-focal cognitive disturbance, with preserved picture naming, suggesting less widespread deterioration than in other dementia-producing disorders (Butters et al. 1978). The communication disorder in Huntington's disease is a combination of dysarthria with particular difficulty in phonation and an altered ability to understand both affective and linguistic prosody (see Chua and Chiu 2000).

Parkinson's disease

Parkinson's disease (PD) is characterized by disturbance of motor function, in particular muscular rigidity and/or tremor. It is most likely to begin around 60 years of age and affects men and women equally. It is a common disease, with a prevalence of approximately 110 per 100 000, of whom 15–43% may have cognitive impairment (Mayeux et al. 1992, Aarsland et al. 2001). For idiopathic Parkinson's disease and adjusting for age-related cognitive changes, the figure is estimated to be probably 15–20% (Brown and Marsden 1984). There is also co-occurrence of Alzheimer's disease and Parkinson's disease. Alzheimer-type cortical changes have been found in neuropathological studies of Parkinson's disease patients. Some studies have suggested that advancing age in a Parkinson's disease population may account for the Alzheimer-type changes (Heston 1981). The dementia associated with Parkinson's disease has been described as subcortical but there is ample evidence that both cognition and language functions show deficits. The average dementia prevalence in Parkinson's disease is thought to be just over 35%, but Parkinson's disease patients show impairments on tasks which require them to use their own internal cues, performing much better when external cues are provided (Brown and Marsden 1988). Tasks which require set shifting are more difficult for Parkinson's disease patients than normal controls despite the absence of dementia (Taylor et al. 1986). Tweedy et al. (1982) found difficulty in the ability of their PD group to utilize semantic cues as memory aids. Several studies have investigated whether increasing cognitive loads, while keeping motoric aspects of the task constant, cause difficulties for Parkinson's disease patients. The majority of these studies show no evidence of processing decrements with increased cognitive load when age-matched groups of Parkinson's disease and normal subjects are used (Brown and Marsden 1986, Rogers et al. 1987) although one study found a decrement in an older but not younger group of PD patients (Wilson et al. 1980). Kulisevsky (2000) reviewed the evidence for cognitive improvement with drug therapy and found that three patterns emerged:

• in early Parkinson's disease there may be some improvement, particularly on executive function (initiation) and memory
• in established Parkinson's disease, drug therapy improves speed of response but not other areas of cognitive skill
• in people who are responding poorly to drug therapy, the increased dose needed to decrease motor difficulties may cause a cognitive deterioration.

The features of parkinsonian dysarthria may convey an impression of slowness of thought and cognitive dysfunction which is not necessarily confirmed on testing. Slowing of the processing of auditory, visual and tactile sensory information is called bradyphrenia. Bradykinesia (slowness of movement) may have an impact on language performance because there may be slowed initiation of motor acts, motor responses may be carried out slowly or motor planning may be slowed (Brown and Marsden 1991).

Damage to subcortical structures may in itself affect language processing in Parkinson's disease, but the language deficit may be caused by reduced cortical functioning as shown in more recent metabolic scanning studies (Kuhl et al. 1984). Language skills in Parkinson's disease may show deficits in complex areas of language processing. Scott et al. (1984) found that their Parkinson's disease patients had difficulty in appreciating intonation and facial expression but showed no language deficits on a shortened aphasia test battery.

There is some evidence of difficulty in interpreting linguistic information in PD. Although Scott et al. (1984) found no impairment of auditory comprehension, either at single word, sentence or paragraph level, McNamara et al. (1992) suggested that Parkinson's disease patients are less able to monitor their own language errors. Using language produced when describing the Boston Cookie Theft picture (Goodglass and Kaplan 1983), they found that Parkinson's disease patients corrected only 25% of their own errors compared to a normal elderly group whose correction rate was over 82%. The Parkinson's disease group, who had an average age of 61.3 years and had been screened to exclude dementia, had a correction rate similar to an Alzheimer group but there were qualitative differences. The Parkinson's disease group were able to correct single words and make reformulation repairs, i.e. corrections that alter the grammatical structure of the phrase or sentence in which the error occurs, but the Alzheimer group used mainly reformulation type repairs. This evidence corresponds to other evidence on word retrieval in Parkinson's disease. Parkinson's disease patients can make single-word corrections because they have better access to their lexicon, whereas naming disorder and specific word retrieval deficits are pervasive in Alzheimer's disease patients.

McNamara et al. (1992) suggest that the Parkinson's disease group have monitoring difficulties due to frontal system dysfunction. Huber et al. (1989), using a Parkinson's disease group with an average age of 70.4 years and matched for cognitive function on the Mini-Mental State Examination, replicated the findings of many studies (see Knight 1992 for a review) that Parkinson's disease patients are significantly worse at word fluency tasks than normals and, on Huber's study, worse than the Alzheimer group. Hanley (1981) suggests that the significant difference in word fluency disappears if age and vocabulary scores are matched. On a naming test, the Parkinson's disease group performed significantly better than the Alzheimer's disease group although they were significantly worse than the normal controls. No deficits in comprehension of single words and commands were found in the Parkinson's disease group who were tested on the Western Aphasia Battery.

Understanding and production of sentences may show deficits, in particular syntax (Obler and Albert 1981, Lieberman et al. 1989, Grossman et al. 1991). Both spoken and written language have been shown to be different from normal age matched controls, having shorter phrase length in spoken language (Illes 1989) but using more words per theme and more complex sentence structure in written language (Obler and Albert 1981). Sentence comprehension seems to be impaired when syntax becomes more complex but increased length of sentence does not increase comprehension difficulty (Grossman et al. 1991, 1992). The ability of Parkinson's disease patients to understand may be helped by semantic constraints such as non-reversibility of sentences (Grossman et al. 1992).

While medication may alleviate some features of Parkinson's disease, patients demonstrate highly complex patterns of drug response. Medication may be the cause of some learning impairment which is not present when medication is withdrawn (Gotham et al. 1988). Improvement in general mobility with medication does not necessarily carry with it any corresponding change in speech patterns, and vice versa.

Depression is common in Parkinson's disease, with a reported incidence of up to 50% (Gotham et al. 1986). Aarsland et al. (2001) found that, in a group of 42 people with Parkinson's disease, 19 had had hallucinations, 17 depression and 13 anxiety. Obviously depression is not necessarily an abnormal reaction to a degenerative disease, but it may require treatment and needs to be taken into account in assessment and management. Maxim and Bryan (1994) suggest that signs of dementia in Parkinson's disease may, for some people, be no more than an interaction between age, motor dysfunction and drug effects. Careful investigation of drug effects, patterns of performance during the day as well as cognitive performance, needs to be made before dementia is diagnosed.

Progressive supranuclear palsy

Alternatively called Steele–Richardson–Olszewski syndrome after the authors who first described it, progressive supranuclear palsy (PSP) typically includes:

- a gaze palsy
- pseudobulbar palsy
- dysarthria
- dysphagia
- dystonic rigidity of the neck and upper trunk.

It may be diagnosed as Parkinson's disease at first because extrapyramidal signs are prominent and the age range for presentation is similar. The dementia of PSP has been described as consisting of the following (Maher and Lees 1986):

- forgetfulness
- slow mentation
- dysarthria
- emotional or personality changes
- impaired ability to manipulate acquired knowledge in the absence of dysphasia, agnosia and perceptual abnormalities.

The disease is progressive and usually results in death within 6 years, unlike Parkinson's disease which is not necessarily life-threatening. It is a subcortical dementia and most investigations of small groups of PSP patients have shown no definite signs of primary language difficulty although other deficits such as initiation problems and dysarthria may produce a communication disturbance (Le Brun et al. 1986). A study by Maher et al. (1985) examined cognitive deficits in PSP subjects at the time of diagnosis and reported mild word-finding difficulty but no evidence of dysphasia or comprehension difficulties. Podoll et al. (1991) found evidence of language impairment secondary to other cognitive deficits which include increased rates of repair and misnamings. Other deficits in reading and writing appear to be due to visual processing changes or to the gaze palsy. Pillon et al. (1994) suggest that people with PSP show impaired immediate memory span, disturbed learning and consistency of recall, and abnormal number of false alarms at recognition, which could be corrected with semantic cueing.

Sentences are well formed but syntactically simple and memory function equals that of normal controls (Milberg and Albert 1989). Van der Hurk and Hodges (1995) confirmed that episodic memory is relatively spared in PSP but there are deficits on tests of semantic memory (the Boston Naming Test, the ADA Synonym Judgement Test, and the Pyramids and Palm Trees Test) and the PSP group showed a significantly greater deficit on the Synonym Judgement Test than an Alzheimer's disease group.

The dysarthria in PSP is characterized by a slow speech rate, low volume and restricted prosody due to both poor pitch variation and difficulty in altering loudness for stress. Palilalia is sometimes found but as the disease progresses speech is initiated less often and response latencies are great (Albert et al. 1974).

Creutzfeldt–Jakob disease

Creutzfeldt–Jacob disease is one of the prion diseases, which are also called transmissible spongiform encephalopathies. Prion diseases can be sub-divided into three aetiological categories (Collinge 2000):

- inherited forms of CJD have a familial history and can now be classified according to the exact mutation of the *PRNP* gene on chromosome 20 (Collinge 2000)
- sporadic forms of CJD are atypical variants
- acquired prion diseases include iatrogenic CJD and new variant CJD (vCJD).

The clinical profile of CJD is a rapidly progressive multifocal dementia (Neary and Snowden 2003), usually with myoclonus. Onset between the ages of 45 and 75 is usual, with a mean onset at the age of 60 and a clinical progression to akinetic mutism and death in less than 6 months. Although CJD patients may have a relatively focal onset with occipital blindness, aphasia or a frontal lobe syndrome, there is rapid spread to other cognitive functions and the early and concurrent emergence of neurological signs of sensorimotor deficit, ataxia, extrapyramidal features and myoclonus (Neary and Snowden 2003). Neuropathological confirmation is by demonstration of spongiform change, neuronal loss and astrocytosis (Global Surveillance 1998).

Patients with a probable diagnosis of sporadic CJD usually have progressive dementia with a typical EEG finding of pseudoperiodic sharp wave activity and two of the following clinical features:

- myoclonus
- cortical blindness
- pyramidal, cerebellar or extrapyramidal signs
- akinetic mutism.

The characteristic EEG is present in 70% of cases. Around 10% of cases of CJD are atypical with a more prolonged clinical course of about 2 years, often with more prevalent cerebellar ataxia, cortical blindness or amyotrophic features (prominent early muscle wasting) (Brown et al. 1997). Iatrogenic transmission of CJD is rare but usually involves inadequately sterilized neurosurgical instruments, contamination from dura mater and corneal grafts or use of infected growth hormone (Collinge 2000). New variant CJD (vCJD) is thought to have a link with bovine spongiform encephalopathy exposure, before the removal of specified bovine offal from human foodstuffs in 1989 (Will et al. 1996).

The presentation of vCJD is dominated by psychiatric syndromes, but neurological symptoms precede psychiatric symptoms in 15% of cases and are present in combination with psychiatric symptoms in 22% of cases from the onset of the disease (Spencer et al. 2002). Common early psychiatric features included dysphoria, withdrawal, anxiety, irritability, insomnia and loss of interest. Within 4 months most patients develop neurological symptoms, with pain, memory difficulties, gait disturbance, dysarthria and sensory symptoms being common. Behavioural disturbances can also occur (Will et al. 1996). Initial referral is often to psychiatry with depression, anxiety, withdrawal and behavioural change. Delusions, auditory and visual hallucinations, emotional lability, aggression and emotional lability can also occur (Zeidler et al. 1997). After a few months, neurological features, typically a progressive cerebellar syndrome, then develop with gait and limb ataxia followed by the onset of dementia which progresses to akinetic mutism. Most patients with vCJD develop swallowing and speech difficulties. A case described by de Vries et al. (2003) showed hypersensitivity to sound and touch which also affected communication. The mean age at onset for the first 100 patients with vCJD was 26, with a range of 12–74 years. The median duration of illness was 13 months, with a range of 6–39 months (Spencer et al. 2002).

There is still uncertainty as to whether the number of vCJD cases will rise sharply. As care for these patients is improved and patients live longer, the role of therapists such as speech and language therapists in terms of both rehabilitation and palliative care will need to be developed and evaluated.

Depression, confusion and dementia

There is a complex interaction between dementia and depression, a common symptom in older populations. Alexopoulos et al. (1993) found that people with a co-existing major depression and cognitive impairment went on to develop a dementia within 5 years, compared with those who had a major depression only. Communication in an elderly person with endogenous (i.e. of unknown origin) depression is often impaired, with reduced intonation range and slow response latency. Language is often impoverished, the patient giving brief replies which are unlikely to lead on to further discussion. On specific tasks, however, depressed patients may do well. Descriptions of the Cookie Theft picture by depressed elderly people may be as good as or better than those given by the normal healthy elderly (Maxim 1991). On the Western Aphasia Battery, Emery (1989) reported that depressed elderly subjects performed significantly better than Alzheimer's disease patients on all measures and were only scoring significantly lower than normal controls on measures which involved errors on the most complex items.

There is a chance of misdiagnosis of the clinically depressed elderly person who presents with a history of cognitive impairment, sleep disturbance, appetite loss, psychomotor slowing, depressed affect and poor memory (Jarvik 1982, Cummings and Benson 1992). Accurate diagnosis of the dementia syndrome of depression from organic causes is obviously essential, because appropriate drug intervention and therapy may be successful (Grossberg and Nakra 1988). Early on in the course of Alzheimer's disease, patients may have a co-occurring depression (Reifler 1986) or may be referred with a diagnosis of depression which is then found to be a primary dementing illness (Feinberg and Goodman 1984), sometimes called pseudodepression. Depression can also be a major feature in the dementias associated with subcortical damage such as Parkinson's disease and Huntington's disease.

HIV-associated cognitive impairment

Navia et al. (1986) described two forms of dementia in AIDS, one being steadily progressive at times punctuated by accelerated deterioration, and the other, occurring in 20% of cases, having a much slower and protracted course. McArthur and Grant (1998), in a review of HIV-associated impairment, suggest four types of difficulty:

• abnormality on only one cognitive domain
• underperformance on two or more cognitive domains
• minor cognitive/motor disorder (MCMD) which affects everyday functioning to at least a mild degree
• HIV dementia where there is marked cognitive impairment.

They also discuss the criteria for diagnosis in each category. Heaton et al. (1995) put forward a neuropsychological test battery which includes language domains and takes into account the younger age profile of this group.

Van Gorp et al. (1992) found that subcortical functions were more affected in AIDS encephalopathy than those in the cortex. In the early stage there may be a dysarthria and motor problems with speech and writing. Mild word-finding problems were found in some subjects and language was affected by slowness of thought and mood changes. As the dementia progresses, verbal responses become slower and less complex with virtual mutism in the final stage of the disease. Most patients with AIDS develop dementia associated with an HIV encephalopathy, but a smaller percentage develop a dementia before AIDS has been diagnosed (Cummings and Benson 1992). The AIDS dementia complex usually includes lethargy, progressive cognitive impairment and slowing of movement and speech (Bannister 1992).

Dementia associated with alcoholism

Wernicke–Korsakoff syndrome, the condition most frequently associated with chronic alcoholism, is an amnesia rather than a dementia. Wernicke's encephalopathy is caused by a thiamine deficiency secondary to chronic alcohol abuse. Victor et al. (1989) found that, despite being given thiamine, 84% of those with Wernicke's encephalopathy went on to develop the amnesia associated with Korsakoff's syndrome. Murdoch (1990) describes the relationship between the two conditions as follows:

> Wernicke's encephalopathy represents the acute stage of this process and Korsakoff's syndrome the residual mental deficit that usually occurs in the late stages of Wernicke's encephalopathy (p. 172).

The conditions are characterized by an isolated loss of recent memory in an otherwise alert person with little other evidence of remote memory, immediate recall or other cognitive changes. The brain may show small haemorrhages and necrotic lesions, and neurotransmitter systems also show disruption.

Chronic alcohol abuse and an associated head trauma can lead to alcohol dementia. As head injury has a peak of incidence in old age, it is important for clinical management that these two conditions are understood to be linked and that an underlying or frank Korsakoff's psychosis may complicate subsequent recovery from head injury. Alcoholic dementia has been described as being more severe in the elderly, and clinically the progression is slow with impairment in abstracting ability, short-term memory and verbal fluency (Cutting 1982). If the patient ceases to consume alcohol there is usually an improvement in cognitive abilities, but return to pre-alcoholic levels is unusual (Grant et al. 1984). Saxton et al. (2000) found that people with alcoholic dementia were more impaired than age-matched normal controls on initial letter fluency, fine motor control, and free recall but did not differ from controls on tests of verbal recognition memory. Kopelman (1991) suggests that frontal lobe dysfunction causes a disorganization of retrieval processes and that this in turn contributes to the retrograde amnesia.

Communication ability is reduced because memory for recent events is poor but language may remain intact. Because of damage to neurotransmitter and subcortical systems, there may be an associated dysarthria.

Down's syndrome and dementia

Down's syndrome is the most common biological cause of developmental delay and is due to a chromosome disorder. Most people with Down's syndrome experience moderate to severe levels of learning disability, various medical problems and language impairments. For a detailed review of language impairments in Down's syndrome, see Laws and Bishop (2004). General improvements in health and more effective treatments for congenital heart disease and infections have resulted in life expectancy for people with Down's syndrome increasing to nearly 50 years (Malone 1988). However, there is now convincing evidence of an age-related increase in the prevalence of dementia, which appears to be of an Alzheimer's disease type in people with Down's syndrome, and which matches that found in the general population but occurring 30–40 years earlier in life. Tyrrell et al. (2001) suggest a prevalence of Alzheimer's disease in people with Down's syndrome of 13.3%, although rates reported vary from 10% to 75% (Zigman et al. 1997). Longitudinal studies are tracking patterns of ageing in people with Down's syndrome and will hopefully clarify normal ageing patterns for them (Carr 2003).

The pattern of cognitive decline in people with Down's syndrome who develop Alzheimer's disease initially involves deterioration in memory, learning and orientation with aphasia, agnosia, and apraxias becoming apparent. Motor slowing is also apparent from an early stage. However, any age-related decline in people with Down's syndrome needs to be investigated carefully, with a possible differential diagnosis of:

- depression
- life events
- sensory impairments
- hypothyroidism
- other cerebral pathologies such as confusional states and B_{12} deficiency.

The diagnosis of dementia in a person with pre-existing cognitive and possibly language difficulty is problematic and the problem of 'diagnostic overshadowing' when either physical or psychiatric disorder is present in someone with a learning disability is a major concern (Holland 2000). An expert working group (Aylward et al. 1997) identified key diagnostic criteria for dementia in people with learning disabilities:

- Evidence of change of function from baseline.
- Functional decline must be present.
- Decline on psychological test scores alone is insufficient evidence.
- The nature of the decline may differ depending on the level of pre-morbid disability.
- The extent of the decline must be greater than would be accounted for by normal ageing.
- Other possible causes of decline must be excluded.

It is essential that information is gained from a carer or family member who has known the person for at least a few months. Evidence of functional decline can then be sought. More formal scales are being developed to assist with the diagnosis of dementia in people with Down's syndrome. The expert working party (Aylward et al. 1997) considered that the ICD-10 diagnostic criteria for Alzheimer's disease were preferable to other criteria because of their greater weighting on behavioural and personality changes.

The CAMDEX informant interview has been modified for use with the main carers of people with Down's syndrome and combined with the CAMDEX diagnostic tests (CAMCOG) has been found to be a useful tool in diagnosing Alzheimer's disease in people with Down's syndrome (Ball et al. 2004). However, use of the CAMCOG tests is limited by the need for participants to score above the floor of the test at baseline.

The Prudhoe Cognitive Function Test (Margallo-Lana et al. 2003) is a relatively brief test, taking approximately 35 minutes with a carer present, and was designed for use by clinicians and other health professionals. The test examines the cognitive functions of orientation, recall, language, praxis and calculation. At the end of the interview, the examiner also rates speech, hearing and vision on four-point scales from normal, through mild and severe to profound impairment. The Prudhoe test has been found to be reliable in diagnosing dementia in people with learning disabilities but again its use with people with profound pre-existing intellectual disability is limited (Kay et al. 2003). The Severe Impairment Battery (Saxton et al. 1993) has also been used with people with Down's syndrome, with most of them being able to score above the floor (Witts and Elders 1998).

There are few studies evaluating interventions for people with Down's syndrome who develop dementia. However, issues of service provision have been documented. There are a number of questions arising, such as should people have access to specialist dementia services, or should existing learning disability services incorporate such provision so that people with Down's syndrome do not lose vital continuity of care? Also, referral to older age services may be inappropriate for someone in their early 40s with Down's syndrome (although the same may be said for anyone with young-onset dementia). Dodd and Christmas (2001) suggest that local authorities should build into their budgets the necessary changes to allow flexible packages of care, particularly for people with Down's syndrome who live at home with carers who may have specific needs of their own. These issues are discussed in Watchman (2003).

Conclusions

Communication disability and specific language impairment are a component of most dementias but do not necessarily co-occur. Someone with

Alzheimer's disease may have a communication disability but very little evidence of language deficits. Another person with a progressive aphasia may show a very specific language deficit but be able to communicate effectively. Intervention and management of language and communication problems in the dementias now needs to differentiate between the needs of people with different forms of dementia.

References

Aarsland D, Cummings JL, Larson JP (2001) Neuropsychiatric differences between Parkinson's disease with dementia and Alzheimer's disease. International Journal of Geriatric Psychiatry 16: 184–191.

Ala TA, Yang KH, Sung JH Frey WH 2nd (1997) Hallucinations and signs of parkinsonism help distinguish patients with dementia and cortical Lewy bodies from patients with Alzheimer's disease at presentation: a clinicopathological study. Journal of Neurology, Neurosurgery and Psychiatry 62(1): 16–21.

Alathari L, Trinh Ngo C, Dopkins S (2004) Loss of distinctive features and a broader pattern of priming in Alzheimer's disease. Neuropsychology 18(4): 603–612.

Albert ML, Feldman RG, Willis AL (1974) The 'subcortical dementia' of progressive supranuclear palsy. Journal of Neurology, Neurosurgery and Psychiatry 37: 121–130.

Alexopoulos GS, Myers BS, Young RC, Mattis S, Kakuma T (1993) The course of geriatric depression with 'reversible dementia': a controlled study. American Journal of Psychiatry 150: 1693–1699.

Almor A, Kempler D, MacDonald MC et al. (1999) Why do Alzheimer patients have difficulty with pronouns? Working memory, semantics, and reference in comprehension and production in Alzheimer's disease. Brain and Language 67(3): 202–227.

Altmann LJ, Kempler D, Andersen ES (2001) Speech errors in Alzheimer's disease: reevaluating morphosyntactic preservation. Journal of Speech, Language and Hearing Research 44(5): 1069–1082.

APA (2000) Diagnostic and Statistical Manual of Mental Disorders, 4th edn, Text Revision. American Psychiatric Association, Washington, DC.

Appell J, Kertesz A, Fisman M (1982) A study of language functioning in Alzheimer's patients. Brain and Language 17: 73–91.

Aylward EH, Burt DB, Thorpe LU et al. (1997) Diagnosis of dementia in individuals with intellectual disability. Journal of Intellectual Disability Research 41: 152–164.

Ball SL, Holland AJ, Huppert FA et al. (2004) The modified CAMDEX informant interview is a valid and reliable tool for use in the diagnosis of dementia in adults with Down's syndrome. Journal of Intellectual Disability Research 48: 611–620.

Bannister R (1992) Brain and Bannister's Clinical Neurology, 7th edn. Oxford University Press, Oxford.

Bayles KA (1981) Comprehension deficits in several dementing diseases. Paper given at Linguistic Society of America 56th Annual Meeting, New York.

Bayles KA (1991) Age at onset of Alzheimer's disease: relation to language dysfuntion. Archives of Neurology 48(2): 155–159.

Bayles KA (2003) Effects of working memory deficits on the communicative functioning of Alzheimer's dementia patients. Journal of Communication Disorders 36(3): 209–219.

Bayles KA, Tomoeda CK (1983) Confrontation naming impairment in dementia. Brain and Language 19: 98–114.

Bayles KA, Tomoeda CK (1993) Arizona Battery for Communication Disorders in Dementia. Canyonlands Publishing, Tucson, AZ.

Bayles KA, Tomoeda CK, Trosset MW (1992) Relation of linguistic communication abilities of Alzheimer's patients to stage of disease. Brain and Language 42: 454–472.

Benson DF (1979) Neurologic correlates of anomia. In: Whitaker H, Whitaker HA (eds) Studies in Neurolinguistics 4. Academic Press, New York, pp. 293–328.

Blanken G, Dittman J, Haas J-C, Wallesch C-W (1987) Spontaneous speech in senile dementia and aphasia: implications for a neurolinguistic model of language production. Cognition 27: 247–274.

Boller F, Becker JT, Holland AL et al. (1991) Predictors of decline in Alzheimer's disease. Cortex 27(1): 9–17.

Brown RG, Marsden CD (1984) How common is dementia in Parkinson's disease? Lancet 2(8414): 1262–1265.

Brown RG, Marsden CD (1986) Visuospatial function in Parkinson's disease. Brain 109: 987–1002.

Brown RG, Marsden CD (1988) Internal versus external cues and the control of attention in Parkinson's disease. Brain 111: 323–347.

Brown RG, Marsden CD (1991) Dual task performance and processing resources in normal subjects and patients with Parkinson's disease. Brain 111: 323–347.

Brown P, Gibbs CJ, Rodgers-Johnson P et al. (1997) Human spongiform encephalopathy: the National Institutes of Health series of 300 cases of experimentally transmitted disease. Annals of Neurology 35: 513–529.

Brun A, Englund B, Gustafson L et al. (1994) Clinical and neuropathological criteria for frontotemporal dementia. Journal of Neurology, Neurosurgery and Psychiatry 57: 416–418.

Bryan K, Binder J, Dann C et al. (2001) Development of a screening test for language in older people (Barnes Language Assessment). Age and Mental Health 5(4): 371–378.

Burns A, Zaudig M (2002) Mild cognitive impairment in older people. Lancet 360: 1963–1965.

Burns A, Luthert P, Levy R, Jacoby R, Lantos P (1990) Accuracy of clinical diagnosis of Alzheimer's disease. BMJ 301: 1026.

Butters N, Sax D, Montgomery K, Tarlow S (1978) Comparison of the neuropsychological deficits associated with early and advanced Huntington's disease. Archives of Neurology 35: 585–589.

Byrne E, Lennox G, Lowe J, Godwin-Austen RB (1989) Diffuse Lewy body disease: clinical features in 15 cases. Journal of Neurology, Neurosurgery and Psychiatry 52: 709–717.

Camus JF, Nicolas S, Wenisch E et al. (2003) Implicit memory for words presented in short texts is preserved in Alzheimer's disease. Psychology in Medicine 33(1): 169–174.

Canning SJ, Leach L, Stuss D, Ngo L, Black SE (2004) Diagnostic utility of abbreviated fluency measures in Alzheimer disease and vascular dementia. Neurology 62: 556–562.

Carr J (2003) Patterns of ageing in 30–35 year olds with Down's syndrome. Journal of Applied Research in Intellectual Disability 16: 29–40.

Chawluk JB, Mesulam MM, Hurtiz H et al. (1986) Slowly progressive aphasia without generalized dementia: studies with positron emission tomography. Annals of Neurology 19: 68–74.

Chertkow H, Bub D (1990) Semantic memory loss in Alzheimer's type dementia. In: Schwartz MF (ed.) Modular Deficits in Alzheimer-type Dementia. MIT Press, Cambridge, MA, pp. 207–244.

Chertkow H, Bub D, Seidenberg M (1989) Priming and semantic memory loss in Alzheimer's disease. Brain and Language 36: 420–446.

Chua P, Chiu E (2000) Huntington's disease. In: O'Brien J, Ames D, Burns A (eds) Dementia, 2nd edn. Arnold, London, pp. 827–837.

Chui HC, Teng EL, Henderson VW, Moy AC (1985) Clinical subtypes of dementia of the Alzheimer type. Neurology 35: 1544–1550.

Chui HC, Lyness S, Sobel E, Schneider LS (1992) Prognostic implications of symptomatic behaviours in AD. In: Florette F, Khachaturian Z, Poncet M, Christen Y (eds) Heterogeneity of Alzheimer's Disease. Springer, Berlin.

Clark CM, Ewbank D, Lerner A et al. (1997) The relationship between extrapyramidal signs and cognitive performance in patients with Alzheimer's disease enrolled in the CERAD Study. Neurology 49(1): 70–75.

Collinge J (2000) Creutzfeldt–Jakob disease and other prion diseases. In: O'Brien J, Ames D, Burns A (eds) Dementia, 2nd edn. Arnold, London, pp. 863–876.

Corkin S (1982) Some relationships between global amnesias and the memory impairments in Alzheimer's disease. In: Corkin S, Davis KL, Growdon JH et al. (eds) Alzheimer's Disease: a report of progress in research. Raven Press, New York.

Cortese MJ, Balota DA, Sergent-Marshall SD, Buckner RL (2003) Spelling via semantics and phonology: exploring the effects of age, Alzheimer's disease, and primary semantic impairment. Neuropsychologia 41(8): 952–967.

Cummings JL, Benson DF (1992) Dementia: a clinical approach. Butterworths, Boston.

Cummings JL, Houlihan JP, Hill MA (1986) The pattern of reading deterioration in dementia of the Alzheimer type: observations and implications. Brain and Language 29: 315–323.

Cutting J (1982) Alcoholic dementia. In: Benson D, Blumer D (eds) Psychiatric Aspects of Neurologic Disease, Vol 2. Grune & Stratton, New York.

Dalla Barba G, Wong C (1992) Encoding specificity and confabulation in Alzheimer's disease and amnesia. Journal of Clinical and Experimental Neuropsychology 3: 378–392.

Dalla Barba G, Wong C, Parlato V, Boller D (1992) Encoding specificity, anosagnosia and confabulation in Alzheimer's disease and depression. Neurobiology of Aging 13: 4–5.

Davis HS, Rockwood K (2004) Conceptualization of mild cognitive impairment: a review. International Journal of Geriatric Psychiatry 19(4): 313–319.

De Vries K, Sque M, Bryan K, Abu-Saad H (2003) Variant Creutzfeldt–Jakob disease: need for mental health and palliative care team collaboration. International Journal of Palliative Nursing 9(12): 512–520.

Dodd K, Christmas M (2001) Down's Syndrome and Dementia: briefing for commissioners. Mental Health Foundation, London.

Duinkerke A, Williams MA, Rigamonti D, Hillis AE (2004) Cognitive recovery in idiopathic normal pressure hydrocephalus after shunt. Cognitive and Behavioral Neurology 17(3): 179–184.

Dumont C, Ska B, Joanette Y (1995) Conceptual apraxia and semantic memory deficit in Alzheimer's disease: two sides of the same coin? Journal of the International Neuropsychological Society 6(6): 693–703.

Emery OB (1989) Language deficits in depression: comparisons with SDAT and normal aging. Journal of Gerontology 44: M85–M92.

Emery VO, Gillie EX, Smith JA (2005) Noninfarct vascular dementia and Alzheimer dementia spectrum. Journal of the Neurological Sciences 229/230: 27–36.

Erkinjuntti T (2000) Vascular dementia: an overview. In: O'Brien J, Ames D, Burns A (eds) Dementia, 2nd edn. Arnold, London, pp. 623–634.

Faber-Langendoen K, Morris JC, Knesevich JW et al. (1998) Aphasia in senile dementia of the Alzheimer type. Annals of Neurology 23: 365–370.

Fearnley JM, Revesz DJ, Frackowiak RSJ, Lees AJ (1991) Diffuse Lewy body disease presenting with a supranuclear gaze palsy. Journal of Neurology, Neurosurgery, and Psychiatry 54: 159–161.

Feinberg T, Goodman B (1984) Affective illness, dementia, and pseudodementia. Journal of Clinical Psychiatry 45: 99–103.

Fisher NM, Rourke BP, Bieliauskas LA et al. (1997) Unmasking the heterogeneity of Alzheimer's disease: case studies of individuals from distinct neuropsychological subgroups. Journal of Clinical and Experimental Psychology 19: 713–754.

Folstein MF, Anthony JC, Parhad I, Duffy B, Gruenberg EM (1985) The meaning of cognitive impairments in the elderly. Journal of the American Geriatrics Society 33(4): 228–235.

Forstl H (2000) What is Alzheimer's disease? In: O'Brien J, Ames D, Burns A (eds) Dementia, 2nd edn. Arnold, London, pp. 371–383.

Foster NL, Chase TN, Patronas NJ, Gillespie MM, Fedio P (1986) Cerebral mapping of apraxia in Alzheimer's disease by positron emission tomography. Annals of Neurology 19: 139–143.

Fromm D, Holland AL, Nebes RD, Oakley MA (1991) A longitudinal study of word-reading ability in Alzheimer's disease: evidence from the National Adult Reading Test. Cortex 27: 367–376.

Funnell E, Hodges J (1990) Progressive loss of access to spoken word forms in a case of Alzheimer's disease. Proceedings of the Royal Society of London B243: 173–179.

Galloway PH (1992) Visual pattern recognition memory and learning deficits in senile dementias of Alzheimer and Lewy body types. Dementia 3: 101–107.

Garrard P, Lambon-Ralph MA, Patterson K et al. (2005) Semantic feature knowledge and picture naming in dementia of Alzheimer's type: a new approach. Brain and Language 93(1): 79–94.

Garrard P, Maloney LM, Hodges JR, Patterson K (2005) The effects of very early Alzheimer's disease on the characteristics of writing by a renowned author. Brain 128(2): 250–260.

Global Surveillance (1998) Diagnosis and Therapy of Human Spongiform Encephalopathies. Report of a WHO consultation. Geneva, Switzerland. WHO/EMC/ZDI/98.9 *www.who.int/emc*

Godbolt AK, Cipolotti L, Watt H et al. (2004) The natural history of Alzheimer disease: a longitudinal presymptomatic and symptomatic study of a familial cohort. Archives of Neurology 61(11): 1743–1748.

Godbolt AK, Cipolotti L, Anderson VM et al. (2005) A decade of pre-diagnostic assessment in a case of familial Alzheimer's disease: tracking progression from asymptomatic to MCI and dementia. Neurocase 11(1): 56–64.

Goodglass H, Kaplan E (1983) Assessment of Aphasia and Related Disorders, 2nd edn. Lea & Febiger, Philadelphia.

Gotham AM, Brown RG, Marsden CD (1986) Depression in Parkinson's disease. A quantitative and qualitative analysis. Journal of Neurology, Neurosurgery and Psychiatry 49: 79–89.

Gotham AM, Brown RG, Marsden CD (1988) 'Frontal' cognitive function in patients with Parkinson's disease 'on' and 'off' levadopa. Brain 111: 299–321.

Graff-Radford NR, Damasio AR, Hyman BT et al. (1990) Progressive aphasia in a patient with Pick's disease: a neuropsychological, radiologic and anatomic study. Neurology 40(4): 620–626.

Graham NL, Emery T, Hodges JR (2004) Distinctive cognitive profiles in Alzheimer's disease and subcortical vascular dementia. Journal of Neurology, Neurosurgery and Psychiatry 75(1): 61–71.

Grant I, Adams KM, Reed R (1984) Aging, abstinence and medical risk factors in the prediction of neuropsychologic deficit among long-term alcoholics. Archives of General Psychiatry 47: 710–718.

Grist E, Maxim J (1992) Confrontation naming in the elderly: the Build-up Picture Test as an aid to differentiating normals from subjects with dementia. European Journal of Disorders of Communication 27: 197–207.

Grossberg GT, Nakra R (1988) The diagnostic dilemma of depressive pseudodementia. In: Strong R (ed.) Central Nervous System Disorders of Aging: clinical intervention and research. Raven Press, New York.

Grossman M, Rhee J (2001) Cognitive resources during sentence processing in Alzheimer's disease. Neuropsychologia 39(13): 1419–1431.

Grossman M, Carvell S, Gollomp S et al. (1991) Sentence comprehension and praxis deficits in Parkinson's disease. Neurology 41: 1620–1626.

Grossman M, Carvell S, Stern MB, Gollomp S, Hurtig HI (1992) Sentence comprehension in Parkinson's disease: the role of attention and memory. Brain and Language 42: 347–384.

Grossman M, Smith EE, Koenig PL et al. (2003) Categorization of object descriptions in Alzheimer's disease and frontotemporal dementia: limitation in rule-based processing. Cognitive, Affective and Behavioral Neuroscience 3(2): 120–132.

Grundman M, Petersen RC, Ferris SH et al. (2004) Alzheimer's Disease Cooperative Study. Mild cognitive impairment can be distinguished from Alzheimer disease and normal aging for clinical trials. Archives of Neurology 61(1): 59–66.

Gupta SR, Naheedy MH, Young JC et al. (1988) Periventricular white matter changes and dementia: clinical neuropsychological, radiological and pathological correlation. Archives of Neurology 45: 637–641.

Hachinski VC, Lassen NA, Marshall J (1974) Multi-infarct dementia. A cause of mental deterioration in the elderly. Lancet ii: 207–210.

Hanley IG (1981) The use of signposts and active training to modify ward disorientation in elderly patients. Journal of Behaviour Therapy and Experimental Psychiatry 12: 241–247.

Hart S, Smith CM, Swash M (1986) Intrusion errors in Alzheimer's disease. British Journal of Clinical Psychology 25: 149–150.

Heaton RK, Grant I, Butters N, White DA et al. (1995) The HNRC 500: Neuropsychology of HIV infection at different disease stages. Journal of the International Neuropsychological Society 1(3): 231–251.

Heindel WC, Salmon DP, Butters N (1990) Pictorial priming and cued recall in Alzheimer's and Huntington's disease. Brain and Cognition 13: 282–295.

Herlitz A, Adolfson R, Backman L, Wilson L-G (1991) Cue utilization following different forms of encoding in mildly, moderately and severely demented patients with Alzheimer's disease. Brain and Cognition 15: 119–130.

Heston L (1981) Genetic studies of dementia with emphasis on Parkinson's disease and Alzheimer's neuropathology. In: Mortimer J, Schuman L (eds) The Epidemiology of Dementia. Oxford University Press, Oxford.

Hier DB, Hagenlocker K, Shindler AG (1985) Language disintegration in dementia: effects of aetiology and severity. Brain and Language 25: 117–133.

Hodges JR (2000) Pick's disease: its relationship to progressive aphasia, semantic dementia and frontotemporal dementia. In: O'Brien J, Ames D, Burns A (eds) Dementia, 2nd edn. Arnold, London, pp. 747–758.

Hodges JR, Patterson K (1995) Is semantic memory consistently impaired early in the course of Alzheimer's disease? Neuroanatomical and diagnostic implications. Neuropsychologia 33(4): 441–459.

Hodges JR, Salmon DP, Butters N (1991) The nature of the naming deficit in Alzheimer's and Huntington's disease. Brain 114: 1547–1558.

Hodges JR, Salmon DP, Butters N (1992) Semantic memory impairment in Alzheimer's disease: failure of access or degraded knowledge? Neuropsychologia 30(4): 301–314.

Holland AL, McBurney DH, Moossy J, Rernmirth OM (1985) The dissolution of language in Pick's disease with neurofibrillary tangles: a case study. Brain and Language 24: 36–38.

Holland H (2000) Down's syndrome and dementia. In: O'Brien J, Ames D, Burns A (eds) Dementia, 2nd edn. Arnold, London, pp. 813–819.

Horner J, Heyman A, Dawson D, Rogers H (1988) The relationship of agraphia to the severity of dementia in Alzheimer's disease. Archives of Neurology 45: 760–763.

Huber SJ, Shuttleworth EC, Freidenberg DL (1989) Neuropsychological differences between the dementias of Alzheimer's and Parkinson's diseases. Archives of Neurology 46: 1287–1291.

Huff FJ, Corkin S, Crowdon J (1986) Semantic impairment and anomia in Alzheimer's disease. Brain and Language 280: 235–249.

Hutchinson JM, Jensen M (1980) A pragmatic evaluation of discourse communication in normal and senile elderly in a nursing home. In: Obler LK, Albert ML (eds) Language and Communication in the Elderly. D. Heath and Co., Lexington, MA.

Illes J (1989) Neurolinguistic features of spontaneous language dissociate three forms of neurodegenerative disease: Alzheimer's, Huntington's and Parkinson's. Brain and Language 37: 628–642.

Imai Y, Hasegawa K (2000) Services for dementia: a Japanese view. In: O'Brien J, Ames D, Burns A (eds) Dementia, 2nd edn. Arnold, London, pp. 321–328.

Iseki E (2004) Dementia with Lewy bodies: reclassification of pathological subtypes and boundary with Parkinson's disease or Alzheimer's disease. Neuropathology 24(1): 72–78.

Ishii N, Nishahara Y, Imamura T (1986) Why do frontal lobe symptoms predominate in vascular dementia with lacunes? Neurology 36: 340–345.

Janssen JC, Schott JM, Cipolotti L et al. (2005) Mapping the onset and progression of atrophy in familial frontotemporal lobar degeneration. Journal of Neurology, Neurosurgery and Psychiatry 76(2): 162–168.

Jarvik LF (1982) Pseudodementia. Consultant 22: 141–146.

Joanette Y, Ska B, Poissant A, Beland R (1992) Neuropsychological aspects of Alzheimer's disease: evidence for inter and intra-function heterogeneity. In: Florette F, Khachaturian Z, Poncet M, Christen Y (eds) Heterogeneity of Alzheimer's Disease. Springer, Berlin.

Johnson DK, Storandt M, Balota DA (2003) Discourse analysis of logical memory recall in normal aging and in dementia of the Alzheimer type. Neuropsychology 17(1): 82–92.

Jorm A (2000) Risk factors for Alzheimer's disease. In: O'Brien J, Ames D, Burns A (eds) Dementia, 2nd edn. Arnold, London, pp. 383–390.

Junque C, Pujol J, Vendrell P et al. (1990) Leuko-araiosis on magnetic resonance imaging and speed of mental processing. Archives of Neurology 47: 151–156.

Kay DWK, Tyrer SP, Margallo-Lana ML et al. (2003) Preliminary evaluation of a scale to assess cognitive function in adults with Down's syndrome: the Prudhoe Cognitive Function Test. Journal of Intellectual Disability Research 47: 155–168.

Kemper S, Marquis J, Thompson M (2001) Longitudinal change in language production: effects of aging and dementia on grammatical complexity and propositional content. Psychology and Aging 16(4): 600–614.

Kempler D (1988) Lexical and pantomime abilities in Alzheimer's disease. Aphasiology 2: 147–159.

Kempler D (1995) Language changes in dementia of the Alzheimer type. In: Lubinski R (ed.) Dementia and Communication. Singular Publishing Group, San Diego, CA, pp. 98–114.

Kempler D, Curtis S, Jackson C (1987) Syntactic preservation in Alzheimer's disease. Journal of Speech and Hearing Research 30: 343–350.

Kim M, Thompson CK (2004) Verb deficits in Alzheimer's disease and agrammatism: implications for lexical organization. Brain and Language 88(1): 1–20.

Knight RG (1992) The Neuropsychology of Degenerative Brain Diseases. Lawrence Erlbaum Associates, London.

Kontiola P, Laaksoner R, Sulkawa R, Erkinjunsi T (1990) Pattern of language impairment in Alzheimer's disease and multi-infarct dementia. Brain and Language 38: 364–383.

Kopelman MD (1986) Recall of anomalous sentences in dementia and amnesia. Brain and Language 29: 154–170.

Kopelman MD (1991) Frontal dysfunction and memory deficits in the alcoholic Korsakoff syndrome and in Alzheimer-type dementia. Brain 114: 117–137.

Kramer JH, Jurik J, Sha SJ et al. (2003) Distinctive neuropsychological patterns in frontotemporal dementia, semantic dementia, and Alzheimer disease. Cognitive and Behavioral Neurology 16(4): 211–218.

Kramer SI, Reifler BV (1992) Depression, dementia and reversible dementia. Clinical Geriatric Medicine 8(2): 289–297.

Kuhl DE, Metter EJ, Reige WH (1984) Patterns of local cerebral glucose utilization determined in Parkinson's disease by [^{18}F]flurodeoxyglucose method. Annals of Neurology 15: 419–424.

Kulisevsky J (2000) Role of dopamine in learning and memory: implications for the treatment of cognitive dysfunction in patients with Parkinson's disease. Drugs and Aging 16: 365–379.

Lahey M, Feier CD (1982) The semantics of verbs in dissolution and development of language. Journal of Speech and Hearing Research 25: 81–95.

Lambon-Ralph MA, Patterson K, Hodges JR (1997) The relationship between naming and semantic knowledge for different categories in dementia of Alzheimer's type. Neuropsychologia 35(9): 1251–1260.

Lambon-Ralph MA, Powell J, Howard D et al. (2001) Semantic memory is impaired in both dementia with Lewy bodies and dementia of Alzheimer's type: a comparative neuropsychological study and literature review. Journal of Neurology, Neurosurgery and Psychiatry 70(2): 149–156.

Lambon-Ralph MA, Patterson K, Graham N, Dawson K, Hodges J (2003) Homogeneity and heterogeneity in mild cognitive impairment and Alzheimer's disease: a cross sectional and longitudinal study of 55 cases. Brain 126(11): 2350–2362.

Laws G, Bishop DVM (2004) Verbal deficits in Down's syndrome and specific language impairment: a comparison. International Journal of Language and Communication Disorder 39: 423–451.

Le Brun Y, Devreux F, Rousseau JJ (1986) Language and speech in a patient with a clinical diagnosis of progressive supranuclear palsy. Brain and Language 27: 247–256.

Lesser R (1989) Selective preservation of oral spelling without semantics in a case of multi-infarct dementia. Cortex 25(2): 239–250.

Lieberman P, Friedman J, Feldman LS (1989) Syntax comprehension in Parkinson's disease. Journal of Nervous and Mental Disease 178: 360–366.

Lishman WA (1987) Organic Psychiatry: The Psychological Consequences of Cerebral Disorder, 2nd edn. Blackwell Scientific, Oxford.

McArthur JC, Grant I (1998) HIV neurocognitive disorders. In: Gendelman HE, Lipton SA, Epstein L, Swindells S (eds) The Neurology of AIDS. Chapman & Hall, New York, pp. 499–523.

McKeith IG, Burn DJ, Ballard CG et al. (2003) Dementia with Lewy bodies. Seminars and Clinics in Neuropsychiatry 8(1): 46–57.

McNamara P, Obler LK, Au R et al. (1992) Speech monitoring skills in Alzheimer's disease, Parkinson's disease and normal aging. Brain and Language 42: 38–51.

Maher ER, Lees AJ (1986) The clinical features and natural history of the Steele–Richardson–Olszewski syndrome (progressive supranuclear palsy). Neurology 36: 1005–1008.

Maher ER, Smith EM, Lees AJ (1985) Cognitive deficits in the Steele–Richardson–Olszewski syndrome. Journal of Neurology, Neurosurgery and Psychiatry 48: 1234–1239.

Mahler ME, Cummings JL (1991) Behavioural neurology of multi-infarct dementia. Alzheimer Disease Association Disorders 5(20): 122–130.

Malone Q (1988) Mortality and survival of the Down's syndrome population in Western Australia. Journal of Mental Deficiency Research 32: 59–65.

Manenti R, Repetto C, Bentrovato S et al. (2004) The effects of ageing and Alzheimer's disease on semantic and gender priming. Brain 127(10): 2299–2306.

Margallo-Lana ML, Moore PB, Tyrer SP et al. (2003) The Prudhoe Cognitive Function Test: a scale to assess cognitive function in adults with Down's syndrome. II Inter-rater and test-retest reliability and reappraisal. Journal of Intellectual Disability Research 47(6): 488–492.

Martin A (1987) Representations of semantic and spatial knowledge in Alzheimer's patients: implications for models of preserved learning in amnesia. Journal of Clinical and Experimental Neuropsychology 9: 121–224.

Martin A (1990) Neuropathology of Alzheimer's disease: the case for subgroups. In: Schwartz MF (ed.) Modular Deficits in Alzheimer-type Dementia. MIT Press, Cambridge, MA, pp. 144–178.

Martin A, Brouwers P, Cox C, Fedio P (1985) On the nature of the verbal memory deficit in Alzheimer's disease. Brain and Language 25: 323–341.

Mast BT, Azar AR, Murrell SA (2005) The vascular depression hypothesis: the influence of age on the relationship between cerebrovascular risk factors and depressive symptoms in community dwelling elders. Aging and Mental Health 9(2): 146–152.

Maxim J (1991) Can elicited language be used to diagnose dementia? Work in Progress 1: 13–21. NHCSS, London.

Maxim J, Bryan K (1994) Language of the Elderly. Whurr, London.

Maxim J, Bryan K (1996) Language, cognition and communication in the older mentally infirm. In: Bryan K, Maxim J (eds) Communication Disability and the Psychiatry of Old Age. Whurr, London, pp. 37–78.

Maxim J, Bryan K, Zabihi K (2000) Semantic processing in Alzheimer's disease. In: Best W, Bryan K, Maxim J (eds) Semantic Processing. Whurr, London, pp. 150–179.

Mayeux R, Stern Y, Sano M (1992) A comparison of clinical outcome and survival in various forms of Alzheimer's disease. In: Florette F, Khachaturian Z, Poncet M, Christen Y (eds) Heterogeneity of Alzheimer's Disease. Springer, Berlin.

Mendez MF, Ashla-Mendez M (1991) Differences between multi-infarct dementia and Alzheimer's disease on unstructured neuropsychological tasks. Journal of Clinical and Experimental Neuropsychology 13(6): 923–932.

Mesulam M (1982) Slowly progressive aphasia without generalized dementia. Annals of Neurology 11: 592–598.

Mesulam MM, Weintraub S (1992) Primary progressive aphasia: sharpening the focus on a clinical syndrome. In: Florette F, Khachaturian Z, Poncet M, Christen Y (eds) Heterogeneity of Alzheimer's Disease. Springer, Berlin.

Meyer JS, McClintic KL, Rogers RL et al. (1988) Aetiological considerations and risk factors for multi-infarct dementia. Journal of Neurology, Neurosurgery and Psychiatry 51: 1489–1497.

Milberg W, Albert M (1989) Cognitive differences between patients with progressive supranuclear palsy and Alzheimer's disease. Journal of Clinical and Experimental Neuropsychology 11(5): 605–614.

Miller N (1986) Dyspraxia and its Management. Croom Helm, London.

Moreaud O, David D, Charnallet A, Pellat J (2001) Are semantic errors actually semantic?: evidence from Alzheimer's disease. Brain and Language 77(2): 176–186.

Moretti R, Torre P, Antonello RM et al. (2005) Frontal lobe dementia and subcortical vascular dementia: a europsychological comparison. Psychological Reports 96(1): 141–151.

Morris JC, Edland S, Clark C et al. (1993) The consortium to establish a registry for Alzheimer's disease (CERAD), part IV: rates of cognitive change in the longitudinal assessment of probable Alzheimer's disease. Neurology 43(12): 2457–2465.

Munoz-Garcia D, Ludwin SK (1984) Classic and generalized variants of Pick's disease: a clinicopathological, ultra structural and immunocytochemical comparative study. Annals of Neurology 16: 467–480.

Murdoch BE (1990) Acquired Speech and Language Disorders. A neuroanatomical and functional approach. Chapman & Hall, London.

Navia BA, Jordan BD, Price RW (1986) The AIDS dementia complex: I. Clinical features. Annals of Neurology 19: 517–524.

Neary D, Snowden JS (2003) Sorting out subacute spongiform encephalopathy. Practical Neurology 3: 268–281.

Neary D, Snowden JS, Gustafson L et al. (1998) Frontotemporal lobar degeneration: a consensus on clinical diagnostic criteria. Neurology 51(6): 1546–1554.

Nebes RD, Martin DC, Horn LC (1984) Sparing of semantic memory in Alzheimer's disease. Journal of Abnormal Psychology 93: 321–330.

Nebes RD, Boller F, Holland A (1986) Use of semantic context by patients with Alzheimer's disease. Psychology and Ageing 1: 261–269.

Nelson J, O'Connell P (1978) Dementia: the estimation of premorbid intelligence levels using the New Adult Reading Test. Cortex 14: 234–244.

Obler LK (1980) Narrative discourse style in the elderly. In: Obler L, Albert M (eds) Language and Communication in the Elderly. D.C. Heath and Co., Lexington, MA.

Obler L, Albert M (1981) Language and aging: a neurobehavioral analysis. In: Beasley D, Davis GA (eds) Aging Communication Processes and Disorders. Grune & Stratton, New York.

Olichney JM, Galasko D, Salmon DP et al. (1998) Cognitive decline is faster in Lewy body variant than in Alzheimer's disease. Neurology 51(2): 351–357.

Orange JB, Kertesz A, Peacock J (1998) Pragmatics in frontal lobe dementia and primary progressive aphasia. Journal of Neurolinguistics 11(1/2): 153–177.

Ott A, Breteler MMB, van Harsclamp F et al. (1995) Prevalence of Alzheimer's disease and vascular dementia: association with education. BMJ 310: 970–972.

Patterson K, Graham N, Hodges J (1994) Reading in dementia of the Alzheimer type: a preserved ability? Neuropsychologia 8: 395–407.

Paulsen JS, Ready RE, Hamilton JM et al. (2001) Neuropsychiatric aspects of Huntington's disease. Journal of Neurology, Neurosurgery and Psychiatry 71: 310–314.

Perri R, Carlesimo GA, Zannino GD et al. (2003) Intentional and automatic measures of specific-category effect in the semantic impairment of patients with Alzheimer's disease. Neuropsychologia 41(11): 1509–1522.

Pick A (1892) Ueber die beziehungen der senilen hirnatrophie zur aphasie. Präger Medizinische Wochenschrift 17: 165–167.

Pillon B, Deweer B, Michon A et al. (1994) Are explicit memory disorders of progressive supranuclear palsy related to damage to striatofrontal circuits? Comparison with Alzheimer's, Parkinson's, and Huntington's diseases. Neurology 44(7): 1264–1270.

Piolino P, Desgranges B, Belliard S et al. (2003) Autobiographical memory and autonoetic consciousness: triple dissociation in neurodegenerative diseases. Brain 126(10): 2203–2219.

Podoll K, Caspary P, Large HW, Noth J (1988) Language functions in Huntingdon's disease. Brain 3: 1475–1503.

Podoll K, Schwarz M, Noth J (1991) Language functions in progressive supranuclear palsy. Brain 114: 1457–1472.

Poeck K, Luzzatti C (1988) Slowly progressive aphasia in three patients. The problems of accompanying neuropsychological deficit. Brain 3: 151–168.

Powell AL, Cummings JL, Hill MA, Benson DF (1988) Speech and language alterations in multi-infarct dementia. Neurology 38: 717–719.

Reichman WE, Cummings JL, McDaniel KD, Flynn F, Gornbein J (1991) Visuoconstructive impairment in dementia syndromes. Behavioural Neurology 4: 153–162.

Reifler B (1986) Mixed cognitive-affective disturbances in the elderly: a new classification. Journalof Clin Psychiatry 47: 354–356.

Reisberg B, Ferris SM, Leon M de, Crook T (1982) The global deterioration scale for assessment of primary degenerative dementia. American Journal of Psychiatry 139: 1136–1139.

Ripich DN, Terrell BY (1988) Patterns of discourse cohesion in Alzheimer's disease. Journal of Speech and Hearing Disorders 53: 8–15.

Ripich DN, Vertes D, Whitehouse P, Fulton S, Ekelman B (1991) Turn-taking and speech act patterns in the discourse of senile dementia of the Alzheimer's type patients. Brain and Language 40: 330–343.

Rochford G (1971) A study of naming errors in dysphasic and in demented patients. Neuropsychologia 9: 437–43.

Rochon E, Waters GS (1994) Sentence comprehension in patients with Alzheimer's disease. Brain and Language 46: 329–349.

Rochon E, Waters GS, Caplan D (2000) The relationship between measures of working memory and sentence comprehension in patients with Alzheimer's disease.Speech Language and Hearing Research 43(2): 395–413.

Rogers D, Lees AJ, Smith E, Trimble M, Stern GM (1987) Bradyphrenia in Parkinson's disease and psychomotor retardation in depressive illness: An experimental study. Brain 110: 761–776.

Roman G (2000) Therapeutic strategies for vascular dementia. In: O'Brien J, Ames D, Burns A (ed) Dementia, 2nd edn. Arnold, London, pp. 667–682.

Roman GC, Sachdev P, Royall DR et al. (2004) Vascular cognitive disorder: a new diagnostic category updating vascular cognitive impairment and vascular dementia. Journal of the Neurological Sciences 226(1/2): 81–87.

Ross ED (1981) The aprosodias: functional organization of the affective components of language in the right hemisphere. Archives of Neurology 38: 561–9.

Rosser A, Hodges JR (1994) Initial letter and semantic category influence in Alzheimer's disease, Huntington's disease and progressive supranuclear palsy. Journal of Neurology Neurosurgery and Psychiatry 57(11): 1389–1394.

Sampson JD, Warren JD, Rossor MN (2004) Young onset dementia. Postgraduate Medical Journal 80: 125–139.

Saxton J, McGonigle KL, Swihart AA, Boller F (1993) Severe Impairment Battery. Thames Valley Test Company, Bury St Edmunds.

Saxton J, Munro CA, Butters MA, Schramke C, McNeil MA (2000) Alcohol, dementia, and Alzheimer's disease: comparison of neuropsychological profiles. Journal of Geriatric Psychiatry and Neurology 13(3): 141–149.

Scheltens P, Hazenberg GJ, Lindeboom J, Valk J, Wolters EC (1990) A case of progressive aphasia without dementia: 'temporal' Pick's disease? Journal of Neurology, Neurosurgery and Psychiatry 53: 79–80.

Schwartz MF (1990) Modular Deficits in Alzheimer-type Dementia. MIT-Bradford, Cambridge, MA.

Schwartz MF, Marin OS, Saffran EM (1979) Dissociation of language function in dementia: a case study. Brain and Language 7: 277–306.

Schwartz MF, Saffran EM, Marin OS (1980) Fractionating the reading process in dementia: evidence for word specific print-to-sound associations. In: Coltheart M, Patterson KE, Marshall JC (eds) Deep Dyslexia. Routledge, London.

Schwartz MF, Saffran EM, Williamson S (1981) The breakdown of lexicon in Alzheimer's dementia. Paper given at Linguistic Society of America 56th Annual Meeting, New York.

Scott S, Caird FI, Williams BO (1984) Evidence for an apparent sensory speech disorder in Parkinson's disease. Journal of Neurology, Neurosurgery and Psychiatry 47: 840–843.

Seltzer B, Sherwin I (1983) A comparison of clinical features in early and late onset primary degenerative dementia. One entity or two? Archives of Neurology 40: 143–146.

Shuttleworth EC, Huber SJ (1989) A longitudinal study of the naming disorder of dementia of the Alzheimer type. Neuropsychiatry, Neuropsychology and Behavioural Neurology 1: 267–282.

Ska B, Guenard D (1993) Narrative schema in dementia of the Alzheimer's type. In: Brownell HH, Joanette Y (eds) Narrative Discourse in Neurologically Impaired and Normal Aging Adults. Singular Publishing Group, San Diego, CA, pp. 299–316.

Ska B, Joanette Y, Poissant A, Beland R, Lecours AR (1990) Language disorders in dementia of the Alzheimer type: contrastive patterns from a multiple single case study. Abstract of the Academy of Aphasia 28th Annual Meeting Baltimore, USA, pp. 21–23.

Skelton-Robinson M, Jones S (1984) Nominal dysphasia and the severity of senile dementia. British Journal of Psychiatry 145: 168–171.

Small JA, Kemper S, Lyons K (1997) Sentence comprehension in Alzheimer's disease: effects of grammatical complexity, speech rate, and repetition. Psychology and Aging 12(1): 3–11.

Small JA, Kemper S, Lyons K (2000) Sentence repetition and processing resources in Alzheimer's disease. Brain and Language 75(2): 232–258.

Smith C, Bryan K (1992) Speech and swallowing dysfunction in multi-system atrophy. Clinical Rehabilitation 6: 291–298.

Smith SR, Murdoch BE, Chenery HJ (1989) Semantic abilities in dementia of the Alzheimer type: I Lexical semantics. Brain and Language 36(2): 314–324.

Snowden JS, Goulding PJ, Neary D (1989) Semantic dementia: a form of circumscribed atrophy. Behavioural Neurology 2: 167–182.

Snowdon DA, Kemper SJ, Mortimer JA et al. (1996) Linguistic ability in early life and cognitive function and Alzheimer's disease in late life. Findings from the Nun Study. JAMA 275(7): 528–532.

Speedie LJ, Brake N, Folstein SE et al. (1990) Comprehension of prosody in Huntington's disease. Journal of Neurology, Neurosurgery and Psychiatry 53: 607–610.

Spencer MD, Knight RSG, Will RG (2002) First hundred cases of variant Creutzfeldt–Jakob disease: retrospective case note review of early psychiatric and neurological features. BMJ 324: 1479–1482.

Stebbins GT, Wilson RS, Gilley DW et al. (1990) Use of the NART to estimate premorbid IQ in dementia. Clinical Neurologist 4: 18–24.

Stevens SJ (1985) The language of dementia: a pilot study. British Journal of Disorders of Communication 20: 181–190.

Swinburn K, Maxim J (1996) Multi-infarct dementia – a suitable case for treatment? In: Bryan K, Maxim J (eds) Communication Disability and the Psychiatry of Old Age. Whurr, London, pp. 206–220.

Tallberg IM, Almkvist O (2001) Confabulation and memory in patients with Alzheimer's disease. Journal of Clinical and Experimental Neuropsychology 23(2): 172–184.

Tatemichi TK (1990) How acute brain failure becomes chronic. A view of the mechanisms of dementia related to stroke. Neurology 40: 1652–1659.

Taylor AE, Saint-Cyr JA, Lang AE (1986) Frontal lobe dysfunction in Parkinson's disease: the cortical focus of neostriatal outflow. Brain 109: 845–883.

Traykov L, Baudic S, Raoux N et al. (2005) Patterns of memory impairment and perseverative behavior discriminate early Alzheimer's disease from subcortical vascular dementia. Journal of Neurological Science 229/230: 75–79.

Troster AI, Salmon DP, McCullough D, Butters N (1989) A comparison of the category fluency deficits associated with Alzheimer's and Huntington's disease. Brain and Language 37: 500–513.

Tweedy JR, Langer KG, McDowell FH (1982) The effect of semantic relations on the memory deficit associated with Parkinson's disease. Journal of Clinical and Experimental Neuropsychology 4: 235–247.

Tyrrell J, Cosgrave M, McCarron M et al. (2001) Dementia in people with Down's syndrome. International Journal of Geriatric Psychiatry 16: 1168–1174.

Tyrrell PJ, Warrington EK, Frackowiak RSJ, Rossor MN (1990) Heterogeneity in progressive aphasia due to focal cortical atrophy. Brain 113: 1321–1336.

Van der Hurk PR, Hodges JR (1995) Episodic and semantic memory in Alzheimer's disease and progressive supranuclear palsy: a comparative study. Journal of Clinical and Experimental Neuropsychology 17(3): 459–471.

Van Gorp WG, Mandelkern MA, Gee M et al. (1992) Cerebral metabolic dysfunction in AIDS: findings in a sample with and without dementia. Journal of Neuropsychiatry and Clinical Neuroscience 4: 280–7.

Victor M, Adams RD, Collins GH (1989) The Wernicke-Korsakoff Syndrome and Related Neurological Disorders Due to Alcoholism And Malnutrition, 2nd edn. F. A. Davis and Co., Philadelphia.

Vogel A, Gade A, Stokholm J, Waldemar G (2005) Semantic memory impairment in the earliest phases of Alzheimer's disease. Dementia and Geriatric Cognitive Disorders Disord 19(2/3): 75–81.

Watchman K (2003) Critical issues for service planners and providers of care for people with Down's syndrome and dementia. British Journal of Learning Disabilities 31: 81–84.

Waters G, Caplan D (2002) Working memory and online syntactic processing in Alzheimer's disease: studies with auditory moving window presentation. Journal of Gerontology B, Psychological Sciences and Social Sciences 57(4): P298–311.

Wechsler AF, Verity MA, Rosenschein S, Fried I, Scheibel AB (1982) Pick's disease: a clinical computed tomographic and histologic study with golgi impregnation observations. Archives of Neurology 39: 287–290.

Weintraub S, Rubin NP, Marsel-Mesulam MM (1990) Primary progressive aphasia: longitudinal course, neuropsychological profile and language features. Archives of Neurology 47: 1329–1335.

Westbury C, Bub D (1997) Primary progressive aphasia: a review of 112 cases. Brain and Language 60: 381–406.

Whitaker H (1976) A case of the isolation of the language function. In: Whitaker H, Whitaker HA (eds) Studies in Neurolinguistics 2. Academic Press, New York.

Will RG, Ironside JW, Zeidler M et al. (1996) A new variant of Creutzfeldt–Jakob disease in the UK. Lancet 347: 921–925.

Wilson RS, Kasniak AW, Klawans HL, Garron DG (1980) High speed memory scanning in parkinsonism. Cortex 16: 67–72.

Witts P, Elders S (1998) The severe impairment battery: assessing cognitive ability in adults with Down's syndrome. British Journal of Clinical Psychology 37: 213–216.

Yesavage JA, Brooks JO 3rd, Taylor J, Tinklenberg J (1993) Development of aphasia, apraxia, and agnosia and decline in Alzheimer's disease. American Journal of Psychiatry 150(5): 742–747.

Zeidler M, Johnstone EC, Bamber RWK (1997) New variant Creutzfeldt Jakob disease: psychiatric features. Lancet 350: 908–910.

Zigman W, Schupf N, Haveman M, Silverman W (1997) The epidemiology of Alzheimer disease in intellectual disability: results and recommendations from an international conference. Journal of Intellectual Disability Research 41: 76–80.

CHAPTER 5

Diagnosing semantic dementia and managing communication difficulties

JULIE SNOWDEN, JACKIE KINDELL AND DAVID NEARY

Introduction and overview of semantic dementia

Semantic dementia is a distinctive and highly disabling disorder, characterized by a progressive loss of understanding of the meaning of words, concepts and knowledge about the world. It results from progressive degeneration of the temporal lobes of the brain. Although often confused with Alzheimer's disease, the two conditions are both clinically and pathologically distinct. Semantic dementia (SD) is a relatively rare disorder compared to other forms of dementia. Nevertheless, its recognition is crucially important. People with semantic dementia have specific needs and require novel approaches to management, reflecting their unique pattern of disability. Understanding the precise nature of deficits in people with dementia, as well as recognizing the domains of function that are preserved, are essential steps towards meeting the needs of people with dementia. This chapter describes the syndrome of semantic dementia in terms of its cognitive, physical and behavioural characteristics, and its pathological substrate. The specific features that point to a diagnosis of semantic dementia and differentiate semantic dementia from other forms of dementia are then highlighted and a guide to management is outlined.

Clinical overview

Semantic dementia is an insidiously progressive and yet selective loss of semantic knowledge (Snowden et al. 1989, 1996, Hodges et al. 1992). A central component of the disorder is loss of word meaning, so the person can no longer name or understand the meaning of words. The semantic impairment is not confined to the verbal domain, but may encompass all sensory modalities. Thus, people with SD may have difficulty recognizing the identity of familiar faces and objects, of non-verbal familiar sounds such as a telephone ringing, of tactile stimuli, tastes and smells. Despite

125

the pervasive nature of the semantic loss, the disorder is circumscribed in the sense that non-semantic aspects of cognitive functioning remain remarkably well preserved. People with SD do not have difficulty in processing the sounds of language and do not make phonological errors in speech. Sentences are grammatically well formed. Moreover, people with dementia have no problems perceiving visual, tactile, gustatory and olfactory stimuli. They are able to distinguish whether two sensory stimuli are alike and therefore perform well on perceptual matching tasks. The problem lies at the level of assigning identity (meaning) to a stimulus that is apparently perceived normally. Thus, people with SD are able to repeat words that they do not understand and can reproduce drawings of objects that they cannot recognize. Spatial skills are well preserved. People with SD are able to find their way without becoming lost and may use spatial cues to compensate for object recognition difficulties (for example, by recalling the spatial location of food items on a supermarket shelf). The day-to-day memory of people with SD also remains relatively well preserved, so they may remember appointments and daily events, such as a visit from a friend, and keep track of time. Their preserved spatial orientation and day-to-day memory are important features that contribute to the differentiation between semantic demenia and Alzheimer's disease. These domains of preserved function undoubtedly contribute to the capacity of people with SD to retain a high degree of functional independence well into the course of disease despite severe semantic loss. An additional contributory factor is the fact that people with SD typically remain physically well and show few neurological signs until late in the disease. When physical signs emerge in advanced disease these are usually limited to mild Parkinsonian features of akinesia and rigidity.

The course of the disease is one of insidious progression, with gradual increase in severity of semantic impairment. The repertoire of vocabulary of people with dementia becomes increasingly restricted, so that eventually only a few stereotyped phrases remain. At no time, however, is speech output effortful or non-fluent. People with SD fail increasingly to recognize the visual environment and may no longer know the function of common objects. Inappropriate behaviours may arise as an integral part of the disease and may occur in part because of semantic recognition failures.

Demographic features

Semantic dementia is a disorder predominantly of late middle age, with onset typically occurring between the ages of 50 and 70. The disorder affects both men and women, apparently with relatively equal frequency, although the relative rarity of the disorder complicates the assessment of relative prevalence. The rate of progression varies. At one extreme there may be a very rapid decline, with death occurring 3 years after onset of symptoms. At the other extreme, some people with SD show a very slow, insidious deterioration and have a total illness duration as long as 15 or 20 years. The average illness duration is about 8 years. Semantic dementia in its pure form is usually sporadic and there is no known family history of a similar disorder. However, in some people with SD with familial forms of frontotemporal lobar degeneration, semantic deficits may represent a prominent characteristic along with prominent behavioural change (Pickering-Brown et al. 2002), indicating a mixed picture of frontotemporal dementia and semantic dementia. In these familial cases mutations have been identified in the tau gene on chromosome 17, indicating the importance of genetic factors in giving rise to the disease. In sporadic cases there may be genetic risk factors, as yet unidentified, that predispose certain individuals towards the development of semantic dementia. Cases of semantic dementia have been reported worldwide. There are no known geographical or socio-economic determinants of disease.

Overview of neuropathology

Anatomy

Semantic dementia is one of a spectrum of clinical disorders that result from focal degeneration of the anterior parts of the brain and fall under the umbrella of 'frontotemporal lobar degeneration' (Snowden et al. 1996, Neary et al. 1998). Other related disorders are frontotemporal dementia and primary progressive non-fluent aphasia. In semantic dementia the atrophy is greatest in the anterior parts of the temporal neocortices. The inferior and middle temporal gyri are particularly affected, whereas the superior temporal gyri, which include the traditional language region of Wernicke's area, are relatively spared. The medial parts of the temporal lobes, including the hippocampi, which are known to be involved in the laying down of new memories, are also relatively spared, accounting for the relative preservation of day-to-day memories of people with SD. In 'pure' cases of semantic dementia the atrophy of the inferior and middle temporal gyri is remarkable for its selectivity. The frontal lobes of the brain may be strikingly spared. However, in some cases there is extension of atrophy into the frontal cortices, particularly the orbital portions. In all cases, the posterior regions of the brain, the parietal and occipital cortices, are relatively preserved.

The temporal lobe atrophy is invariably bilateral, although often asymmetrical. The left- or right-sided emphasis of atrophy determines the precise pattern of symptomatology (Snowden et al. 2004). In people with SD with predominantly left temporal atrophy the semantic impairment is most apparent in the verbal domain, so that they initially present with problems in word comprehension and naming. In people with SD with right-sided predominance there is greater emphasis in the history on problems with recognition of familiar faces and objects. There are reports in the literature of people with dementia with 'progressive prosopagnosia' associated with degeneration of the right anterior temporal lobe (Tyrrell et al. 1990, Evans et al. 1995, Gainotti et al. 2003). These people with dementia are likely to have semantic dementia, presenting with a face recognition disorder. Indeed, follow-up of these people with dementia invariably demonstrates the emergence of a more widespread loss of semantic knowledge.

Histology

Affected areas of the brain have a spongy appearance (microvacuolation) due to loss of large pyramidal nerve cells (Lund and Manchester groups 1994). There is also a reactive astrocytosis typically of mild degree. Ballooned neurones and inclusion bodies, conventionally considered pathological hallmarks of Pick's disease, are typically absent. Moreover, the pathological hallmarks of Alzheimer's disease are also absent.

The pathological changes in semantic dementia are identical to those seen in other forms of frontotemporal lobar degeneration, namely the behavioural disorder of frontotemporal dementia and the language disorder of progressive non-fluent aphasia. The difference between these conditions lies in the anatomical distribution of pathological change within the anterior cerebral hemispheres: predominantly the temporal lobes in semantic dementia, the frontal lobes in frontotemporal dementia and the perisylvian regions of the left hemisphere in progressive aphasia.

Diagnosing semantic dementia

Clinical diagnostic features for semantic dementia have been published (Neary et al. 1998) and are summarized in the box below. Core features are those that are central to the disorder and must be present for the diagnosis to be made. Supportive features are those that add weight to the diagnosis, but are not invariably present. Each feature will be discussed in turn.

Clinical diagnostic features of semantic dementia

I Core diagnostic features

A Insidious onset and gradual progression
B Language disorder characterized by
    (i) progressive, fluent, empty spontaneous speech
    (ii) loss of word meaning, manifested by impaired naming and comprehension
    (iii) semantic paraphasias

and/or

C Perceptual disorder characterized by:

(i)   prosopagnosia: impaired recognition of identity of familiar faces
and/or

(ii) associative agnosia: impaired recognition of object identity

D Preserved perceptual matching and drawing reproduction

E Preserved single-word repetition

F Preserved ability to read aloud and write to dictation orthographical-
ly regular words

II Supportive diagnostic features

A Speech and language

(i)   press of speech

(ii)   idiosyncratic word usage

(iii) absence of phonemic paraphasias

(iv)   surface dyslexia and dysgraphia

(v)   preserved calculation

B Behaviour

(i)   loss of sympathy and empathy

(ii)   narrowed preoccupations

(iii) parsimony

C Physical signs

(i)   absent or late primitive reflexes

(ii)   akinesia, rigidity and tremor

D Neuropsychological testing

(i)   profound semantic loss, manifest in failure of word comprehension and naming and/or face and object recognition

(ii)   preserved phonology and syntax, elementary perceptual processing, spatial skills and day-to-day memorizing

E Electrophysiology
normal

F Brain imaging (structural and/or functional)
predominant anterior temporal abnormality (symmetric or asymmetric)

Source: Neary et al. (1998)

Insidious onset and gradual progression

The disorder emerges insidiously and is gradually progressive. This feature distinguishes semantic dementia from disorders with acute onset
such as stroke. Care is required in history-taking to establish the gradual
evolution of symptoms. Relatives of people with semantic dementia might
occasionally claim an abrupt onset, on the basis that they were made

aware of the existence of a problem by a specific episode or event (e.g. 'We went to a restaurant. There was broccoli on the menu. My wife said "What's broccoli?" even though she's eaten it hundreds of times before. I knew there must be something wrong'). Probing will elicit the fact that there was no sudden illness or weakness associated with the event and that symptoms have gradually increased over time.

Fluent, empty spontaneous speech

Output is fluent and effortless, with normal articulation and prosody. These features may give the superficial impression that language is normal, contrasting with the very profound impairment in naming that becomes evident on formal naming testing. Closer examination of conversational speech will reveal an empty quality to the speech of the person with dementia, reflecting a dearth of nominal terms. People with SD may substitute generic terms for precise substantives and rely on stock words and phrases. The repertoire of conversational topics on which people with SD embark is typically limited to a few themes, invariably pertaining to their own life. The superficial facility that they have with language is diagnostically important. It shows that people with SD are not actively searching for words. They do not pause or hesitate, and they show none of the frustration that accompanies impaired word-finding in many aphasic people with dementia. The reason is that the problem is not merely one of lexical retrieval; words are systematically becoming lost from the vocabulary of the person with SD and therefore are no longer available to be sought. Thus, people with SD speak (fluently and effortlessly) within the confines of the vocabulary that is available to them. Like a young child, whose vocabulary is limited, they may be aware that others use words that they themselves do not understand, yet in their own conversation they do not search for those words as they are not available to be sought.

Loss of word meaning, manifested by impaired naming and comprehension

As noted above, the fluent, effortless speech output of people with SD may mask the underlying problem. As a consequence the semantic impairment is often very considerable by the time they come to medical referral. It is not uncommon for people in whom there is only a hint of a problem in conversational speech to perform virtually at floor level on standard naming tasks, such as the Graded Naming Test (McKenna and Warrington 1983) and Boston Naming Test (Kaplan et al. 1983). This is an important clue to diagnosis. Naming skills are typically dramatically impaired, contrasting with their preserved abilities in other areas of function. This contrasts with the naming deficit in Alzheimer's disease, which is typically commensurate with deficits in other areas of cognitive function.

Responses are produced at a normal rate, whether correct or incorrect, and there are never indications of effortful word search or frustrated attempts at word retrieval (tip-of-the-tongue phenomena). Moreover, there is no benefit from provision of phonemic or semantic cues. This reflects the fact that the problem is not one of accessing vocabulary that is potentially available: there is a central loss of the vocabulary itself. Naming performance is consistent across testing occasions. A failure to name an item on one occasion predicts failure on that same item on future occasions.

A semantic disorder, by definition, affects both naming and word comprehension. Therefore a diagnosis of semantic dementia would need to demonstrate impairment not only in naming but also in single-word comprehension. A characteristic feature of people with semantic dementia, and a powerful clue to the presence of a semantic deficit, is their demonstrable incomprehension of individual words in conversation. For example, a question such as 'Have you ever been to France?' might elicit the response 'What's France?'; an instruction 'Can you pass me the jam' the response 'What's jam?'. Formal testing procedures commonly used to assess word comprehension include word definition and word–picture matching (e.g. PALPA, Kay et al. 1992) and semantic association tasks (e.g. Pyramids and Palm Trees, Howard and Patterson 1992). People with SD typically show a high degree of consistency of performance from one testing session to another; words that are not understood on one occasion will not be understood on another.

It should be emphasized that deficits in comprehension, although present, may appear to be of a lesser magnitude than the problem in naming. The reason is that semantic impairment is not all or none: people with SD may have degraded semantic information that is sufficient to permit accurate performance on many comprehension tests, but insufficient to support naming. Naming tasks require access to the precise term and refined discrimination between concepts. By contrast, word comprehension tests typically involve forced-choice alternatives, so that accurate performance might be achieved on the basis of partial information and by a process of elimination.

In keeping with the fact that information loss may be partial, comprehension test performance is influenced by the particular demands of the task. A person with SD might, for example, successfully match the word 'tiger' with a picture of a tiger, when the alternative pictures are of a tomato and comb, but be unable to match correctly when the alternative pictures are of a giraffe and kangaroo. That is, the word 'tiger' may be recognized as meaning an animal rather than something to eat or an object, but not understood as referring to the particular animal that is striped and dangerous.

At any one time in the course of the disease, the person with SD will know some words and not others. What is retained is influenced by word frequency: commonly used words are better understood than words not in common usage. Knowledge is, moreover, particularly influenced by personal familiarity and use (Snowden et al. 1994, 1995). Thus, people with SD may understand and use entirely appropriately vocabulary relevant to their personal experience, while failing to understand comparable vocabulary that is not personally linked. Word comprehension and naming tests should therefore not be restricted to the common objects that are in daily use but should include names of animals, foods and objects that would, under normal circumstances, be expected to be known, yet do not relate directly to the daily routine of the person with dementia.

Some people with semantic dementia show disproportionate degrees of impairment for certain types or categories of information. In particular, they may be more impaired in their understanding of the names of animals and foods than object names. This is an added reason why assessment of comprehension should go beyond simple clinical bedside tests such as asking the person with dementia to point to objects or body parts, to include assessment of words relating to different categories of information. Tests are available that are explicitly designed to tap differences across semantic categories (McKenna 1998). The basis for category differences is a continuing subject for debate. A prominent view is that biological and non-biological concepts place different weights on sensory and functional properties in their differentiation. Biological concepts are heavily defined by visual/sensory properties: the conceptual differentiation between an apple and banana lies in their shape and colour. Their function (something to eat) is very similar. By contrast, non-biological concepts are defined more by their function. A glass and a vase may be visually very similar, but have quite distinct functions. The parts of the temporal lobes that are preferentially affected in semantic dementia appear to be particularly important for the representation of visual/sensory aspects of knowledge. However, different categories also inevitably vary in terms of personal relevance. Common objects are encountered in the daily life of the person with SD, whereas wild animals are not.

The problem in comprehension for people with SD lies at the level of word meaning. Understanding of syntax is well preserved. Standard tests of comprehension of grammar, such as the revised Token Test (De Renzi and Faglioni 1978) and the Test for the Reception of Grammar (TROG) (Bishop 1989), may be performed surprisingly well, compromised only by a failure to understand individual lexical terms. This pattern differs from that of Alzheimer's disease: people with Alzheimer's disease typically show relatively preserved comprehension at a single-word level but poor comprehension at a sentence level. Thus, the finding of relatively preserved performance on sentence comprehension tasks in the context of impaired performance in single-word comprehension is of considerable diagnostic value in identifying people with semantic dementia.

Semantic paraphasias

A prominent clue to the presence of a semantic disorder is the presence of semantic errors (e.g. 'dog' for 'tiger'; 'sock' for 'glove'). People with SD may use such words overinclusively (e.g. 'dog' to refer to a variety of animals; 'water' to refer to a range of liquids). Semantic errors may be present in spontaneous speech, although typically infrequently in the early stages. They are more likely to be elicited on formal naming tests, particularly picture naming tests covering a range of semantic categories (e.g. animals, fruits and vegetables, articles of clothing) that require precise differentiation between exemplars of a category. Initially errors are typically semantically close to the target, but deviate progressively in semantic proximity over the course of the disease (Hodges et al. 1995).

Perceptual disorder characterized by prosopagnosia and agnosia

People with semantic dementia most commonly present with problems in the verbal domain. However, the semantic disorder is not confined to language. People with dementia develop difficulty, not only in understanding what words mean, but also in recognizing who familiar people are (prosopagnosia) and what objects are for (agnosia). Indeed, in some people with SD, in whom there is greater atrophy of the right than the left temporal lobe, breakdown in these visual aspects of meaning predominates over impairments in word semantics. Thus, diagnostic assessment of people with dementia needs to include examination of face and object recognition.

A set of photographs of famous people who are easily recognized by most adults in the population provides a valuable clinical tool. It is important to determine whether difficulties in identification genuinely reflect a loss of face identity or are simply due to difficulties in name retrieval. This can normally be established by requesting information about why the person is famous or by providing alternative names or occupations, from which the person with dementia is asked to find a 'match' for the face.

Many people with semantic dementia have difficulty recognizing both famous faces and their corresponding name (e.g. a photograph of Margaret Thatcher and the name Margaret Thatcher). However, there can be dissociations (Snowden et al. 2004). People with SD with greater atrophy in the left compared to the right hemisphere tend to be better at recognizing faces than names, whereas people with SD with greater right-sided atrophy show the opposite pattern.

Object recognition is typically a less sensitive measure of semantic impairment than face or word recognition. The reason is that objects and pictures of objects provide clues to meaning in a way that words or faces do not. For example, a jug suggests that it is a form of container, that the contents are poured out and that it is an object to be handled simply by virtue of its physical properties. The word 'jug' provides no such information. A rabbit provides clues to the fact that it is a living creature by the fact that it has legs, eyes and a mouth and that it moves independently. By contrast, there are no intrinsic characteristics of the word 'rabbit' that inform whether the word refers to an animal or, for example, an article of clothing. This feature of objects does not of course mean that understanding of their meaning is necessarily entirely intact. Rather it implies merely that people with dementia may have sufficient information to distinguish and use objects appropriately (e.g. distinguish between an edible and non-edible item) at a time when they have no apparent comprehension of the corresponding word.

Object and/or picture recognition tasks are nevertheless a vital component of the assessment for semantic dementia. The fact that such tasks are so apparently easy means that when recognition failures do occur they are particularly instructive. People with SD who look with perplexity at a toothbrush or razor and deny knowing what those objects are for provide a striking demonstration of semantic memory loss.

Preserved perceptual matching and drawing reproduction

Problems in face and object recognition in semantic dementia occur at a semantic level, in the assignation of meaning. The ability to perceive stimuli is entirely normal. Demonstration that the deficit is indeed occurring at a semantic rather than pre-semantic, perceptual level is typically achieved using perceptual matching tests (i.e. tasks that require the subject to judge whether two perceptually similar stimuli are precisely the same or different) and drawing tasks (i.e. copying line drawings of objects or abstract figures). The ability to copy accurately shows that the person with dementia is able to perceive the stimulus, despite being unable to recognize its identity.

Drawings tasks are valuable in differential diagnosis. In Alzheimer's disease failures of object recognition are most likely to result from problems in perception, which inevitably compromises the ability to copy.

Preserved single-word repetition

Just as visual perception is preserved in semantic dementia, so is auditory perception; people with SD can hear words and reproduce them, even when they do not understand their significance. Inevitably problems in understanding words will have some secondary impact on repetition performance, at least for lengthy utterances (contrast the task of repeating a sentence in one's native language compared to an unfamiliar foreign language). Nevertheless, asking people with dementia to repeat words that they do not understand provides a valuable means of ensuring that a problem in comprehension is not merely a result of hearing loss or phonological processing.

Preserved ability to read aloud and write regular words to dictation

The problem in semantic dementia is in deriving meaning from a spoken or written word. However, the rules for transcoding between phonology and orthography are well preserved. Thus, people with SD can pronounce written words (and non-words) and write words (and non-words) to dictation, albeit without understanding. It should be noted, though, that this accuracy applies only to words with regular pronunciations and spellings (see below, section on surface dyslexia and dysgraphia).

Press of speech

People with semantic dementia always speak effortlessly. Sometimes they are frankly garrulous and it is difficult to interrupt the flow.

Idiosyncratic word usage

Incorrect word substitutions may seem idiosyncratic (e.g. the word 'plate' used to refer to a wide range of objects including books, combs and spoons; the word 'twisting' to refer to all action words, including the action of sitting, running and jumping).

Absence of phonemic paraphasias

The absence of phonemic paraphasias reinforces the evidence that the disorder arises at a semantic and not a phonological level. The reason that this is not cited as a core feature is that some sound-based errors might potentially be elicited, for example on demanding repetition tasks, as a secondary effect of a semantic disorder.

Surface dyslexia and dysgraphia

In English many words do not have regular pronunciations or spellings. They cannot be read or written using conventional conversion rules between phonology and orthography. Models of reading and writing assume that such words depend upon semantic mediation. Thus, the phonological word form elicits meaning, which in turn accesses the appropriate orthographic form. When meaning is impaired then people with SD become reliant on standard phonological–orthographic conversion rules (Patterson et al. 1985, Funnell 1996). The result is that people with SD 'regularize' irregular words. They may pronounce the written word 'pint' in a way that rhymes with 'mint'. They may write 'caught' as 'cort'. The presence of such 'surface dyslexic' and 'surface dysgraphic' errors provides supportive evidence that their disorder arises at a semantic level.

Preserved calculation

A useful diagnostic feature in semantic dementia is the relative preservation of number concepts (Diesfeldt 1993, Cappelletti et al. 2001, Crutch and Warrington 2002). People with SD have no difficulty appreciating the significance of spoken and written numerals and, unlike people with Alzheimer's disease, may tell the time accurately, count money and reckon change. Commonly they enjoy number games such as the television quiz show 'Countdown'. The general procedures for carrying out additions and subtractions are well preserved. Relatives' comments that the person with dementia is 'good with numbers' despite having difficulty with words are a useful pointer to the presence of semantic dementia rather than Alzheimer's disease. Where problems relating to number emerge in semantic dementia, these are typically in terms of identity: people with dementia may no longer recognize the significance of a coin or banknote and may not recognize arithmetical signs. In the late stages, people with SD may no longer recognize the meaning of spoken and written numbers.

Changes in behaviour

The diagnosis of semantic dementia is based principally on the distinctive cognitive disorder. Nevertheless, people with SD also show a characteristic pattern of behavioural change (Snowden et al. 1996, 2001), which can sometimes constitute the major challenge for their management.

Loss of sympathy and empathy

People with SD commonly show changes in their expression of emotions. In particular, they show a reduction in sympathy and empathy towards others. They become more self-centred and are less able to see other points of view. This is likely, in part, to relate to their semantic loss: people with SD no longer retain concepts of the world beyond their own personal experience and therefore are unable to put themselves in another person's shoes. The result is a progressive narrowing of world-view and egocentric behaviour.

Narrowed preoccupations

One manifestation of this narrowing of world view is that people with dementia commonly become preoccupied with a narrow range of activities, which they pursue relentlessly, to the exclusion of all else. Thus a housewife might do jigsaws or word puzzles all day, neglecting domestic responsibilities, or else clean the house constantly. Perhaps the most striking aspect of the narrowed behaviour of people with SD is that it has a compulsive quality. They frequently clockwatch. They may have to do things at precisely the same time each day, and become distressed if their routine is upset. They are highly inflexible to change, and resist disruption to an adopted pattern of behaviour.

Parsimony

A feature that is present in some but not all people with SD is a decrease in generosity and an unwillingness to spend money. The clinical impression is that this feature is more common in people with SD with predominant left-sided temporal lobe atrophy, and that in some people with SD with more right-sided atrophy the reverse behavioural pattern is present.

Physical signs

Semantic dementia occurs in the context of physical well-being. A total absence of neurological signs or signs limited to mild parkinsonian features would be in keeping with the diagnosis.

Neuropsychological testing

A diagnosis of semantic dementia may be suspected by careful history-taking and observation of the person with dementia in a clinical setting. However, as noted above, the fluent speech of people with SD frequently masks the underlying deficit at superficial interview. Formal assessment by a neuropsychologist or speech and language therapist is therefore essential to elicit the phenomena of semantic loss, in the context of preserved phonology and syntax, elementary perceptual processing, spatial skills and day-to-day memorizing.

Standard tests of spatial abilities include the test of Line Orientation (Benton et al. 1978), and the Dot Counting, Position Discrimination, and Cube Estimation sub-tests of the Visual Object and Space Perception battery (VOSP) (Warrington and James 1991). People with semantic dementia typically perform well on these spatial sub-tests of the VOSP, while performing poorly on perceptual sub-tests such as Silhouettes and Object Decision, which require recognition of object identity. This is the opposite pattern to that typically shown by people with Alzheimer's disease.

Although preservation of autobiographical memory in semantic dementia may be striking on clinical grounds, this preserved area of function is less easily captured by standard memory tests. Standard memory tests typically involve lists of words, faces or line drawings that may have little meaning for the person with SD, so that memory performance is inevitably less good than normal. Visually based recognition tests such as

Recognition Memory for faces (Warrington 1984) and picture recognition tasks are useful and can elicit well preserved performance in semantic dementia people when the atrophy is predominantly left-sided. However, performance on these visually based tests may be impaired in sematic dementia with right-sided temporal atrophy. Evaluation of the status of the memory needs of people with SD should include questions regarding personal orientation and autobiographically relevant events, supported by ecological observation of them in their daily lives.

Investigations

Electrophysiology

The routine electroencephalogram in semantic dementia is usually reported as normal. This is a useful diagnostic feature because in most forms of dementia, including Alzheimer's disease, there is slowing of wave forms.

Brain imaging (structural and/or functional)

Structural brain imaging in semantic dementia reveals cerebral atrophy. The presence of atrophy per se does not distinguish semantic dementia from other forms of cerebral degeneration. However, neuroradiological reports that the atrophy is circumscribed and involves particularly one or more temporal lobes would provide strong support for the diagnosis. Sometimes a predominance of atrophy in the temporal lobes is demonstrable on computed tomography (CT) scanning, although CT is not always sufficiently sensitive to reveal clear anatomical differences in the distribution of atrophy between the two cerebral hemispheres and between the different lobes of the brain. Temporal lobe atrophy is more consistently demonstrated on magnetic resonance imaging (MRI), and this may be obviously asymmetric, affecting the left or right temporal lobe preferentially. Functional brain imaging using positron emission tomography (PET) or single-photon emission computed tomography (SPECT) shows abnormal function of the anterior cerebral hemispheres, particularly the temporal regions. Appearances may be bilateral and symmetrical or markedly asymmetric affecting disproportionately the left or right hemisphere.

Managing communication difficulties in semantic dementia

Semantic dementia has some features in common with other language disorders. For example, people with SD are more likely to understand common than uncommon words. Thus, in attempting to communicate with people with SD the use of simple, high-frequency vocabulary is advisable. As for many aphasic people with dementia, the disorder of language affects both spoken and written language, so that the one medium cannot provide a substitute for impairment in the other. There are, however, ways in which people with semantic dementia differ from those with other aphasic syndromes and which have specific implications for management.

Length of utterance

For many aphasic people with dementia, communication is optimal when sentences are short and structurally simple. However, in semantic dementia the problem in language arises at a single-word level. Understanding of grammar is relatively well preserved. That means that the rule 'syntactic simplicity is best' does not necessarily apply. Indeed, for people with semantic dementia comprehension may be poorest when words are presented in isolation and enhanced when presented in the context of a full grammatical sentence. The more contextual support, the better.

Partial knowledge

It is usual to regard the appropriate conversational usage of particular words as a reliable indicator that the person with dementia understands those words. It is worth emphasizing that breakdown of meaning in semantic dementia can be partial. The person with SD may certainly understand the meaning of a word in the very specific sense in which they use that word, but may not have full understanding of that concept (Snowden et al. 1995). Thus, one sematic dementia person understood the word 'licence' to refer to her own driving licence, but had no understanding of the more generic meaning of 'licence' as something that gives leave or permission. For her, the word had a very precise, personal meaning. Her understanding did not generalize to other examples of 'licence'. One should be careful, therefore in making assumptions about the depth of understanding of the person with SD. Even normal word usage does not necessarily mean that a concept is preserved.

Gesture and pantomime

In people with semantic dementia, semantic loss is not confined to words. It can affect understanding of meaning in other sensory modalities, including the ability to understand the meaning of symbolic gestures and mimed actions. It can come as a surprise to a clinician who puts his hand out to shake hands when the person with dementia does not offer a hand in return. It is not a question of antisocial behaviour. Rather, the handshake posture may simply carry no meaning for the person with SD. Similarly, a pointing action, designed to direct a person's attention to a particular visual stimulus, may fail to elicit a change in direction of eye gaze because the pointing action carries no meaning to the person with semantic dementia.

Just as comprehension of gestures can be impaired, so too is their production. Thus, semantic dementia people cannot easily 'act out' actions as a substitute for words, as might be the case in aphasic people with dementia whose naming difficulties reflect impaired lexical retrieval. Not surprisingly, use of non-verbal communication techniques may be less successful in semantic dementia than in other forms of aphasia. That does not mean, however, that gesture and pantomime are of no value.

Loss of meaning in semantic dementia is, however, not all-or-none. The use of gesture, action pantomime and pointing can be important in providing additional contextual information to support the spoken utterance. People with SD who have only partial conceptual understanding of a word may benefit from the addition of these extra non-verbal clues. It is also important not to abandon attempts at gestural communication after an initial failed attempt. Sometimes repeated demonstrations can help. A semantic dementia person who initially does not understand may suddenly grasp what is required. In general, the more sources of information (spoken words, verbal expression, facial expression, gestural demonstration) the better.

Link to personal experience

There is strong evidence that in semantic dementia understanding is particularly poor for abstract concepts. It is significantly better for information relevant to the person with dementia's daily life (Snowden et al. 1994, 1995). Thus, for example, a highly educated semantic dementia person whom we studied knew that the word 'oil' referred to the commodity that was delivered to her home in a large lorry and stored in her outhouse for use in her radiators to keep her warm in winter. She had no knowledge of where oil came from before arriving at her home, and had no understanding of other potential uses of oil. Another person with SD was unable to recognize a drawing of a clockface, yet had no difficulty recognizing her own grandfather clock and could tell the time on it despite its use of roman numerals. We have found that personal belongings are consistently recognized better than alternative examples of the same object. Moreover, objects that the person with SD uses on a daily basis are better recognized in their normal surroundings than in an alternative context.

We have argued that this feature results from the preserved autobiographical memory in people with SD: concepts which are lost in their abstract sense have some meaning to the person with SD if they are framed within the context of their ongoing daily experience. By implication, input from speech and language therapists is more likely to be beneficial if this takes place in the person's own surroundings using their own belongings as referents, than in the abstract setting of a clinical consulting room using standard pictorial materials.

Using key terms

People with semantic dementia may recognize words only within the specific context in which they are normally used. Thus a person with SD might know that 'Auntie Maggie' is the person who visits every Thursday, yet might show no sign of familiarity to that person's alternative appellations, such as 'Auntie Margaret' or 'Maggie'. Use of terms in a consistent way (and in the precise way used by the person with dementia) is therefore essential. Moreover, as noted above, words are understood most poorly in the abstract and best when linked to an event or routine in the life of the person with SD. Thus, a reference to 'Auntie Maggie who comes on Thursdays' is more likely to be understood than 'Auntie Maggie' alone. Similarly a common noun 'chicken' might be understood when qualified as 'chicken that you have for your tea', but met with incomprehension when used in isolation. Thus, both consistency of usage and linkage of words to personally relevant events or routines are prerequisites for optimal comprehension.

Understanding the person with dementia

The foregoing has focused principally on optimizing the understanding of other speakers by the person with SD. However, communication is a two-way process. Idiosyncratic word usage by people with semantic dementia has the potential to create misunderstanding on the part of the listener. A person with SD who says 'Can we go to the bank to buy chocolate?' may actually be referring to the local shop along the road, yet uses the word 'bank' generically to refer to any shop or high-street building. Another person who reports that he will put on his pyjamas to go out might actually be using the word 'pyjamas' to refer to his overcoat. Understanding the way in which terms are used is crucial to avoid misunderstanding.

Re-learning of lost words

It has been argued here that therapeutic intervention is optimal in surroundings familiar to the person with SD. There are additional reasons why this is important. There is clinical evidence in SD that re-learning is possible, including verbal learning. People with SD may, for example, effectively learn the names of new acquaintances and the names of medicines prescribed to them. They may succeed in re-learning some lost vocabulary (Graham et al. 1999, Snowden and Neary 2002). However, this does not necessarily mean that they will be able to generalize to other instances. Learning that their own comb is called a 'comb' depends only on establishing a verbatim link between the object and word. By contrast, knowing that other examples of combs are also called 'comb' depends on recognition of semantic identity. It is worth reinforcing the point here that the semantic disorder affects the ability of people with SD to recognize objects as well as words. The implication is that attempts at re-training should be directed at the specific instances that are relevant to the person with SD in their daily life.

Learning and forgetting

Although people with semantic dementia can learn and re-learn, retention of that knowledge is tenuous and depends on regular use and rehearsal. To illustrate, a semantic dementia person attending our clinic who was in the process of moving home had no difficulty learning the names of the prospective purchasers of her house, retained and used spontaneously those names throughout the period of the house sale, yet 3 months later showed no recognition whatever of those names. Another person who went into respite care for 2 weeks did not recognize, on his return, the boiled egg that his wife gave him each morning for breakfast (he had not eaten boiled eggs during his period of respite). He was able to re-learn what to do with the egg after a demonstration. It is essential for the person with SD to participate directly in activities in order to maintain at least partial understanding. Ensuring that people with SD maintain a range of experience in their daily lives is vital in helping to resist the narrowing of conceptual knowledge in people with dementia.

Understanding and context

Conceptual understanding of words and objects is not all or none and is influenced by context. A person with SD, when living in his own home, might recognize his own razor and use it appropriately to shave each morning, yet when he moves to residential care might show no recognition of the razor and resist all attempts by staff to shave him with it. Changes of environment require careful re-training and re-establishment of routine. Behavioural problems that arise in the context of altered environment can be reduced significantly by putting into place a highly organized and rigid routine.

Explaining concepts that are not understood

People with semantic dementia may spontaneously ask what a particular word means or what an object is for. The challenge is to provide an explanation in terms that the person understands. The problem is well illustrated by a common scenario: people with semantic dementia may spontaneously consult a dictionary to discover the meaning of a word that they do not understand. Typically, they do not understand the dictionary definition, and have to look up the meaning of words provided in the definition. They do not understand those definitions either and the process is one of infinite regression. The best approach is to try to link the unrecognized word or object to something with which the person is known to be familiar that is relevant to them or their daily life, even if this is at the expense of precise accuracy of definition. For example, explanations that a 'sundial' is 'for telling the time, like your clock in the living room' is likely to convey a notion of the sundial's function more successfully than precise explanations in terms of shadows cast by the sun. Sometimes a person with SD will be preoccupied by certain words or concepts and request explanations from multiple people. Consistency of response is vital. Different responses will only add to the confusion.

Taking advantage of preserved domains of function

It has already been indicated that the preserved day-to-day memory of people with SD may provide a source of compensation for their deficits and support their residual semantic knowledge. There are two other aspects of function that people with semantic dementia have to draw upon: time and space. As noted here, their concept of number is relatively well preserved; they may understand days, dates and times while failing to understand word and object concepts. Time provides people with SD with a meaningful reference point. It is likely that this is one reason why they are often time-bound. They may spontaneously clockwatch and have to do certain activities at specific times of the day. It is important for service providers to accommodate and adapt to an established routine and not disrupt it. If the person with SD is expecting a visit at 1 o'clock, then the visit needs to take place at 1 o'clock and not half an hour later. Maintaining routine helps preserve the level of functioning of the person with SD. Disruption of routine creates distress and anxiety and leads to breakdown of function.

Not only does time provide a meaningful reference point for the person with SD, so too does spatial location. People with semantic dementia are able to find their way without becoming lost and may use spatial cues to compensate for object recognition difficulties (for example, by looking for specific foods in a particular location in the supermarket). Moreover, spatial information may provide specific clues to the object's meaning, which are not available from the object alone. A kettle seen out of context might not be recognized, whereas when seen in its usual position in the kitchen presents no difficulty (Snowden et al. 1994). Keeping objects in the same place in the home helps people with SD to recognize those objects' functions. They are often exceptionally tidy and dislike things being out of place. This trait is of practical value: it helps maintain under-standing of the environment.

Educating professionals

Perhaps the greatest obstacle in managing people with semantic demen-tia arises from prior conceptions of the characteristics of dementia. The 'model' that most professionals have arises from their experience of peo-ple with Alzheimer's disease. They may expect people with semantic dementia to forget when they do not, and to understand when they do not. Professionals may be perplexed by the finding that semantic demen-tia people accomplish with ease apparently demanding feats such as finding their way unaccompanied round their neighbourhood, yet fail ostensibly easier tasks such as recognizing a comb. This apparently para-doxical behaviour may make it difficult for service providers to evaluate need because people with SD cannot be measured along conventional dimensions of severity. Speech and language therapists can play a crucial role in this regard because of their understanding of the semantic system and of the repercussions of its breakdown.

Conclusion

Semantic dementia is a striking disorder, clinically distinct from Alzheimer's disease and other forms of dementia. People with SD exhibit unique patterns of cognitive and behavioural symptomatology, which demand novel approaches to treatment and management. The following is a summary of key points relevant for professionals involved in the care of people with semantic dementia:

- Identify words and phrases that the person with SD uses idiosyncrati-cally, and ensure that all relevant people know how they are being used to reduce misunderstanding.
- Link words and people's names to events or routines in the daily life of the person with SD and use this linked information in conversation (e.g. 'Auntie Maggie, who comes on Thursdays') to aid comprehension. Encourage others to use the same links.
- Increase information redundancy by combining speech with gesture and pointing to relevant objects.
- Teach words and use of objects in a naturalistic, familiar setting, not an unfamiliar clinic environment.
- Preserve the daily routine of people with SD. Encourage others to rec-ognize the routine and to adapt to it.
- Educate other professionals and carers in the nature of semantic dementia. People with semantic dementia do not conform to general expectations of dementia, which are typically based on experience of Alzheimer's disease.

Accurate diagnosis of semantic dementia is a prerequisite for appropriate management. Moreover, a clear understanding of the person with semantic dementia's impairment of conceptual knowledge, its clinical manifestations and associated behavioural changes can have a significant impact in optimizing communication and preserving function in daily life for people with semantic dementia.

References

Benton AL, Varney NR, Hamsher K de S (1978) Visuo-spatial judgement: a clinical test. Archives of Neurology 35: 364–367.

Bishop D (1989) Test for the Reception of Grammar. Thomas Leach, Abingdon.

Cappelletti M, Butterworth B, Kopelman MD (2001) Spared numerical abilities in a case of semantic dementia. Neuropsychologia 39: 1224–1239.

Crutch SJ, Warrington EK (2002) Preserved calculation skills in a case of semantic dementia. Cortex 38: 389–399.

De Renzi E, Faglioni P (1978) Normative data and screening power of a shortened version of the token test. Cortex 14: 41–49.

Diesfeldt HFA (1993) Progressive decline of semantic memory with preservation of number processing and calculation. Behavioural Neurology 6: 239–242.

Evans JJ, Heggs AJ, Antoun N, Hodges JR (1995) Progressive prosopagnosia associated with selective right temporal lobe atrophy: a new syndrome? Brain 118: 1–13.

Funnell E (1996) Response biases in oral reading: an account of the co-occurrence of surface dyslexia and semantic dementia. Quarterly Journal of Experimental Psychology 49A: 417–446.

Gainotti G, Barbier A, Marra C (2003) Slowly progressive defect in recognition of familiar people in a patient with right anterior temporal atrophy. Brain 126: 792–803.

Graham KS, Patterson K, Pratt KH, Hodges JR (1999) Relearning and subsequent forgetting of semantic category exemplars in a case of semantic dementia. Neuropsychology 13: 359–380.

Hodges JR, Patterson K, Oxbury S, Funnell E (1992) Semantic dementia. Progressive fluent aphasia with temporal lobe atrophy. Brain 115: 1783–1806.

Hodges JR, Graham N, Patterson K (1995) Charting the progression of semantic dementia: implications for the organization of semantic memory. Memory 3: 463–495.

Howard D, Patterson K (1992) Pyramids and Palm Trees: a test of semantic access from pictures and words. Thames Valley Test Company, Bury St Edmunds.

Kaplan E, Goodglass H, Weintraub S, Segal H (1983) Boston Naming Test. Lea and Febiger, Philadelphia.

Kay J, Lesser R, Coltheart M (1992) Psycholinguistic Assessments of Language Processing in Aphasia (PALPA). Lawrence Erlbaum Associates, Hove.

Lund and Manchester groups (1994) Consensus Statement. Clinical and neuropathological criteria for fronto-temporal dementia. Journal of Neurology, Neurosurgery and Psychiatry 4: 416–418.

McKenna P (1998) The Category Specific Names Test. Lawrence Erlbaum Associates, Hove.

McKenna P, Warrington EK (1983) Graded Naming Test. NFER-Nelson, Windsor.

Neary D, Snowden JS, Gustafson L et al. (1998) Frontotemporal lobar degeneration. A consensus on clinical diagnostic criteria. Neurology 51: 1546–1554.

Patterson KE, Marshall JC, Coltheart M (1985) Surface Dyslexia: neuropsychological and cognitive studies of phonological reading. Lawrence Erlbaum Associates, Hove.

Pickering–Brown SM, Richardson AM, Snowden JS et al. (2002) Inherited frontotemporal dementia in 9 British families associated with intronic mutations in the tau gene. Brain 125: 732–751.

Snowden JS, Neary D (2002) Relearning of verbal labels in semantic dementia. Neuropsychologia 40: 1715–1728.

Snowden JS, Goulding PJ, Neary D (1989) Semantic dementia: a form of circumscribed atrophy. Behavioural Neurology 2: 167–182.

Snowden JS, Griffiths H, Neary D (1994) Semantic dementia: autobiographical contribution to preservation of meaning. Cognitive Neuropsychology 11: 265–288.

Snowden JS, Griffiths HL, Neary D (1995) Autobiographical experience and word meaning. Memory 3: 225–246.

Snowden JS, Neary D, Mann DMA (1996) Frontotemporal Lobar Degeneration: frontotemporal dementia, progressive aphasia, semantic dementia. Churchill-Livingstone, London.

Snowden JS, Bathgate B, Varma A et al. (2001) Distinct behavioural profiles in frontotemporal dementia and semantic dementia. Journal of Neurology, Neurosurgery and Psychiatry 70: 323–332.

Snowden JS, Thompson JC, Neary D (2004) Knowledge of famous faces and names in semantic dementia. Brain 127: 860–872.

Tyrrell PJ, Warrington EK, Frackowiak RSJ, Rossor MN (1990) Progressive degeneration of the right temporal lobe studied with positron emission tomography. Journal of Neurology, Neurosurgery and Psychiatry 53: 1046–1050.

Warrington EK (1984) Recognition memory test. NFER-Nelson, Windsor.

Warrington EK, James M (1991) The Visual Object and Space Perception Battery. Thames Valley Test Company, Bury St Edmunds.

CHAPTER 6

Assessment of language and communication difficulties in the dementias

SUSAN STEVENS

Assessment is the starting point for all decisions about diagnosis, therapy and management, and therefore needs to be as rigorous as the circumstances will allow. In the field of mental health, the patient, the pathology and the circumstances in which the assessment is carried out may all contribute to the challenge. Indeed, even recently, patients were sometimes said to be 'unable to be assessed', because of either the severity of the communication problem or their challenging behaviour. These challenges in assessment have been compounded by the lack of appropriate validated and targeted test measures.

Given the gold standard of multidisciplinary work, all members of a mental health team should be able to contribute to the assessment process, some via formal assessment and others by informal assessment and observation of behaviour. All members will be aware of the difficulties of carrying out assessment, as well as interpreting observations and responses.

Such life-changing diagnostic labels as 'dementia' should be applied with great care. Although some drug treatments for dementia are now available, their main aim is to slow the process of deterioration and mitigate cognitive impairment: only rarely can the process be reversed and cure achieved. It is crucial, however, that such potentially curable conditions as depression are fully considered before a diagnostic decision is reached. Conversely, because there are treatments available which slow the progress of some types of dementia and which may mitigate symptoms, it is important that accurate diagnostic decisions facilitate prescribing.

Because assessment remains an imprecise science, with a significant number of false positive and negative diagnoses (a diagnosis of a dementia may be made where there is none = false positive, or no diagnosis may be made when a dementia is present = false negative), reassessment after an appropriate length of time is always advisable. O'Neill et al. (1992) concluded that a stable diagnosis could be achieved in patients attending a memory clinic (i.e. with early pathology) after four assessments over a 2-year period. Such an extended assessment period allows for the elimination of such variables as other medical conditions, fatigue, stress and the establishment of any pattern of change over time.

This chapter aims to highlight what assessments of cognition, language and communication are available, primarily to speech and language therapists but also to others, what diagnostic pointers may be evident, and how some of the assessment information may be interpreted. Although the main focus is on assessing language and communication in the dementias, consideration is also given to other mental health problems.

The assessment process

Although most readers will be practised in the science and skill of assessment, it may be helpful to reconsider the following components of the assessment process in relation to work in the mental health field:

- obtaining case history information (biographical, medical and social)
- observation, especially in communicative situations
- physical examination
- informal assessment
- formal assessment
- interpretation of results against known norms after collating team members' reports
- considering all likely diagnostic possibilities against research findings
- formulation of possible/probable diagnosis hypothesis
- audited implementation of management
- reassessment over time.

Some of these stages have inherent problems; for example, there may be difficulties in obtaining case history information from a distressed older person, living alone, unknown to neighbours and social services, and with no obvious family. Information obtained may need verification from other sources such as the GP or past medical records. Even an unexpected visitor, friend or family can be of value in this context. Observation of an individual on a ward or in a day centre, for example, can often provide useful pointers to functional communication ability.

Although there are assessments targeted at all levels of dementia severity, and formal assessment of people with moderate to severe problems may be limited, the current availability of appropriately targeted and structured assessment tools means that the information and results obtained are of use, especially in planning management. Because research about all types of dementia is continually being published, comparison with such recent findings is advisable in order to achieve the most accurate diagnosis possible.

Consideration should also be given to the influence of other health problems and the presence of any possible infection, dehydration or malnutrition, all known to heighten risk of acute confusion. Re-evaluation of initial findings are crucial to best practice and are part of the audited process of service provision. More detailed consideration of the assessment process is to be found in Eastley and Wilcock (2000).

Reasons for assessment

The reasons for assessment will drive the process in terms of format and extent. The most likely reasons are:

- to establish a diagnosis
- to provide the basis for informed management
- to identify deficits and retained skills
- to facilitate legal processes, e.g. Power of Attorney, ability to drive, ability to give consent
- to establish suitability for a particular type of residential/day care, or participate in a rehabilitation or management programme
- to establish suitability for a research project.

The role of the speech and language therapist in team assessment

In mental health practice, doctors, nurses, psychologists, occupational and speech and language therapists (SLTs) all have an interest in, and the skills to assess, cognitive functions, of which language and communication are a crucial part. Indeed the great majority of cognitive assessments are language based, which means that any individual with a communication deficit (be it language breakdown, a speech problem, a hearing loss or not having English as a first language) may be disadvantaged. There is therefore some advantage in having a SLT involved in the process, as she is likely to identify which deficits may be due to any communication problem and which deficits to a more general cognitive breakdown. It is important that assessments, in whole or part, are not repeated unnecessarily as this is a waste of limited staff time and is likely to cause distress and annoyance to patients. The team should agree:

- who will carry out general cognitive measures
- at what point in the assessment process such measures are used
- why each assessment will be done
- what form assessments should take
- what scoring parameters should be used.

The criteria for success and scoring parameters on any test item should be agreed by the team. For example, if a patient only remembers part of an address, is the scoring changed to reflect the partial recall? The commonly used Mini-Mental State Examination (Folstein et al. 1975) can be carried out by any member of the team but it exists in a number of versions: for example, in the Attention section, do you get individuals to spell *world* backwards or count backwards in 7s from 100? Someone who does not have English as their first language or has poor literacy skills may find the second task easier than the first and could therefore be penalized by a version which uses spelling. Inter-rater agreement and reliability, therefore, need to be established in clinical work, as well as in research. Although some assessments require the tester to be registered with a company or organization before they can be used (notably those used by psychologists such as the Wechsler Adult Intelligence Scale), the most commonly used communication assessments are available to all. Some difficulties may arise in the interpretation of responses if, for example, knowledge of semantic, syntactic and phonological processing and breakdown is limited. A sub-test of the Barnes Language Assessment (Bryan et al. 2001) requires analysis of confrontation naming errors by the test administrator, a task at which SLTs are well practised, but others may find challenging.

Language and communication performance is, therefore, probably best assessed by SLTs. If perceptual/spatial skills are the focus of assessment, an occupational therapist has valuable knowledge and experience, while an old age psychiatrist will have extensive knowledge of mental health problems and the interpretation of depression scores, and a nurse will have a knowledgeable overview of general health problems. But in the absence of any one team member, another is likely to have the skills and experience to administer an assessment and the team should work together to ensure that such a skill mix is possible. The more stable a team is over time and the more robust their protocols, the greater is the likelihood of transferable skills and knowledge being shared. In such a team, the administration of assessments may be more flexible.

Places of assessment

As mental health services cover a wide spectrum of site provision, assessments may be carried out in:

- acute units
- day centres/hospitals
- residential/nursing homes
- peoples' own homes
- specialist clinics, e.g. memory clinics.

Wherever assessment is carried out, some considerations are constant and there should be:

- a quiet environment, with no or few distractions

- good lighting, natural or artificial
- comfortable and practical facilities, e.g. tables and chairs
- appropriate timing of assessments, preferably earlier in the day
- access to functioning hearing aid and glasses
- a minimum of interruptions.

While the patient may be more relaxed in their own home, and there is a greater chance of the assessor picking up helpful clues about the case history and background information, distractions may be less easily controlled, and the therapist may find not everything required is to hand. A disorientated individual is likely to achieve better results when tested in a familiar, rather than a strange, environment. However, improved performance on retest could be because the individual has become familiar with the environment and the assessor, rather than because the condition has actually improved. The converse might also be true, with apparent deterioration being due to a change in place or personnel for assessment. It is therefore advisable to avoid formal testing or retesting too soon after a change in the patient's circumstances, such as a move from their own home to residential care.

Other cognitive, perceptual and social issues

A number of other considerations are pertinent to the cognitive assessment process, some of them especially relevant to older people such as:

- sight and hearing problems
- other medical conditions
- dental status
- fatigue and pain
- alcohol and drug considerations
- psychiatric history, past and present behaviour
- language status (English not being the first language)
- educational and social status
- social situation.

If flexibility is possible, it may be better to assess an older individual in the morning or early afternoon in order to maximize performance and reduce the effect of fatigue. Individuals may have good and bad days and, for those with probable vascular dementia or Lewy body disease, the daily swings may be more marked (see Chapter 2, p. 41).

One issue which is becoming more common as the immigrant populations age in the UK is the interpretation of results in people whose first language is not English; especially if, as is often the case, the assessor has little knowledge of the other language (Obler et al. 1991). It is helpful to use an interpreter or bilingual co-worker, but this may cause difficulties in relation to test validity and the accuracy of response interpretation.

Assessing the dementias

It is thought that there are about 70 different types of pathology which can cause dementia or chronic cognitive impairment. Because patients may present at any stage during the disease process, the approach to assessment is, of necessity, variable. This section of the chapter will be divided into two parts which reflect the different rationales and assessment procedures required in the assessment of mild to moderate dementia and of moderate to severe dementia. Such a division does not mean, however, that there is no overlap between the two:

• What may be considered severe in the context of a memory clinic, designed to facilitate diagnosis of early pathology, is moderate in a residential home setting.
• The length of time since observed onset does not dictate where, on the disease spectrum, any patient may fall.
• Symptoms may only have been identified at a time of crisis, such as the death of a spouse, when in reality they may have been present for some time before that event.
• Different disease processes progress at different rates.

Table 6.1 presents a template of communication performance relative to the Dementia Global Deterioration Scale, adapted from Reisberg et al. (1982), to provide some framework for the assessment of language deterioration.

Table 6.1 Global Deterioration Scale

Clinical phase (modified GDS)	Clinical characteristics	Language
Normal (1)	No evidence memory deficit	Normal
Forgetful (2)	Subjective memory complaints No objective evidence	Normal
Early confusional (3)	Some deficits: – lost way, lost object of value – concentration	Naming problems
Mild-late confusional (4)	Less knowledge recent events Personal history confusion Financial/travel management problems Difficulty with complex tasks Depression/denial/situation avoidance	Syntax intact Comprehends but forgets Less sensitive to context Word-finding problems Follows 2/3-stage commands

Table 6.1 continued

Clinical phase (modified fast/GDS)	Clinical characteristics	Language
Moderate early dementia (5)	Some assistance needed Disorientated time/place Limited current life knowledge Self-knowledge maintained Wandering	Syntax intact Naming problems Vocabulary reduced Less output/cohesion Tangential/less gesture Problems with related ideas Poor 3-stage commands Multiple choice: Yes/no questions easier Good oral reading Written comprehension impaired
Middle dementia (6)	Unaware of most events Needs ADL assistance Personality/emotional changes Anxiety Forgets family names Urinary incontinence	Syntax simplified Vocabulary reduced Empty speech Little cohesion Concrete Still read/write words 1/2-stage commands Adds to conversation Matches pictures/objects
Severe dementia (7)	Disorientated time/place/person Reduced intellectual function Memory systems all limited Doubly incontinent	Syntax deviant Nonsensical output Might give name/read some words Limited comprehension Some social speech Repetitive utterances
Very severe dementia (8)	Global deterioration Not walking/bedridden	Almost no language Occasional social speech Agitation on communication

Assessing mild to moderate dementia

The main aim of assessing the language and communication function of individuals presenting with mild, or mild to moderate, cognitive problems (often in the context of a memory clinic or combining clinical and research services) is to contribute to a differential diagnosis, with the following options being considered:

- normal/abnormal ageing
- different types of dementia (see Chapter 2)

- a dementia/dysphasia
- a dementia/depression
- a dementia/confusion
- a dementia/delirium.

Although the 'worried well' are sometimes able to refer themselves, many individuals with a possible dementia pathology do not gain access to appropriate services. The working hypothesis, often formed by the team after acquiring initial case history and observation information, will inform the choice of assessment tools. The aim should be to acquire maximum pertinent information in the most time-efficient and patient-friendly manner. The accuracy of the initial diagnosis has become more crucial in recent years, with the advent of drugs, such as Aricept and rivastigmine for use in mild to moderate dementia of Alzheimer's disease, and more recently, memantine for use in moderate to severe Alzheimer's disease. Therefore the greater the accuracy of the diagnosis, the better the chance of appropriate prescribing and optimum benefit to the patient. As will be shown in this chapter, assessment of language and communication can be more sensitive in the early stages of pathology than many of the general cognitive measures in widespread usage (Stevens et al. 1992).

Until the late 1980s there were few standardized language assessments available which gave values for the normal older population, so the differential diagnosis between normal and abnormal ageing was an informed guess, rather than a decision based on evidence. It is, for example, easy to be misled by an individual performing poorly on tasks with a visuo-spatial component such as Unusual Angle Photograph Naming (photographs of objects taken from unusual angles), but adequately in other areas of cognition. If that individual had earned their living as an architect (a profession in which sophisticated use of such skills would be required) it could well be a symptom of significant cognitive decline; if, however, he had been a journalist, it is possible that such tasks were never easy and that any decline is non-existent or, at most, not significant. Now that there are standardized assessments for which normed ageing values are available, diagnosis is more informed.

General cognitive measures

Although there is assessment material available which charts some of the changes in language performance occurring with age, material addressing the effect of age on general cognition is limited. Piguet et al. (2002) argue that age itself does not affect executive function significantly, but that when combined with pathology, the effect is measurable. The most commonly used and available general cognitive assessments are listed in Table 6.2.

The Mini-Mental State Examination (MMSE), in common with the majority of such assessments, is based on language, and therefore the performance of anyone with a deficit such as dysphasia (difficulty with

Table 6.2 General cognitive measures

Assessment	Author(s)	Time taken (min)	Brief description
Mini-Mental State Examination (MMSE)	Folstein et al. (1975)	5–10	30-point scale covering STM, orientation, registration, recall, language, spatial perception
Mental Test Score (MTS)	Hodkinson (1973)	5	10 questions covering STM, orientation, self-knowledge, general information
CAMCOG	Roth et al. (1986)	40	All areas of cognition
Rivermead Behavioural Memory Test (RBMT)	Wilson et al. (1991)	15	Tests functional memory with everyday objects
Middlesex Elderly Assessment Mental State (MEAMS)	Golding (1989)	30	All areas of cognition, designed for older people
Ruchill Memory and Information Test	Caird and Judge (1974)		Tests memory, recall, orientation, calcul-ation, self-knowledge
Clifton Assessment Procedures for the Elderly (CAPE)	Pattie and Gillard (1979)	15–20	Short cognitive scale, behavioural rating scale gives independence rating
Kendrick Cognitive Tests for the Elderly	Kendrick (1985)	15–20	Object learning, digit copying
Raven's Coloured Progressive Matrices (RCPM)	Raven (1965)	15	Non-verbal test using shape/design matching

understanding and using language) may be compromised. Conversely, although language is used as the medium through which cognitive assessment is undertaken, the ability of these tools to assess language is limited, with, for example, the MMSE requiring only the naming of two extremely common objects (a pen and a watch). Age-related deficits such as hearing loss and factors such as limited educational status and not having English as a first language may lead to poor scores and therefore a misdiagnosis. The CAMCOG (Roth et al. 1986), which includes the MMSE, has been translated into Spanish, Dutch, Italian and German, but even in translation, bias may exist. The diagnosis of cognitive problems needs to be judiciously made, especially when the compounding variables such as age-related deficits and cultural issues are present.

Most of the general cognitive measures listed in Table 6.2 cover similar areas of function, namely orientation, registration, recall, attention, calculation, praxis, visuo-spatial skills and language. The relative importance of any one area of function within any test may vary, as may the type, size and format of presentation. Work reported by the Hammersmith Hospital Memory Clinic (Stevens et al. 1992) found that a considerable number of well-educated individuals who were concerned by their declining memory abilities did not fall below the cut-off point delineating diagnosis on such measures as CAMCOG and MMSE, but language and computerized assessments were more sensitive to their declining function.

Language assessments

The most common types of dementia likely to be seen for communication assessment are: Alzheimer's disease, vascular dementia, Lewy body dementia, semantic dementia/progressive aphasia and other presentations of frontotemporal dementia, all of which, apart from Lewy body dementia, are likely to present with significant communication deficits. Possibly the most commonly used communication assessment in the English-speaking world, used either in whole or in part, is the Arizona Battery for Communication Disorders in Dementia (ABCD) (Bayles and Tomoeda 1993). This test battery has 14 sub-tests which cover the constructs of linguistic comprehension and expression, mental status, episodic memory and visuo-spatial construction. The test has been standardized on normal elderly, mild dementia of Alzheimer type, moderate dementia of Alzheimer type, normal Parkinson's disease and Parkinson's disease with dementia. The disadvantage of the test is that it takes about 90 minutes to complete, a length of time not always available to the assessor and potentially tiring for the person being tested. If the test is not completed, information about the comparative breakdown of the targeted constructs may not provide an accurate profile for diagnosis, although the norms available for each sub-test still provide useful diagnostic comparators. The ABCD is the only available test to provide information about language performance in Parkinson's disease, both with and without dementia, a topic that will be revisited later in the chapter. The ABCD standardization information indicates which sub-tests are most sensitive to early change, notably Delayed Story Recall and Word Learning. The Hammersmith Hospital Memory Clinic team, brought together in 1986, was the first in the UK to include a SLT, and, as the ABCD was not available in its complete form at that time, the SLT compiled an eclectic battery designed to detect changes in semantic language function in early pathology. The battery is shown in full in Table 6.3.

Table 6.3 Hammersmith Hospital Memory Clinic Battery

Auditory Comprehension	10 active/passive and 10 comparative questions
Word Learning	Recognition and recall of 48 presented words (Arizona Battery for Communication Disorders in Dementia: Bayles and Tomoeda 1993)
Word Fluency	Semantic (animals and towns) and phonemic ('s'), production of as many words as possible in a minute
Written Picture Description	Written description of a composite picture in 2 minutes (Whurr 1996/Reich 1982)
Dictation Homophone Pairs	Dictation of 10 pairs of homophones, e.g. nose/knows, presented with a semantic link
Paragraph Reading Comprehension	5 short paragraphs each followed by 2 factual and 2 inferential questions: timed (Aphasia Reading Battery: La Pointe and Horner 1998)
What's Wrong?	10 pictures with visual errors with error described. Scored for recognition and explanation
Story Retelling	Short story is read to the patient who has to retell it immediately and after a delay (ABCD: Bayles and Tomoeda 1993)
Sentence Disambiguation	5 ambiguous sentences presented as a picture matching task, and 5 presented orally for explanation
Unusual Angle Photograph Naming	10 black and white unusual angle photos for naming
Boston Naming Test	60 black and white drawings ranging from frequent to infrequent (Kaplan et al. 1983)

Tests are listed in the order in which they were presented.

Because of their diagnostic potential, the Story Retelling and Word Learning sub-tests from the prototype version of the ABCD were used together with other sub-tests drawn from research studies, and a scoring system based on Reich's (1982) abstraction ability hypothesis. When the clinic was established, normal scoring and standard deviation values were available for the Boston Naming Test (Kaplan et al. 1983) and Word Fluency tasks, facilitating the normal/abnormal ageing distinction. The scoring systems for some of the other sub-tests had a qualitative as well as quantitative dimension to them (e.g. What's Wrong?, Unusual Angle Photograph Naming and the Boston Naming Test), which had the potential to aid diagnostic decisions between different types of dementia.

In this battery several tests, such as Written Picture Description, Boston Naming Test and What's Wrong?, have a visuo-spatial component. Therefore groupings of perceptual errors (for example, interpreting an open suitcase lid as a mirror in the Written Picture Description) can be indicative of possible site of lesion. These errors may link to case history information, obtained from the patient or their family or friends, of misusing objects and getting lost. This battery takes about an hour to administer, but, as the totality is not validated, sub-tests can be readily used and will provide valuable information. Although it has not been published, many of the components will be available to therapists. Further information and commentary can be found in Stevens et al. (1996).

One of the most readily accessible items is the Boston Naming Test (Kaplan et al. 1983), originally designed for use with people who may have a focal aphasia, but in recent years often used in research projects and clinical practice with people who have a dementia of varying ages and cultures (Margolin et al. 1990, Nicholas et al. 1996). There is now a considerable amount of published work on the effect of gender, age, educational and cultural background on performance on the Boston Naming Test (BNT). In 1986 Van Gorp et al. published norms and standard deviations showing that the mean score between 59 and 80 years drops by just over 5 points. It is also of note that the standard deviation for the over-80-year-old subjects was 7, much greater than the 3 for the youngest group, denoting greater variability in the performance of older people. More recently Worrall et al. (1995) published normative data for an Australian population, while Fillenbaum et al. (1997) compared the performance of elderly white and African American community dwellers, finding that even when gender, education, age and word frequency factors were controlled the African American group performed significantly worse. These researchers used one of the shortened versions of the BNT now available. This type of background information provides an improved basis upon which to make judgements about normal/abnormal ageing, while highlighting the complexity of the situation.

Although not so widely used in published work, the Armstrong Naming Test (Armstrong 1997) is validated on a British population and aims to differentiate the normal elderly from those with mild aphasia and those with Alzheimer's disease. Like the BNT, it provides baseline measures of word-finding and cueing responsiveness, together with error type analysis. While the BNT takes account of frequency, Armstrong's test considers stimulus name length. It can therefore be of value in the dementia/dysphasia diagnostic paradigm as well as the normal/abnormal ageing question. Table 6.4 gives comparative information on naming tests.

The Graded Naming Test (McKenna and Warrington 1983), although shorter than the BNT, is of value with highly literate individuals, when there may be a ceiling effect on other tests. A number of stimulus items are extremely uncommon – e.g. periscope, tutu – therefore biasing results to an unacceptable degree against those with limited, or even average,

Table 6.4 Confrontation naming tests

Test name	Time (min)	Comments
Boston Naming Test (Kaplan et al. 1983)	10–15	60 black/white pictures of varied frequency. American bias but cultural adaptions/shortened versions developed. Norms for 50+ years. Can give semantic/phonemic cues
Armstrong Naming Test (Armstrong 1997)	10–15	British. 50 items. Developed for differential diagnosis DAT, aphasia and normal elderly. Cueing, error analysis. Stimulus length controlled
Graded Naming Test (McKenna and Warrington 1983)	15	30 items, many very uncommon. Suitable for highly literate people with mild problems

vocabularies. In the USA lexical comprehension (naming) is sometimes assessed using the Peabody Picture Vocabulary Test (Dunn and Dunn 1981) but this is not common clinical practice in the UK, although a form of this test (the English Picture Vocabulary Test, EPVT) is used in research.

While confrontation naming can be affected early in the disease process, it has been suggested that generative naming, a task of executive function, is impaired at an even earlier point. Word fluency tests can be carried out quickly and with little equipment, thereby in some respects being less stressful to the person being tested. In addition, they can be easily used with those with sight and/or hearing problems, the former being especially disadvantaged by the confrontation naming tasks listed above. The most common version of the test is when the individual is given a minute in which to produce as many words as possible in a certain category (semantic fluency), or beginning with a certain letter (phonemic fluency). Such a semantic fluency test (using the category of animals) is included in one general cognitive assessment; the CAMCOG (Roth et al. 1986). If the CAMCOG is administered by a different member of the team, it may be more useful for the SLT to carry out a different fluency test, using 'towns' for example, found to be more sensitive to mild pathology in some studies (Hart et al. 1988, Stevens et al. 1996). Stevens et al. (1996) hypothesized that this may be due to the early acquisition of animal names in the vocabulary and their high frequency, unlike the names of towns, which are likely to be acquired later in life.

Several authors have highlighted evidence of semantic language breakdown using semantic word fluency tasks (Hart et al. 1988, Bschor et al. 2001) and its role in differential diagnosis (Basso et al. 1988, Phillips et al. 1996). Although it is semantic fluency tasks which are most likely to highlight deficits in early dementia (Salmon et al. 2002), it is worth doing a phonemic word fluency task as a comparator. Indeed, phonemic (letter) fluency has been found to be comparatively impaired in a group of subjects with progressive non-fluent aphasia, compared to a group with early Alzheimer's disease (Mendez et al. 2003).

The problem with certain assessments is their length, with limited professional time available and older people likely to tire more easily, especially later in the day. A screening test is therefore advantageous, for while it is structured and may be validated, all pertinent areas are covered in a rational and ordered way. It may cause less distress to the patient and is practical for the assessor. Helm-Estabrooks (2001) developed the Cognitive Linguistic Quick Test which enables the assessor to determine a severity rating for attention, memory, executive functions, language and visuo-spatial skills as well as a composite severity rating, and takes less than 30 minutes to administer. The Alzheimer's Quick Test (Wiig et al. 2002) is designed to detect early dementia by assessing parietal lobe function, so it may be a useful adjunct to other tests that focus on language. Tests in common use are shown in Table 6.5.

The Barnes Language Assessment (BLA) (Bryan et al. 2001) is a British-based screening test, which is in the process of being validated on a normal elderly population. The BLA covers most areas already mentioned, together

Table 6.5 Mild–moderate dementia: possible tests

Assessment	Time (min)	Areas covered	Comments
Arizona Battery for Communication Disorders in Dementia (ABCD) (Bayles and Tomoeda 1993)	60	Comprehension, expression, mental status, episodic memory, visuo-spatial/construction	Standardized, norms for elderly, DAT, PD. Long, but sub-tests /constructs stand alone
Hammersmith Hospital Memory Clinic Battery (Stevens et al. 1996)	45	Semantic expressive tasks, episodic memory, visuo-spatial skills	Certain sub-tests available and standardized
Peabody Picture Vocabulary Test (Dunn and Dunn 1981)	15–20	Lexical comprehension	Designed for children. Used in USA in dementia
Cognitive Linguistic Quick Test (CLQT) (Helm-Estabrooks 2001)	30	Attention, memory, executive functions, language, visuo-spatial skills	American. 50% tasks make minimal language demands. Severity rating
Alzheimer's Quick Test (AQT) (Wiig et al. 2002)	10–15	Parietal lobe function	Designed to support early diagnosis with imaging/other tests

Table 6.5 continued

Assessment	Time (min)	Areas covered	Comments
Barnes Language Assessment (BLA) (Bryan et al. 2001)	45	Comprehension, expression, memory, visuo-spatial skill, executive functions	British screening test, available on disc
Repeatable Battery for the Assessment of Neuropsychological Status (RBANS) (Randolph 1998)	30	Attention, immediate/delayed memory, visuo-spatial, construction, language	Adapted for UK use. Can be core test, or screening battery

with assessments of working memory by testing forward digit span and story retelling. Both these tasks are acknowledged to detect early cognitive change (Bschor et al. 2001, Salmon et al. 2002). Results from this screening test produce a clear pattern of performance which can be compared against that of normals, and gives pointers as to which areas may be usefully further investigated. It is therefore helpful in informing the differential diagnosis between people with normal and abnormal function, providing comparative patterns of performance for different pathologies such as vascular dementia, semantic dementia and probable Alzheimer's disease.

Some research has considered the potential of computerized assessments. One such in use in a number of clinics and services in the UK is the Cognitive Drug Research Programme (CDR) (Simpson et al. 1991); others include the Cambridge Neuropsychological Test Automated Battery (CANTAB) (Robbins and Sahakian 1994) and the Memory Assessment Clinic System (MAC) (Crook et al. 1986). These assessments cover some areas of language function, but not in such depth as the language assessments mentioned above. Experience at the Hammersmith Hospital Memory Clinic suggests that computerized assessment was no problem to older people, and as computers become more widely used in all spheres of life any deleterious effect is likely to diminish. Computerized testing does have the advantage of being able to time performance precisely, and as slower response times might be a possible indicator of early pathological change as well as a potential diagnostic indicator for depression, it may well provide a more complete picture.

Some shorter tests available for those with a mild to moderate dementia focus on specific areas of language function. One, which aims to assess pragmatic function, is the Discourse Abilities Profile (DAP) (Ripich 1991). The DAP is quick and easy to use, taking the form of a structured conversation; it requires no equipment, and has the advantage of seeming relevant to the person being tested. Terrell and Ripich (1989) and Ulatowska et al. (1998) have both emphasized the value of analysing

discourse in early pathology because of its relevance to functional conversation. The latter group concentrated particularly on the potential of
this type of assessment for differential diagnosis between a dementia and
dysphasia. The Right Hemisphere Battery (Bryan 1995) also contains a
discourse sub-test, with discourse being defined as a two-way interaction
or conversation. It looks at parameters such as supportive and assertive
routines, questions, narrative, variety, formality and turn taking all pertinent to pragmatic change in dementia pathology.

Assessment information, whether acquired early or late in the disease
process, is only as good as the interpretations which are made from it, as
the following two case histories illustrate.

Case history 1

Mrs P is a 64-year-old retired schoolteacher, living with her husband,
with no significant sensory deficits, medical, psychiatric or family history. She was referred to a memory clinic with a 2-year history of memory
loss. At the time of referral Mrs P was able to live independently, even
when her husband went away. She could follow complex knitting patterns and manage Scottish dancing competently.

1st assessment
MMSE   22 (cut off for normal = 24)
CAMCOG   60 (cut off for normal = 79)
No evidence of depression, with a test performance severely limited
because of communication problems.
Putative diagnosis by psychogeriatrician: PRESENILE DEMENTIA

Language assessment
Comprehension Comparative Questions: Score (10) 6
Repetition needed despite good hearing. Evident loss of semantic concept for certain, often common, words, e.g. banana, feather. Simpler
sentences were no better understood than complex ones as a result.

Story Retelling: Immediate (25) 7, Delayed (25) 7
Although registration was limited, information that was registered was
retained, a pattern not typical of probable Alzheimer's disease.

Homophone Pair Dictation: Score (10) 0
A surprisingly low score, given her previous educational ability and her
relatively competent social function.

Paragraph Reading:
Task could not be completed because of marked deficits, rather than
anxiety.

Written Picture Description: Score: Whurr (5) 4, Reich (A) C
Limited evidence of ability to draw inferences, but as syntax and
phonology were intact relatively high scoring on the Whurr scale. No evidence of visual misinterpretation.

What's Wrong?:   Recognition (10) 9, Explanation (10) 1
Although there was no significant deficit in visuo-perceptual skill, marked semantic deficits were evident in her explanations.

Word Fluency: Animals 7, Towns 3, Letter 's' 1
Frontal lobe deficits evident affecting both types of fluency task. Given her educational and occupational background, performance must be considered severely impaired.

Boston Naming Test: Score (60) 6
Extreme difficulty demonstrated, with only the most common names being correctly produced, a deficit out of proportion to her age and background and relatively fluent conversation.

Unusual Angle Photograph Naming: Score (10) 0
Errors were apparently due to access problems, rather than difficulties with recognition, a pattern that fits with BNT and What's Wrong? performance.

Conclusion
Language assessment identified the following areas of skill and deficit:

* severe anomia
* reduced vocabulary
* impairment of single-word comprehension
* relatively preserved comprehension of more complex syntactic structures
* preserved phonology/syntax
* preserved autobiographical/day-to-day memory.

All these are characteristic of semantic dementia (see Chapter 5).

The differential distinction between Alzheimer's disease (of which presenile dementia is a variant) and semantic dementia is important in three respects:

* Drugs now available for the management of dementia of Alzheimer type may not be appropriate in semantic dementia.
* Some re-learning is possible in individuals with mild–moderate semantic dementia if programmes are carefully targeted (Funnell 1995), so a short course of therapy may be appropriate.
* More pertinent information can be given to family and patient as the course of the disease is different from Alzheimer's disease, with other cognitive skills being preserved over a longer period of time, and a longer average disease duration.

Case history 2

Mrs R is a 78-year-old Frenchwoman, living with her husband, who had worked as an import/export agent and spoke fluent English and Spanish. She had no relevant medical, family or psychiatric history, wore reading glasses as appropriate and had a probable high-frequency hearing loss. She was referred to a memory clinic because of the sudden onset of mislaying items.

1st assessment
MMSE   27 (cut off for normal = 24)
CAMCOG   89 (cut off for normal = 79)
There was no evidence of depression.
Putative initial diagnosis by psychogeriatrician: MINIMAL COGNITIVE IMPAIRMENT

Language assessment
Word Learning (from ABCD):   Recall (16) 8, Recognition (48) 3
Indicating considerable encoding and retrieving problems.

Story Retelling: Immediate (25) 19, Delayed (25) 0
Although immediate recall is within normal limits, no facts were recalled on delayed performance indicating a lack of working memory, a common pattern in dementia of Alzheimer type.

Word Fluency: Animals 16, Towns 22, Letter 's' 8
All scores within normal ranges.

Paragraph Reading: Factual (10) 9, Inferential (10) 10
No significant difference between the two scores, with the task done within the expected time range.

Boston Naming Test: Score (60) 46
Although below the mean score for her age range, Mrs R's score is within the appropriate scoring range. As English was not her first language, a lower than mean score might not be significant, with a greater number of errors on less familiar words. It was of interest that 33% of her responses were, although correct, in French, suggesting that some semantic breakdown may be occurring in the acquired, but not the original language.

Homophone Pair Dictation: Score (10) 3
Errors appeared to be due to semantic rather than phonemic difficulties.

Written Picture Description: Whurr (5) 3, Reich (A) C
Limited ability to make inferences. Syntax was correct, if simplified, and there was no evidence of visual misinterpretation. Writing was rather disorganized and there was evidence of language switching (French/ English).

Conclusion
Although the original putative diagnosis following general cognitive assessment had been minimal cognitive impairment, implying some deficits but none which could be considered as denoting pathology, language assessment results indicated a greater degree of difficulty in certain areas, but not across the board. Suggestions of some semantic language breakdown can possibly be detected earlier in those tested in

their acquired not their first language, which might indicate the early stages of dementia. However, the reported sudden onset of memory symptoms and the patchy nature of performance might indicate early vascular dementia rather than Alzheimer's disease. Recent research has shown considerable overlap between the two conditions, and refers to a category of 'mixed dementia' (Kalaria 2003, Rockwood 2003), highlighting the complexity of clinical diagnosis.

Points to note in this case were:

- inappropriate switching of languages
- poor delayed recall
- seeming lack of awareness and concern about communication problems
- presence of some language deficits in the presence of 'normal' function on general cognitive measures
- appropriate behaviour.

In such circumstances, reassessment is essential. Mrs R's communication was reassessed 42 months later (ideally it should have been sooner than this). In the interim she had been taking aspirin (for stroke prevention) and Aricept (donepezil), a drug used in mild dementia. Her husband reported her speech had been slurred at one point, indicating a possible vascular event. Although her recent memory was extremely poor, she continued to manage the household without help.

Communication reassessment showed:

- marked deterioration in all tasks, apart from Picture Description and Dictation Homophone Pairs
- a slight decrease in the amount of French naming responses, although her score was now well below expected for her age range
- use of French in phonemic word fluency, previously not noted.

A CT scan showed cerebral and cerebellar atrophy, and evidence of small-vessel disease. On review, the diagnoses of Binswanger's disease or lacunar disease need to be considered, in which dysarthria may feature as part of the syndrome, although semantic deficits are uncharacteristic.

The patchy performance and variable scoring, exacerbated by language background, would appear to make a diagnosis of vascular dementia more likely. Certainly language assessment, especially earlier on, was detecting deficits before general cognitive measures did so, contributing to potentially more accurate diagnosis.

Assessing moderate to severe dementia

The issues of assessment for those with a more advanced dementia pathology differ from those mentioned in the context of more mild pathology.

A diagnosis of dementia may have been agreed some time ago, and the present requirement for communication assessment may be to delineate retained skills and areas of deficit so that the most appropriate advice may be given to family and carers to maximize communication function and reduce related stress and incidences of challenging behaviour, sometimes caused by communication breakdown. The semantic and pragmatic changes of early pathology are likely to be compounded by syntactic (grammatical) and phonological (sound) deficits as the disease progresses. Because of deteriorating attention skills, it is unlikely that assessments such as the Arizona Battery for Communication Disorders in Dementia (Bayles and Tomoeda 1993) can be used in their entirety, although certain sub-tests or construct sections may be feasible and of value.

In the past, sub-tests from aphasia assessments were used to assess those with language breakdown in dementia. In Britain, the Whurr Aphasia Screening Test was a useful starting point (Stevens 1989) because it has large print and clear pictures. In a current standardized revised form (Whurr 1996) it may still be of value because it has performance means for older people and because the SLT experience of using it for people with aphasia provides a pertinent framework for comparisons. The Frenchay Aphasia Screening Test (FAST) (Enderby et al. 1987), often used by health professionals other than SLTs, has also been used in this context, although it is of doubtful value at later stages in the disease process. Sub-tests from the Boston Diagnostic Aphasia Examination (now revised: Goodglass et al. 2000) and the Western Aphasia Battery (Kertesz 1982) have been of value in research from the USA (Faber-Langendoen et al. 1988).

As the disease progresses, syntax appears to become simplified and then shows errors. A certain amount of information can be abstracted from performance on assessments already mentioned, such as Written Picture Description and the Discourse Abilities Profile (Ripich 1991) but others which look at syntax in more detail, such as the Token Test (De Renzi and Faglioni 1978) and the Test for the Reception of Grammar (TROG) (Bishop 1989), may be of use (a shortened version of the latter is included in the Barnes Language Assessment; Bryan et al. 2001). Other tests looking at aspects of syntactic skill, but perhaps better known in the USA than the UK, are the Auditory Comprehension Test for Sentences (Shewen 1979) and the Reporter's Test (De Renzi and Ferrari 1978). It is noteworthy that the majority of these tests were developed some time ago, mainly for use with individuals with aphasia.

Some tests developed more recently target the problems resulting from severe or advanced pathology, even in those people thought to be untestable. One is the Severe Impairment Battery (SIB) (Saxton et al. 1993) which provides a baseline measurement of cognitive function and aims to chart subsequent change. It takes about 20 minutes to administer and is presented by means of one-step commands, accompanied by gestural cues. The six sub-scales measured are attention, orientation, language, memory, visuo-spatial ability and construction, so language is only a part of the whole. There are also brief tests of praxis, orientation to name and social interaction. SIB, like the Discourse Abilities Profile (Ripich 1991), addresses pragmatic function, although at a much simpler level.

Table 6.6 charts the assessments available for use with moderate to severe pathology. One of these is the Functional Linguistic Communication Inventory (Bayles and Tomoeda 1994) which aims to quantify the functional communication skills of individuals with such cognitive impairment, determining the level of severity and predicting skills likely to be lost as the disease continues to progress. Uniquely it looks at such pragmatic areas as pantomime and gesture, as well as conversational skills. The Cognitive Linguistic Quick Test (Helm-Estabrooks 2001), the Dementia Rating Scale 2TM (Mattis et al. 2002) and the Modified Ordinal Scales of Psychological Development (M-OSPD) (Auer et al. 1994) all may be of value in assessing those with advanced pathology, although the CLQT is the one likely to be of most interest to those assessing communication function. Benefits of carrying out such assessments in a residential or day care setting are that care staff, often challenged by patients' communication difficulties, can observe positive responses being made, and retained communication skills can be enhanced and maximized by a suitable communication environment.

Table 6.6 Moderate–severe dementia: possible tests

Assessment	Time (min)	Areas covered	Comments
Severe Impairment Battery (Saxton et al. 1993)	20	Attention, orientation, memory, language, visuo-spatial, construction	Also tests orientation to name, praxis and social interaction
Functional Linguistic Communication Inventory (Bayles and Tomoeda 1994)	30	Greeting, naming, comprehension, writing, reading, reminiscing, gesture, conversation	Aims to quantify functional communication skills
Dementia Rating Scale 2TM (DRM-2TM) (Mattis et al. 2002)	15–30	Brief, comprehensive neuropsychological measure	Can track change over time. User friendly
Cognitive Linguistic Quick Test (CLQT) (Helm-Estabrooks 2001)	12–30	Attention, memory, executive functions, language, visuo-spatial skills	50% tasks have minimal language demands. Severity rating
Modified Ordinal Scales of Psychological Development (M-OSPD) (Auer et al. 1994)		Broad-ranging	Specifically designed for severe pathology

Although several of the assessments discussed here have been used in research, some tests have been specifically designed to measure cognition in those subjects participating in drug trials. The best known of these is the Alzheimer's Disease Assessment Scale (ADAS) (Rosen et al. 1984) which assesses a range of cognitive functions, as does the SKT (Erzigkeit 1989), but neither of these tests considers communicative or linguistic function in any detail.

Assessing depression

Functional disorders are frequently seen by mental health teams, the most common of these being depression, with incidence figures varying from 1% to 13% in older people, partly depending on whether classification relates to depressive symptoms or classic depressive illness. The likelihood is that symptoms are underreported by elderly people, therefore underdiagnosed in the population. It is known to be higher in general practice attenders, and much higher in hospital settings (Jackson and Baldwin 1993).

SLTs are less likely to see individuals where the only, or the most obvious, diagnosis is acute depression. They may well, however, wherever they work, see elderly people in whom depressive symptoms are a part of the whole picture, notably when a dementia and vascular disorders are present.

The most common depressive symptoms are:

- disturbances in eating with loss/increase in appetite/weight
- disturbances in sleep patterns resulting in insomnia or hypersomnia
- loss of interest and pleasure, notably in things previously enjoyed
- feelings of worthlessness and guilt
- impaired concentration and memory
- fatigue and loss of energy
- inability to cope
- increased illness/pain and hypochondriasis
- suicidal thoughts
- physical retardation or agitation/anxiety.

All of these symptoms will, directly or indirectly, affect the presentation, amount and content of communication although frequently the effect may be hard to quantify. The causes of depression are potentially varied and numerous covering physical, social, emotional and life changes. The most common are:

- loss events including trauma, e.g. bereavement, independence
- illness and acquired handicaps
- medication
- sleep impairment

- social isolation
- malnutrition
- loss of occupation, opportunities and status, e.g. retirement
- pathological ageing changes in the brain.

Genetic factors are thought to be less important in late-onset depression. There may be a complex interaction between cause and effect when, for example, malnutrition may be a possible cause of depression or a resulting symptom and may complicate management of eating problems which, in turn, may then involve the SLT to whom a referral for assessment is made.

A comprehensive case history, if available, and a physical examination followed by a general cognitive assessment are the starting points for further assessment. There are a variety of screening tools for depression which can be used by any member of a mental health team, but it is essential that a psychiatrist or psychogeriatrician is involved as depression is a potentially treatable condition. Some of the most available and commonly used assessments are listed in Table 6.7.

Table 6.7 Depression screening assessments

Assessment	Time (min)	Comments
Geriatric Depression Scale (GDS) (Yesavage et al. 1983)	4–5	15 items, avoiding somatic questions so good for the elderly. Score 5+ indicates pathology. Useful in mild–moderate dementia
Hamilton Rating Scale for Depression (HRSD) (Hamilton 1960)	10	Widely used, but not so suitable for the elderly because of somatic questions
Montgomery–Asberg Depression Rating Scale (MADRS) (Montgomery and Asberg 1979)	10–15	Sensitive to change in depression, but may not be reliable in dementia
Cornell Depression Scale (CDS) (Alexopoulos et al. 1988)	10–15	Designed and validated for screening for depression in dementia. Uses patient/informant reports. Score 10+ indicates depression. 9 items
Hospital Anxiety and Depression Scale (HADS) (Zigmond and Snaith 1983)	10–15	Self-administered, bidimensional
Brief Assessment Schedule Depression Cards (BASDEC) (Adshead et al. 1992)	5	Statements presented in large print on cards for True/False answers. Useful with hard of hearing, and those with speech problems. Score 7+ indicates depression

The Hamilton Rating Scale for Depression (HRSD) (Hamilton 1960), the Montgomery–Asberg Depression Rating Scale (Montgomery and Asberg 1979) and the Hospital Anxiety and Depression Scale (HADS) (Zigmond and Snaith 1983) are all well established, ask focused questions of clinical relevance and are often used. The Brief Assessment Schedule Depression Cards (BASDEC) (Adshead et al. 1992), designed specifically for use with older people, are a useful tool which can be used by any team member. However, the Cornell Depression Scale (CDS) (Alexopoulos et al. 1988) is the only tool to address the question of differential diagnosis of dementia/depression. The percentage of individuals with early dementia who have depressive symptoms is debatable, with ranges of 0–52% being recorded in the literature. As the incidence of depression in those attending memory clinics ranges from 2% to 44% (Ballard and Eastwood 1999), it should always be excluded before a diagnosis of dementia is considered. There is current debate as to whether depression is more likely to co-exist with a dementia pathology, or whether it is a precursor to dementia (Alexopoulos et al. 1993). It is probable that both scenarios exist and that the presentation of depression and/or dementia may be qualitatively different. There is evidence that the assessment of communication may be of help in this differential diagnosis. Observation of the content of spontaneous communication may be indicative, as may an observed slowness and paucity of speech.

The content of written material, e.g. the sentence in the MMSE, may provide a pointer. Depression also limits communication in a broader sense, because of greater isolation, social withdrawal, reduced concentration and memory deficits. However, more formal assessment using semantic language tests can produce more tangible diagnostic evidence of differences between dementia and depression (Stevens et al. 1996). This study found that, when four matched groups of patients (probable Alzheimer's disease, vascular dementia, depression and worried well) were compared, the depressed group did not present with semantic language deficits as did the dementia groups. There was, however, a wide spread of performance within the depressed group, indicating heterogeneity which might relate to possible clinical differences between depression as an independent clinical entity and depression that is a precursor to dementia. There was minimal overlap between scores in the depressed and dementia groups. One of the most useful tests in this context is the Boston Naming Test (Kaplan et al. 1983). In the study by Stevens et al. (1996), only 3 out of 14 depressed subjects (21%) scored below age-related cut-off points, while 13 out of 19 (68%) test subjects with dementia of Alzheimer type did. Also 50% of the depressed group scored below the mean for their age group, compared to 84% of the dementia groups. It may be that some of the heterogeneity can be accounted for by better naming ability in those depressed people with reversible cognitive impairment (Dessonville et al. 1992), while those in whom depression is a precursor to dementia are already showing some measurable signs of semantic language deficits, known to be common in dementia, especially Alzheimer's disease.

Word fluency also highlights differences between Alzheimer's disease and those with depression. Although there was some overlap in performance when using the 'animals' semantic word fluency task, there was none using 'towns' with group mean scores of 9.6 for the group with dementia of Alzheimer type and 20.6 for the depressed group. As one characteristic of depression is physical slowing, it might be expected that timed tasks would disadvantage those with depression. Paragraph Reading (La Pointe and Horner 1998) results showed that the depressed group, although slightly slower than the worried well group, were quicker than either of the two dementia groups tested. Story Retelling, a test of memory rather than semantic function, and therefore possibly more at risk in depression, showed a similar pattern with the depressed group score falling between the worried well and dementia groups.

The evidence is, therefore, that some language assessment is beneficial in terms of acquiring useful diagnostic information. It is also important in providing a baseline against which change can be measured, either decline, or if antidepressants have been prescribed, possible improvement. Case history 3 demonstrates that improvement in both memory and semantic function can be measured when depression is treated.

Case history 3

Mrs D is a 65-year-old, widowed, retired laboratory technician of Polish origin who was referred to the memory clinic by her GP. No significant medical or family history was found, nor did she have any sensory deficits or history of alcohol abuse, although she did have a history of agoraphobia, for which she was successfully treated with diazepam. She was worried about financial matters and selling her house.

1st assessment
MMSE   28 (cut off for normal = 24)
CAMCOG   96 (cut off for normal = 79)
Computerized testing   slow
BASDEC 9.5 indicating depression

Language assessment
Word Learning: Recall (16) 11, Recognition (48) 36
Both indicating retention deficits.

Story Retelling: Immediate (25) 19, Delayed (25) 19
Indicating that recall and retention were better in a context.

Word Fluency: Animals 17, Towns 18, Phonemic 20
All within or above the normal scoring range.

Boston Naming Test: Score (60) 38
Well below the cut-off point for her age, but her language background might be significant.

The initial hypothesis resulting from the above scores was that, although memory and confrontation naming were impaired, there were no consistent signs of semantic language breakdown that would indicate a dementia pathology. Reassessment was however necessary to confirm this. Meanwhile, Mrs D was treated with an antidepressant (fluoxetine).

On re-assessment (8 months later)
Word Learning: Recall 11, Recognition 41
Indicating some improvement in recognition.

Story Retelling: Immediate 22, Delayed 21
Also indicating improvement in recall, and demonstrating that almost all encoded material could be recalled.

Word Fluency: Animals 17, Towns 22, Phonemic 16
All scores remain within or above the normal range, with slight improvement in semantic fluency, but slight deterioration in phonemic. This is an unusual pattern for dementia, sometimes seen in those for whom English is not the first language, and who may have a more fragile phonemic system.

Boston Naming Test: Score 42
An improvement of 4, still below the cut-off point for her age.
Her BASDEC score was now 3, no longer in the pathological range, and that together with the improved language test results would indicate depression rather than dementia pathology.

2nd re-assessment (33 months later)
General cognition:

MMSE	30
CAMCOG	107
Computerized testing	less slow
BASDEC 5	not depressed

Word Learning: Recall 16, Recognition 45 (within normal range)

Story Retelling (immediate):   Score 19 (no change)

Word Fluency: Animals 20, Towns 23, Phonemic 14
Semantic scores have increased again, and phonemic decreased, but still remain within the normal range.

Boston Naming Test: Score 51 (within age range)
Even deterioration that might have been anticipated due to age was not evident. Although Mrs D was still concerned that her memory was deteriorating in spite of assessment evidence to the contrary, she was now thought to be worried well.

Late-onset schizophrenia and paraphrenia

At present there is a debate about the diagnostic validity of late-onset schizo-phrenia-like psychoses and paraphrenia, as to whether or not there are pathological links to dementia of Alzheimer type and/or dementia with Lewy bodies. Prevalence figures for late-onset paraphrenia in the elderly commu-nity population range from 0.1% to 4%, with the condition being more common in women. A contributory precipitating factor may be hearing loss. Almeida et al. (1995a) estimate that there is a four times greater risk of hear-ing impairment in the condition than with matched controls. Whether or not this is so, hearing needs to be considered when assessing patients of this type.

Whatever the age of onset, patients with chronic schizophrenia appear to have generalized cognitive impairment, paucity of speech and possible thought disorder, some of which would be seen in dementia. However, learning capacity is relatively spared (Almeida et al. 1995b). There is a slightly higher risk that some individuals with schizophrenia will go on to develop dementia (Hymas et al. 1989).

As this is quite a specialized area of work, only a small number of ther-apists may be asked to assess patients of this type. Many of the assessments listed for use with mild to moderate dementia could be used, although there is doubt about how sensitive such structured tests would be in detecting thought disorder. While semantics may be distorted, syntax and phonology remain intact. Poor performance on expressive language tasks may therefore be due to disordered thought rather than defective re-sponses to stimuli. Some pragmatic features of communication can be distorted, and output reduced, while others such as inflection, facial expression and gesture are lacking. Affective blunting may be present, although this is more likely in younger onset patients (Andreasen et al. 1990), while orofacial dyskinesia is frequently evident in older individuals.

The Right Hemisphere Battery (Bryan 1995), which assesses the more subtle and abstract areas of language mediated by the right hemisphere, may be of value. Bryan acknowledges the role of right hemisphere lan-guage processing in psychiatric disorders. None of the sub-tests are dependent on memory skills, but instead focus on use of metaphor, humour, integration of linguistic information, discourse, prosody and stress, and emotional language. Facial recognition deficits and anosog-nosia are also tested.

Certain tasks which require learning, such as the Word Learning Sub-Test (ABCD) (Bayles and Tomoeda 1993) and Story Retelling may be relatively well performed by those with schizophrenia type pathology rather than dementia. The following short case history illustrates this.

Case history 4

Miss R was a 51-year-old unmarried English woman referred to the memory clinic by her GP.

1st assessment

MMSE	27
CAMCOG	95 (both scores above cut-off)

Language assessment

Story Retelling: Immediate (25) 21, Delayed (25) 18
Indicating good retention of material

Word Fluency: Animals 15, Towns 15, Phonemic 11
Scores within the normal ranges.

Written Picture Description: Whurr (5) 5, Reich (A) A
Therefore no deficits in semantics, syntax or spelling, with good ability
to draw appropriate inferences.

Boston Naming Test: Score (60) 44
Below the cut-off point for her age.

Although her confrontation naming score might indicate pathology,
the fact that there were no deficits in other areas of performance makes
it more likely that it is an artefact of limited educational background. The
medical history was the crucial factor in formulating a diagnosis of
schizoaffective disorder.

Alcohol abuse and related conditions (Wernicke–Korsakoff syndrome)

As with the schizophrenia group of pathologies, there is ongoing debate
about the exact pathology of conditions related to alcohol abuse, notably
whether alcohol intake per se can cause cognitive deficits severe enough
to be classed as a dementia. Wernicke's encephalopathy has three main
identifying features:

- global confusion
- gait ataxia
- ocular abnormalities.

It is associated with excessive alcohol intake, but is actually caused by
thiamine deficiency. Although the number of such individuals that a therapist is asked to assess may be limited, alcohol intake may be a
compounding factor in other dementia presentations. Cutting (1978),
using the Weschler Adult Intelligence Scale (WAIS) on groups of
Korsakoff's and alcoholic dementia patients, found no signs of dysphasia
or dyspraxia, although problem solving, abstraction abilities, memory and
psychomotor skills were all affected. However, this test is not geared to
detailed semantic language assessment, but rather to assessing general
intelligence. He concluded that Korsakoff's and dementia were on the

same diagnostic spectrum and that some cognitive improvement was possible when alcohol intake ceased or was reduced, as Case history 5 shows.

Case history 5

Mr B was a 65-year-old English retired driver, referred to the clinic by his GP, living with his wife. He was a heavy drinker, consuming 50 units per week. Relevant medical history: *mitral infarct* 10 years ago. No hearing loss, but evidence of glaucoma.

1st assessment

MMSE	26
CAMCOG	85 (both above cut-off points)

Language assessment

Word Learning:	Recall (16) 4, Recognition (48) 20
Story Retelling:	Immediate (25) 17, Delayed (25) 0
Paragraph Reading:	Factual (10) 10, Inferential (10) 10, Time 5' 32"
Homophone Pair Dictation:	Score (10) 4
What's Wrong?:	Recognition (10) 6, Explanation (10) 4
Word Fluency:	Animals 19, Towns 20, Phonemic 19
Unusual Angle Photograph Naming:	Score (10) 2
Boston Naming Test:	Score (60) 36

From these results there was clear evidence of difficulty with the retention of newly presented material. Although his ability to make appropriate inferences was intact there was poor performance on a number of semantic tasks. However, it would appear that performance was adversely influenced by his visual problem, with all tasks with a visual component being below norms or expectations.

Re-assessment (6 months later)

In the interim Mr B had been drinking less. On retest his general cognitive performance as measured by CAMCOG had declined to 60, below the cut-off point. Of the 13 language measures retested, 5 showed deterioration, 5 were improved and 3 stayed the same. There was no improvement in retention of material, and changes in semantic performance were inconsistent.

The severity and longevity of Mr B's drinking problems, combined with a possible vascular pathology and a significant visual problem, led to a mixed performance, some of which proved to be irreversible. The lack of consistency in semantic deficits differentiates performance from that usually seen in Alzheimer's disease. A primary diagnosis of alcoholic dementia was made.

Patients of this type are likely to have amnesia for recent events, so such tests as Story Retelling and Word Learning will be poorly performed while, in most instances, semantic, syntactic and phonological skills remain intact, unless there are other pathologies.

Dementia in Parkinson's disease

Mayeux et al. (1990) found that 25% of their 249 review patients with Parkinson's disease went on to develop dementia. By 85 years the cumulative incidence of dementia was 65%, with the greatest increase in risk being for those between 65 and 75 years. This is significantly higher than the 29% incidence of dementia in those over 85 years old in the total population, according to EURODEM prevalence figures (Burns and Forstl 1998). Therefore a number of such patients are likely to be seen by a mental health team, rather than a neurologist, or simply remain under GP care.

Available general cognitive measures have been mentioned earlier in this chapter (see Table 6.2) and these are the starting point for assessment. Marinus et al. (2003) have produced a short, reliable and valid cognitive screening assessment for use specifically in this field. It is called the SCOPA-COG (Scales for Outcomes of Parkinson's Disease – Cognition). Using this measure Marinus and his colleagues showed a clear trend towards lower cognition scores for those with more advanced disease. The test's coefficient of variation was higher than the CAMCOG or MMSE, indicating better ability to detect differences between individuals. Others (Green et al. 2002) have concluded that frontal lobe function is frequently impaired in advanced Parkinson's disease in the absence of depression and other signs of dementia. Greater motor problems were related to poorer performance on multiple neuropsychological measures.

Because many individuals with Parkinson's disease have a flat affect and demonstrate psychomotor slowing (bradykinesia), depression may appear to be present and therefore assessment of depression is advisable. A suitable screening test is the BASDEC (Adshead et al. 1992) which requires limited verbal responses and which can be interpreted with greater ease and accuracy if speech is unclear. Another common problem in Parkinson's disease is a dysarthria and a reduction in speech intelligibility, which is one of the most significant difficulties for many people with Parkinson's disease. Because speech will be compromised at some stage in the disease process, an assessment is essential. The Frenchay Dysarthria Assessment (Enderby 1983) and the Robertson (1982) Dysarthria Profile are the most commonly used in the UK.

Any assessment of cognitive skills therefore needs to encompass

- general cognitive skills
- speech, language and pragmatic function
- frontal lobe (executive) function.

Although not designed only for assessment, the Parkinson's Disease Management Pack (Swinburn and Morley 1997) is useful. As would be expected, a dysarthria profile is obtained, and some of the assessment is geared towards assessing frontal lobe cognitive function, an integral part of this type of dementia (Dubois et al. 1990, Green et al. 2002).

Bayles and Tomoeda (1993) provide mean scores and scoring ranges for the performance of demented and non-demented people with Parkinson's disease, which makes the Arizona Battery for Communication Disorders in Dementia a valuable tool, in whole or in part. It presents a clearly identifiable profile of a group of subjects with Parkinson's disease with dementia compared to a matched group of subjects with mild dementia of Alzheimer type. The Parkinson's disease group was characterized by relatively poor generative naming, but word learning and delayed story recall, although impaired compared to normal elderly and Parkinson's disease without dementia, were better than in the group with dementia of Alzheimer type.

Other tests available for assessing frontal lobe function are the Wisconsin Card Sorting Test (Heaton 1991), the Trail Making Test (Reitan 1958) and Word Fluency. Both Trail Making and Word Fluency have been incorporated into the Barnes Language Assessment (Bryan et al. 2001).

Just as it is important to reassess individuals whose condition may be improving, it is also integral to good management to re-evaluate those with a progressive condition, so that skills and deficits can be defined and explained and appropriate advice given to patient, family and carers.

Down's syndrome

Thanks to improved standards of medical care and better public health, people with Down's syndrome are now living to an older age. As long ago as the 1940s, single cases of Down's syndrome who developed dementia were being reported. Goldgarber et al. (1987) localized the gene coding for the amyloid precursor protein to chromosome 21, thus explaining the likely link between Down's and Alzheimer's. On post-mortem both conditions are found to have neurofibrillary tangles and amyloid deposits (see also Chapter 4). Assessment of further cognitive decline in those in whom cognition may already be limited is challenging, with results hard to interpret especially if the individual is unknown to the assessor. Key points to remember are:

- Is there a change from a known or assumed baseline?
- Is functional decline present, not just a decline in psychomotor scores?
- Is the nature of any decline different, and, if so, in what way?
- Is the extent of any decline greater than would be expected through normal ageing?
- Are there any possible illnesses, including sensory problems, which might cause such decline?

Three scales have been designed for use in this area to aid diagnosis: Dementia Questionnaire for Mentally Retarded Persons (Evenhuis 1990), Dementia Scale for Down's Syndrome (Gedye 1995) and Down's Syndrome Mental State Examination (Haxby 1989).

Close questioning, using a structured format, of those who know the individual well may be of value (Holland et al. 1998), as would re-evaluation using previously used communication assessments. Other more functionally based assessments could also help provide care staff and families with information and appropriate management strategies. In many instances the diagnosis may not be in question, but accurate delineation of skills and deficits can help to maximize function, reduce antisocial behaviour, improve quality of life, reduce carer stress and monitor change. Deterioration over time may be anticipated, but regular re-assessment can detect whether that change is as expected, or possibly due to an acute and transient episode such as an infection. Because communication is the currency with which all carers work, accurate information and management strategies based on reasoned assessment are essential.

Conclusion

This overview of the assessment of language and communication in older people with mental health problems has highlighted the scope and variety of assessments available. However, it is worth reiterating the following points:

- Tests continue to be used in situations, and with individuals, for which they were not designed; therefore validity may be compromised and interpretation made harder.
- Many of the tests in common usage were designed and validated some time ago; therefore with changes in knowledge, as well as cultural and social mores, their suitability and sensitivity may be open to question.
- The challenges of using assessments with an interpreter, or in translated form, are likely to increase with the ageing of immigrant populations.
- More tests, in original or revised versions, are being standardized on older people, although the concept of normality in 'normal' ageing is potentially problematic.
- The importance of accurate diagnosis is greater than ever, because of the increasing availability of appropriate drugs.
- A greater number of user-friendly screening or functional assessments are available, providing valuable diagnostic and management information.

The practice of assessment remains a compromise between science and skill, so that although the tools available are improving, they are only as valuable as the assessor's knowledge, skills and interpretation of them allow. It is a detective process where not all clues and forensic information are available, but it is, nevertheless, one which is essential, challenging and satisfying.

References

Adshead F, Cody D, Pitt B (1992) BASDEC: a novel screening instrument for depression in elderly medical inpatients. BMJ 305: 397.

Alexopoulos GS, Abrams RC, Young RC, Shamoian CA (1988) Cornell scale for depression in dementia. Biological Psychiatry 23: 271–284.

Alexopoulos GS, Meyers BS, Young RC et al. (1993) The course of geriatric depression with 'reversible dementia': a controlled study. American Journal of Psychiatry 150(11): 1693–1699.

Almeida OP, Howard RJ, Levy R et al. (1995a) Cognitive features of psychotic states arising in late life (late paraphrenia). Psychological Medicine 25: 685–698.

Almeida OP, Howard RJ, Levy R et al. (1995b) Psychotic states arising in late life – the role of risk factors. British Journal of Psychiatry 166: 215–228.

Andreasen NC, Flaum M, Swayze VW et al. (1990) Positive and negative symptoms in schizophrenia: a critical appraisal. Archives of General Psychiatry 47(7): 615–621.

Armstrong L (1997) Armstrong Naming Test. Psychological Corporation, London.

Auer SR, Sclan SG, Yaffee RA, Reisberg B (1994) Modified ordinal scales of psychological development (M-OSPD): the neglected half of Alzheimer's disease and functional concomitants of severe dementia. Journal of the American Geriatrics Society 42: 1266–1272.

Ballard C, Eastwood R (1999) Psychiatric assessment. In: Wilcock GK, Bucks RS, Rockwood K (eds) Diagnosis and Management of Dementia. Oxford University Press, Oxford.

Basso A, Capitani E, Laiacona M (1988) Progressive language impairment without dementia: a case with isolated category specific semantic deficit. Journal of Neurology, Neurosurgery and Psychiatry 51: 1201–1207.

Bayles KA, Tomoeda CK (1993) Arizona Battery for Communication Disorders in Dementia. Canyonlands Publishing, Tucson, AZ.

Bayles KA, Tomoeda C (1994) Functional Linguistic Communication Inventory. Canyonlands Publishing, Tucson, AZ.

Bishop DVM (1989) Test for the Reception of Grammar, 2nd edn. Medical Research Council, London.

Bryan KL (1995) The Right Hemisphere Battery, 2nd edn. Whurr, London.

Bryan K, Binder J, Dann C et al. (2001) Development of a screening test for language in older people (Barnes Language Assessment). Age and Mental Health 5(4): 371–378.

Bschor T, Kuhl K-P, Reischies FM (2001) Spontaneous speech of patients with dementia of the Alzheimer's type and mild cognitive impairment. International Psychogeriatrics 13(3): 289–298.

Burns A, Forstl H (1998) Alzheimer's disease. In: Butler R, Pitt B (eds) Seminars in Old Age Psychiatry. Royal College of Psychiatrists, London.

Caird FI, Judge T (eds) (1974) Assessment of the elderly patient. Pitman Medical, London.

Crook T, Salama M, Gobert J (1986) A computerised test battery for detecting and assessing memory disorders. In Bes A et al. (eds) Senile Dementias: early detection. John Libbey Eurotext, Paris, pp. 79–85.

Cutting J (1978) The relationship between Korsakov's syndrome and 'alcoholic dementia'. British Journal of Psychiatry 132: 240–251.

De Renzi E, Faglioni P (1978) Normative data and screening power of a shortened version of the Token Test. Cortex 14: 41–49.

De Renzi E, Ferrari C (1978) The Reporter's Test: a sensitive test to detect expressive disturbance in aphasics. Cortex 14: 279–293.

Dessonville C, Stoudemire A, Morris R et al. (1992) Dysnomia in the differential diagnosis of major depression, depression related cognitive dysfunction and dementia. Journal of Neuropsychiatry and Clinical Neuroscience 4: 64–69.

Dubois B, Pillon B, Sternic N et al. (1990) Age-induced cognitive disturbances in Parkinson's disease. Neurology 40: 38–41.

Dunn LM, Dunn LM (1981) Peabody Picture Vocabulary Test – Revised. American Guidance Service, Circle Pines, MI.

Eastley R, Wilcock G (2000) Assessment and differential diagnosis of dementia. In: O'Brien J, Ames D, Burns R (eds) Dementia. Arnold, London.

Enderby P (1983) Frenchay Dysarthria Assessment. NFER-Nelson, Windsor.

Enderby P, Wood V, Wade D (1987) Frenchay Aphasia Screening Test (FAST). NFER-Nelson, Windsor.

Erzigkeit H (1989) The SKT – a short cognitive performance test as an instrument for the assessment of clinical efficiency of cognitive enhancers. In: Bergener M, Reisberg B (eds) Diagnosis and Treatment of Senile Dementia. Springer-Verlag, Berlin, pp. 164–174.

Evenhuis HM (1990) The natural history of dementia in Down's syndrome. Archives of Neurology 47(3): 263–267.

Faber-Langendoen K, Morris JC, Knesevich JW et al. (1988) Aphasia in senile dementia of the Alzheimer type. Annals of Neurology 23: 365–370.

Fillenbaum GG, Huber M, Taussig IM (1997) Performance of elderly white and African American community residents on the abbreviated CERAD Boston Naming Test. Journal of Clinical and Experimental Neuropsychology 19(2): 204–210.

Folstein MF, Folstein SE, McHugh PR (1975) Mini-Mental State: a practical method for grading the cognitive state of patients for the clinician. Journal of Psychiatric Research 12: 189–198.

Funnell E (1995) A case of forgotten knowledge. In: Campbell R, Conway M (eds) Broken Memories. Blackwell, Oxford, pp. 225–236.

Gedye A (1995) Dementia Scale for Down's Syndrome. Gedye Research and Consulting, Vancouver.

Goldgarber D, Lerman MI, McBride WO et al. (1987) Isolation, characterization and chromosomal localization of human brain DNA clones coding for the precursor of the amyloid of brain in Alzheimer's disease, Down's syndrome and aging. Journal of Neural Transmitters Supplement 24: 23–28.

Golding E (1989) Middlesex Elderly Assessment of Mental State (MEAMS). Thames Valley Test Company, Bury St Edmunds.

Goodglass H, Kaplan E, Barressi B (2000) Boston Diagnostic Aphasia Examination, 3rd edn (BDAE-3). Psychological Corporation, London.

Green J, McDonald WM, Vitek JL et al. (2002) Cognitive impairment in advanced Parkinson's disease without dementia. Neurology 59: 1320–1324.

Hamilton M (1960) A rating scale for depression. Journal of Neurology, Neurosurgery and Psychiatry 23: 632–637.

Hart S, Smith CM, Swash M (1988) Word fluency in patients with early dementia of Alzheimer type. British Journal of Clinical Psychology 27: 115–124.

Haxby JV (1989) Neuropsychological evaluation of adults with Down's syndrome: patterns of selective impairment in non-demented old adults. Journal of Mental Deficiency Research 33: 193–210.

Heaton RK (1991) Wisconsin Card Sorting Test. Psychological Assessment Resources, Odessa, FL.

Helm-Estabrooks N (2001) Cognitive Linguistic Quick Test. Psychological Corporation, London.

Hodkinson M (1973) Mental impairment in the elderly. Journal of the Royal College of Physicians 7: 305–317.

Holland AJ, Hon J, Huppert F et al. (1998) Population based study of the prevalence and presentation of dementia in adults with Down's syndrome. British Journal of Psychiatry 172: 493–498.

Hymas N, Naguib M, Levy R (1989) Late paraphrenia, a follow-up study. International Journal of Geriatric Psychiatry 4: 23–29.

Jackson R, Baldwin B (1993) Detecting depression in elderly medically ill patients: the use of the Geriatric Depression Scale compared with medical and nursing observations. Age and Ageing 22: 349–353.

Kalaria RN (2003) Vascular factors in Alzheimer's disease. International Psychogeriatrics 15(1): 47–52.

Kaplan E, Goodglass H, Weintraub S (1983) Boston Naming Test. Lea and Febiger, Philadelphia.

Kendrick DC (1985) Kendrick Cognitive Tests for the Elderly. NFER-Nelson, Windsor.

Kertesz A (1982) Western Aphasia Battery. Psychological Corporation, London.

La Pointe L, Horner J (1998) Reading Comprehension Battery for Aphasia (RCBA-2). Psychological Corporation, London.

McKenna P, Warrington E (1983) Graded Naming Test: Manual. NFER-Nelson, Windsor.

Margolin DI, Pate DS, Friedrich FJ, Elia E (1990) Dysnomia in dementia and in stroke patients: different underlying cognitive deficits. Journal of Clinical and Experimental Neuropsychology 12: 597–612.

Marinus J, Visser M, Verwey A et al. (2003) Assessment of cognition in Parkinson's Disease. Neurology 61: 1222–1228.

Mattis S, Jurica P, Leitten C (2002) Dementia Rating Scale-2TM. Psychological Corporation, London.

Mayeux R, Chen J, Miabello E et al. (1990) An estimate of the incidence of dementia in idiopathic Parkinson's disease. Neurology 40: 1513–1517.

Mendez MF, Clark DG, Shapira JS, Cummings JL (2003) Speech and language in progressive nonfluent aphasia compared with early Alzheimer's disease. Neurology 61: 1108–1113.

Montgomery S, Asberg M (1979) A new depression scale designed to be sensitive to change. British Journal of Psychiatry 134: 382–389.

Nicholas M, Obler LK, Au R, Albert ML (1996) On the study of naming errors in aging and dementia: a study of semantic relatedness. Brain and Language 54: 184–195.

Obler LK, Santi S, Goldberger J (1991) Bilingual dementia: pragmatic breakdown. In: Lubinski R (ed.) Dementia and Communication. BC Decker, Hamilton, chapter 4.

O'Neill D, Surmon DJ, Wilcock GK (1992) Longitudinal diagnosis of memory disorders. Age and Ageing 21: 393–397.

Pattie AH, Gillard CJ (1979) Manual of the Clifton Assessment Procedures for the Elderly (CAPE). Hodder and Stoughton, Sevenoaks.

Phillips LH, Dellasella S, Trivelli C (1996) Fluency deficits in patients with Alzheimer's disease and frontal lobe lesions. European Journal of Neurology 3(2): 102–108.

Piguet O, Grayson DA, Broe A et al. (2002) Normal aging and executive functions in 'old-old' community dwellers: poor performance is not an inevitable outcome. International Psychogeriatrics 14(2): 139–159.

Randolph C (1998) Repeatable Battery for the Assessment of Neuropsychological Status (RBANS). Psychological Corporation, London.

Raven JC (1965) Guide to the Standard Progressive Matrices. HK Lewis, London.

Reich SS (1982) Picture perception, brain damage and dysphasia. British Journal of Disorders of Communication 17: 121–131.

Reisberg B, Ferris SH, DeLeon MJ, Crook T (1982) The Global Deterioration Scale for the assessment of primary degeneration dementia. American Journal of Psychiatry 139: 1136–1139.

Reitan RM (1958) Validity of the Trail Making Test as an indicator of organic brain damage. Perceptual and Motor Skills 8: 271–276.

Ripich DN (1991) Differential diagnosis and assessment. In: Lubinski R (ed.) Dementia and Communication. BC Decker, Hamilton.

Robbins TW, Sahakian BJ (1994) Computer methods of assessment of cognitive function. In: Copeland JRM, Abon-Selah MT, Blazer DG (eds) Principles and Practice of Geriatric Psychiatry. John Wiley & Sons, Chichester, pp. 205–209.

Robertson SJ (1982) Robertson Dysarthria Profile. Winslow Press, Bicester.

Rockwood K (2003) Mixed dementia: Alzheimer's and cerebrovascular disease. International Psychogeriatrics 15(1): 39–46.

Rosen WG, Mons RC, Davis KL (1984) Alzheimer's Disease Assessment Scale (ADAS): a new rating scale for Alzheimer's disease. American Journal of Psychiatry 141: 1356–1364.

Roth M, Tym E, Montjoy CS et al. (1986) CAMDEX: a standardised instrument for the diagnosis of mental disorder in the elderly with special reference to the early detection of dementia. British Journal of Psychiatry 149: 698–709.

Salmon DP, Thomas RG, Pay MM et al. (2002) Alzheimer's disease can be accurately diagnosed in very mildly impaired individuals. Neurology 59: 1022–1028.

Saxton J, McGonigle KL, Swihart AA, Bollen F (1993) Severe Impairment Battery. Thames Valley Test Company, Bury St Edmunds.

Shewen CM (1979) Auditory Comprehension Test for Sentences. Biolinguistics Clinical Institute, Chicago.

Simpson P, Surmon D, Wesnes K, Wilcock G (1991) The cognitive drug research computerized assessment system for demented patients: a validation study. Journal of Geriatric Psychiatry 6: 95–102.

Stevens SJ (1989) Differential naming difficulties in elderly dysphasic subjects and subjects with senile dementia of Alzheimer type. British Journal of Disorders of Communication 24: 77–92.

Stevens SJ, Pitt BMN, Nicholl CG et al. (1992) Language assessment in a memory clinic. International Journal of Geriatric Psychiatry 7(1): 45–52.

Stevens SJ, Harvey RJ, Kelly CA et al. (1996) Characteristics of language performance in 4 groups of patients attending a memory clinic. International Journal of Geriatric Psychiatry 11: 973–982.

Swinburn K, Morley R (1997) Parkinson's Disease Management Pack. Psychological Corporation, London.

Terrell B, Ripich D (1989) Discourse competence as a variable in intervention. Seminars in Speech and Language Disorders 24: 77–92.

Ulatowska HK, Chapman SB, Highley AP, Prince J (1998) Discourse in healthy old-elderly adults: a longitudinal study. Aphasiology 12(7/8): 619–633.

Van Gorp WG, Satz P, Kiersch ME, Henry R (1986) Normative data on the Boston Naming Test for a group of normal older adults. Journal of Clinical and Experimental Neurology 8: 702–705.

Whurr R (1996) Aphasia Screening Test. Wiley, London.

Wiig E, Nielson NP, Minthon L, Waikentin S (2002) Alzheimer's Quick Test. Psychological Corporation, London.

Wilson B, Cockburn J, Baddeley A (1991) The Rivermead Behavioural Memory Test. Thames Valley Test Company, Bury St Edmunds.

Worrall LE, Yin EML, Hickson LMH, Barnett HM (1995) Normative data for the Boston Naming Test for Australian elderly. Aphasiology 9: 541–551.

Yesavage J, Brink T, Rose T et al. (1983) Development and evaluation of a geriatric depression screening scale: a preliminary report. Journal of Psychiatric Research 17: 37–49.

Zigmond AS, Snaith RP (1983) The Hospital Anxiety and Depression Scale. Acta Psychiatrica Scandinavica 67: 361–370.

CHAPTER 7

Environmental and team approaches to communication in the dementias

KATE ALLAN

This chapter seeks to explore the place of communication generally in work with people with dementia, in particular focusing on 'whole team' approaches to communication (particularly applicable in residential and day services), and on the role of the environment in communication.

Dementia, personhood and communication

An account of why communication with persons with dementia must be at the heart of what those of us in a supporting role do, has to start with an examination of ideas about what it means to be a person at all. This argument has been presented most extensively by Kitwood, in all of his writings but most fully in Kitwood (1997). As part of his thesis, challenging the belief that the individual who has dementia has essentially disappeared or disintegrated, Kitwood goes back to what the whole notion of 'personhood' means. He identifies a tradition in Western philosophical thought which sees the quality of personhood as arising out of the possession of certain sorts of abilities on the part of an individual.

Capacities such as the use of language, the ability to think and make judgements in a rational way, and to exercise a moral sense, are examples cited by thinkers such as Quinton (1973). According to such theories, in order for a human being to be a person, he or she must possess and be able to exercise these capacities. It is immediately apparent, however, that this way of thinking about personhood excludes many individuals, for example young children, people who are ill or unconscious, those with severe learning disabilities and, of course, many people who have dementia. Does this mean that we just conclude that persons with dementia are not fully persons? This is unacceptable for various reasons. In response to this, Kitwood described an alternative way of thinking about how human beings come by their personhood, and this was not at all dependent on the sorts of capacities or abilities mentioned above. Instead, Kitwood (1997) proposed, the reality of personhood arises from the ways in which human beings interact and how they regard one another. He wrote:

> It is a standing or status that is bestowed on one human being, by others, in the context of relationship and social being. It implies recognition, respect and trust. (p. 8)

From this we can see that for each of us, whether or not we have dementia, our sense of being a person comes from each other. It is simply not the sort of thing one person, in isolation of anyone else, can possess or hold within themself. Relationships, then, are the critical underpinning of personhood.

How, then, does this link to communication? To answer this we need to take another small step to realizing that for a relationship to be a real thing, it is dependent on communication. We cannot have a relationship with another person without being in communication. So we can see that if, as Kitwood argues, personhood is based on relationships, and relationships are based on communication, then our own and everyone else's sense of being a person is tied up intimately with communication.

The development of interest in communication in dementia

Interest in the subject of communication with people who have dementia is an integral part of Kitwood's approach, particularly in the identification of what he termed 'malignant social psychology'. This is a collective term he used to describe various ways of relating to individuals with the condition. The word 'malignant' is not intended to suggest that they are practised with the intention of doing harm or causing distress; rather, they arise from certain beliefs about the nature of dementia as a condition and the characteristics of those affected. For example, the belief that the fact of having dementia is the most important defining characteristic of a person, could lead to the practice of what Kitwood (1997) called 'labelling':

> using a category such as dementia, or 'organic mental disorder' as the main basis of interacting with a person and explaining their behaviour. (p. 46)

Similarly:

> treating a person as if they were a lump of dead matter . . . without proper reference to the fact that they are a sentient being (p. 47)

is the practice Kitwood (1997) called 'objectification', and is understandable as a consequence of holding the belief that the person with dementia is no longer aware of anything that is happening.

In his book, Kitwood (1997) lists 17 distinct examples of 'malignant social psychology'. It was Kitwood's view that such styles of interaction have a profoundly damaging effect on the individual with dementia; indeed, he saw this as a more powerful influence on how the person feels and is able to function than the effects of the brain damage. It follows, therefore, that if these ways of behaving towards the individual have such a potent negative influence, reversing them and behaving in ways which acknowledge, encourage and celebrate the continued 'personhood' of the individual should have the opposite effect. Kitwood (1997) provides descriptions of positive ways of interacting, which he termed 'positive person work'. Examples of this include 'recognition':

> the caregiver brings an open and unprejudiced attitude, free from tendencies to stereotype or pathologize, and meets the person with dementia in his or her uniqueness. (p. 119)

Another is 'facilitation', which Kitwood (1997) defines as:

> a readiness to respond to the gesture which a person with dementia makes; not forcing meaning upon it, but sharing in the creation of meaning, and enabling action to occur. (p. 120)

Facilitation can be practised in both verbal and non-verbal ways. Accepting, for example, the initiation of touch by a person with dementia, and allowing the interaction to unfold at the person's own pace, while refraining from interpreting such an act solely within one's own frame of reference (perhaps as a demand for attention or as sexually motivated), would be one approach appropriately described as facilitation. An instance of verbal facilitation would be to adopt an encouraging and meaning-seeking demeanour in relation to speech which seems confused, rather than jumping to conclusions about what the person is intending to express or writing off their difficulty with expression as merely a symptom of dementia.

Other significant influences on our way of thinking about dementia as a condition include that of Feil (see for example Feil 1982). Writing during the 1980s and 1990s, and indeed still teaching at present, Feil developed the concept of 'validation', which essentially involves valuing and responding to the person's own subjective reality, and acknowledging feelings expressed, even if these seem very confused. This approach stood in contrast to the dominant ideology of that period which emphasized the need to orientate the person with dementia to a shared reality, for example by continually reminding them of the date and time, and where they are. The work of Miesen (1999) has applied psychological theories of attachment (Bowlby 1969) between adults and children to the situation of people with dementia who demonstrate their sense of wishing to be with long-dead parents.

To return to the theme of communication specifically, work which began independently of Kitwood's came from Killick. His views about the place of communication in our work with persons who have dementia developed through direct experience of encountering individuals living in nursing homes as a writer in residence. His own journey started with complete ignorance of the dementias and the experiences of people living with them, followed by feelings of confusion, distress and alienation, and moved towards the realization that the people he met in the first dementia unit he entered were in fact communicating with him and with each other, but in a way that required a degree of personal immersion in the world in which all this was taking place in order to understand what might be being said. His background as a poet and critic gave him a distinctive perspective on what he experienced in this context, in particular enabling him to appreciate the inherently creative and poetic qualities of the language of the unit's residents. Close observation of the non-verbal dimensions of these people's communication was rewarded by the discovery, again, of a coherence which was hitherto imperceptible. This story, and subsequent experiences and reflections are most fully presented in Killick and Allan (2001), but two books of poems, 'found' and developed by Killick in the speech of people with dementia, most of whom were living in nursing homes, have also been published (Killick 1997, Killick and Cordonnier 2000).

Following on from Kitwood and others, and coming from a research perspective, another significant contributor was Goldsmith. In 1994 he sought the views of a large number of individuals, including people with dementia, their relatives and professionals working within the field of dementia care in many different roles. He gathered these perspectives together in a book (Goldsmith 1996) which has served as a turning point for many people, crystallizing and influencing their own views about the subject of communication. Goldsmith presents the main themes of his data as the individuality of each person with dementia and the importance of appreciating their own unique subjective 'reality'. He explores the crucial role of non-verbal communication and the impact the physical environment can have on people's ways of communicating. He suggested that incidences of so-called 'challenging behaviour' are best reframed as acts of communication, and highlights the crucial dimension of 'pacing' in interactions ('outpacing', consistently moving or talking at a speed which exceeds the capacity of the other person, is another of Kitwood's examples of malignant social psychology). Goldsmith concludes that, although dementia makes it more difficult for people to communicate, it is our responsibility as people without dementia to embrace as inclusive a view of communication as possible, and to provide opportunities for people with dementia to overcome the obstacles that face them.

Since the work of Goldsmith and the continuing contributions of Killick to the field of communication, a major strand of research has investigated ways of involving and consulting people with dementia about their views of services. During the early 1990s a small number of small-scale studies investigated the feasibility of asking people with dementia about their views of the services they were using (for example, Lam and Beech 1994, Sutton and Fincham 1994 and Sperlinger and McAuslane 1994). These studies were carried out within the field of clinical psychology, and concluded that people with dementia do indeed have views and can express them given the right kind of support. However, most of this work involved people who retained good verbal skills. In direct follow-up to Goldsmith's work, and as a continuation to this set of studies, Allan (2001) undertook a study which sought to explore the process of consulting service users with dementia about their views of the support they used, and to investigate how people with more advanced dementia can be helped to express opinions and needs.

The study involved direct care staff in creating situations in which individual service users could be encouraged to share their views, then supported the practitioner participants in reflecting on the experience and outcomes of these initiatives, and planning how successful interactions could be followed up and approaches developed. As well as generating ideas for how people with dementia can be encouraged to express their views, the study highlighted a number of issues about how communication must be integrated with the organization and delivery of the whole service. These issues are discussed in greater detail later in this chapter.

The idea of 'person-centred care'

The term 'person-centred care' for people with dementia is a direct development of Kitwood's ideas about the nature of dementia and now has an established place within the vocabulary of those concerned with understanding dementia as a condition and providing support for those living with it. (The history of the term 'person-centred' and its relationship to the use of the term within the field of psychotherapy are explored by Morton 1999.) However, despite its frequent use, Kitwood never provided a fully comprehensive description of what constitutes person- centred care, and how its successful implementation can be brought about and objectively measured.

Tools such as Dementia Care Mapping (Bradford Dementia Group 1997) have contributed towards this aim and continue to undergo revision as ideas about care practice develop (Brooker 2002). Dementia Care Mapping is a method of capturing information about the activity profile and apparent level of well-being or ill-being of individual service users within a care context. Ratings are made of an individual's activities and apparent emotional state by a trained 'mapper' every few minutes for a period of several hours. This information is processed to reach overall scores, and should be fed back to the team of practitioners providing the care in order that strengths and weaknesses of practice and team function can be recognized and addressed.

However, questions about the robustness of person-centred care as a concept and its feasibility as a practice continue to be raised (for example Baker et al. 2003; Sheard 2004), and form an important part of our developing understanding of how theory relates to practice, and how in turn, behaviour can be changed and enlightened practices can be established and progressed.

Communication and person-centred care

We can see that given the socially constructed nature of 'personhood', it follows that if the absence of communication, and therefore the absence of genuine relationships between the individual who has dementia and those in a supporting role, is damaging to the person with dementia, then it must also have a detrimental effect on the person who is providing the care. This crucial part of the equation is often ignored in systems and organizations which see care workers as depersonalized 'units' with a crucial operative role, but not fully as people requiring consideration and support in their own right. The centrality of communication to practitioners' sense of meaning in what they are doing is illustrated by this comment which came from a care worker taking part in a study carried out by Ekman et al. (1991):

> When you cannot get into contact with the patient you feel insufficient, without hope, dissatisfied or burned out. Care seems meaningless. You lose your commitment. (p. 168)

At this point in the argument we are in a position to recognize that creating opportunities for high-quality communication, both between practitioners/family carers and people with dementia and between people with dementia, forms an essential ingredient in the kind of support people with dementia need. Being able to retain valued relationships and develop new ones through genuine communication will not only enhance the quality of life of people with the condition; it should, if Kitwood's theory is accurate, actually constitute a force which has the potential to counteract the progress of the dementia itself. Also, creating opportunities for genuine communication to take place between service users and those with responsibilities to provide support is an essential part of a meaningful and satisfying experience for workers. Again, we can see the reciprocity of the situation, mirroring Kitwood's ideas about the nature of personhood.

In 1999 Gibson posed the question 'Can we risk person-centred communication?'. Her answer to this question is a resounding 'yes':

> We must employ whatever power we have in the world of dementia care for this purpose. We must use our present knowledge, our skills and feelings to communicate. We are morally obliged to continue working in extending our limited understanding, developing our embryonic skills and taming our deep anxieties. (p. 24)

But, in reaching this conclusion, she presents a thorough consideration of what is required for such an ideal to become reality. She writes of
the ethical dimensions which arise in the pursuit of genuine communication, considering the risks which face persons with dementia themselves,
and those who support them. The 'technical' issues, namely what we have
available in terms of the kinds of approaches which can be used in the
service of communication, are reviewed and difficult questions about
resource implications are confronted. Gibson's article provides a powerful 'taking stock' of where we have reached in terms of thinking about
communication and its costs and benefits. But we are still faced with the
question of how in practice we can achieve the quality of communication
that both persons with dementia and those who support them, either in
family or paid positions, deserve.

Despite our progress in recognizing the place of communication in the
services we provide, there remain considerable obstacles in giving this
aspect of our work the prominence it requires. One frequently mentioned
issue is that of time. Practitioners often complain that they do not have
sufficient time to engage properly with the people in their care. Although
realistically the shortage of human resources in health and social services
imposes limitations, this is not the whole story. Unfortunately, in many
settings there persists a negative attitude towards care staff devoting time
to communication as an activity in its own right. A worker seen sitting
down engaged in a conversation with a service user may not be seen as
doing 'real' work, and may be criticized either explicitly or implicitly. This
way of thinking often forms part of a broader set of attitudes which con-
ceptualize 'care' as a set of discrete tasks to be completed, rather than as
a process which seeks to engage with individuals at deeper levels. Such
attitudes constitute formidable obstacles to the development of services
which recognize and nurture personhood in both users and practitioners.

Another such limitation is our own short-sightedness about what constitutes communication at all. In what the ethicist Post (1995) describes as
our 'hypercognitive culture', 'clarity of mind and economic productivity
determine the value of human life' (p. 3).

This means that we tend to attach greater importance to the use of language than to non-verbal dimensions of communication. It is common to
hear health and social care professionals say that someone with dementia
'can't communicate', when what they really mean is that the person has
largely stopped using verbal language. The fact that they are expressing
their thoughts and feelings through a wide variety of non-verbal means
tends to be overlooked and undervalued. This bias towards the verbal is
something we need constantly to guard against, and we need to challenge
our own powerful predispositions towards verbal communication, on
both the personal and professional levels.

Moving forward

What, then, do we need to think about in enhancing the potential for communication to take up its rightful place in services for people with dementia? Allan's (2001) research exploring the process of consulting and involving persons with dementia in developing services highlighted the following needs.

Person-centredness must apply to workers as well as service users

If we are serious about our commitment to developing practices which truly acknowledge and celebrate the unique needs and experiences of persons with dementia, it is impossible to do this while ignoring and riding roughshod over the needs and experiences of those who provide care. We have seen that in order for workers to have a positive sense of meaning in what they do, they must have genuine opportunities for communication with service users, and this means that their own experiences and needs as individuals come into the equation. A system which calls upon workers' humanity in the very delivery of the services it provides cannot simultaneously deny the needs of staff that arise in the course of the work that they do. What this means in practice will vary from context to context, and will depend on the characteristics of the individuals involved, but at the very least it must involve a commitment to providing training and supporting opportunities for staff to express and reflect on their needs, and in changing arrangements to meet practitioners' needs where at all possible.

Positive values and practices must be supported by every member of the team

Although individual acts of high-quality communication are of great value, for a team to work effectively there must be a collective commitment to a philosophy of care and to helpful practices. It is unfortunately true that even relatively infrequent instances of being undermined in terms of personhood and communication can have a very negative effect overall, especially for people who are vulnerable, such as those with dementia. A collective approach of the kind being envisaged here, however, should not be equated with a situation in which everybody is expected to do the same things in the same ways. Indeed, this would go against the understanding of what it means to be a person upon which we are building this argument. Just as each person with dementia is unique, practitioners are individuals, and this means that each person will have their own ways of doing things, and their own individual styles of relating to people. A 'whole team' approach to communication must support and encourage this diversity while at the same time enabling each practitioner's practice to reflect and sustain a deeper unity. This leads on to our next point.

Practitioners must have opportunities to reflect on their experiences and develop their understanding of what is going on both for them and for their service users

Communication is an extremely complex activity, and the reasons why we do what we do are seldom, if ever, immediately and completely apparent. There is also the fact that whenever any of us communicates with another person the words and actions we use to convey our message are influenced by a multitude of variables. Our personal history, our background and culture, our emotional and physical states all play a part. What we say and do may be influenced by aspects of the physical environment, how well we can see or hear, and what has happened in the recent past. A myriad of assumptions and expectations about other people come into play and influence our behaviour. In addition, all the same sorts of factors affect the person with whom we are trying to communicate. Whatever we may believe about the distinction between our 'professional' and 'private' identities, it is impossible for us to separate the intimacy of the personal from the ways in which we communicate. Nor is it desirable that we should try. New ways of understanding dementia teach us that we must use ourselves – not just a set of attitudes, knowledge and skills – in our attempts to engage positively with persons with dementia. But this makes the practice of reflection essential. By 'reflection' here we mean the attempt to understand the reasons underpinning the actions and words which constitute communication. Without a commitment to supporting practitioners in engaging in genuine reflection, including reflection on the reasons for our own actions and responses as well as those of people with dementia, real communication will prove elusive. Our all too human tendencies to rely on assumptions and 'shortcuts' – which in reality act to short-circuit the potential for connection – will always dominate. Müller-Hergl (2004) talks about this issue in terms of the need to avoid 'depersonalization':

> . . . dementia care is neither a technique nor a medical skill proper but an art and a human skill. . . . Reflection in the act of care delivery (being accepting and observing myself in how I am accepting) is necessary. (p. 9)

He goes on to talk about how a failure to reflect can lead to the potentials which exist in many, if not all, human beings, for negative and destructive patterns of behaviour, for example avoiding contact at a meaningful level, to predominate.

Reflection at a practitioner–practitioner level is also essential

One of the major findings of Allan's (2001) research was the value gained by opportunities for practitioners in a service to come together with the aim of reflecting on issues of communication. These often took the form of discussion of particular incidents or interactions, and proved successful not only in gaining a greater understanding of the experiences of particular service users, but also about themselves as people and practitioners and how they functioned as a team. It was often at these times that members of the team realized that they held different views about particular people, or made different interpretations of the same events or interactions. Sometimes it became apparent that they each held separate pieces of the jigsaw which, when put together, made the reasons for a particular problem obvious, or pointed towards a change which could alleviate difficulties or improve someone's quality of life. It was clear that regular shared reflection between members of a team had to be integrated with the routine of the service, and that activity was distinct from the mere 'handing over' of information arising from one particular shift.

Communication between members of a team can also have the benefit of helping individual members to understand why, for example, some people have more spontaneous or more effective relationships with some service users than others. Again, it is essential that the individuality of each member of the team is appreciated and utilized in creative ways, and that not everyone will approach the same situation or need in identical ways. This need may seem at odds with the increasingly pervasive imperative of establishing 'evidence-based' practice where there is often considered to be one 'best' way of achieving certain outcomes, but this is a dilemma which must be faced and thought through if our commitment to the individuality of our service users is to be made real.

Efforts to improve the quality of communication within a service must be led and supported by those in authority

It may seem too obvious to point out, but it is impossible for the kinds of developments described above to come about if those in managerial roles are not fully behind the effort. Müller-Hergl (2003) has written about this subject in describing the joint nature of a contract between a learner on an educational course, and his or her team and managers.

The main outcome of Allan's research is a learning and development tool called *Finding Your Way: Explorations in Communication* (2002a). It is designed to be used in the context of everyday practice and provides a structure within which to explore communication with people with dementia generally, and to highlight opportunities for service users to be consulted and involved. The central idea of the tool is encapsulated in a series of three steps:

- The first is the practice of **focusing** on an aspect of communication, for example how someone uses eye contact. This kind of observation would be done during the course of normal interaction with the individual.
- The next step, the **reflecting** stage, involves using a set of questions which prompt practitioners to reflect on the variety of possible influences on what they have noticed at the focusing stage: for example, the

contribution of background and culture, emotion and mood, the effects of the environment, physical health and well-being, etc. Integral to this stage are prompts for practitioners to consider what they themselves are bringing to the situation, and what sorts of influences from their own lives could underpin patterns in terms of what they find important or significant.

- The third stage is called **exploring**, and this utilizes what has been learnt during the focusing and reflecting steps by continuing with actions or ideas that could enhance the quality of communication.

In addition to this material there is a source book and a set of leaflets which provide diverse perspectives on many aspects of communication, and suggestions for individualized ways of creating new opportunities and making the most of those which arise naturally. This material includes many quotations from people with dementia, relatives and practitioners. A fuller description of the tool and how it works can be found in Allan (2002b).

The tool can be used in many different ways to enhance communication. Although it is entirely possible for an individual practitioner to work through the material, real benefits to 'whole team' approaches can be gained from people who work alongside each other using the material together, for example by focusing on the communication style of a particular service user, perhaps a new person or someone who presents challenges, or by using the 'reflecting' questions in order to reach a deeper understanding of an incident that has already occurred in the service setting. The ideas presented in the material, and the practice of reflection, as guided by the questions provided, can open up opportunities for much more integrated ways of understanding what is happening within a team and how individuals function within that team. This is essential when working in such complex territory where personal values have such a significant impact on practice and outcomes.

In relation to the involvement of speech and language therapists specifically, the tool could promote more effective team working in at least two respects. Problems can arise where a specialist is involved in working with an individual who is also supported by other practitioners, many of whom may not understand fully the nature of both the assessment and intervention the specialist is providing. *Finding Your Way* could act as a bridge both in terms of enabling care practitioners to collect information regarding an individual's style of communicating which may be useful for an initial assessment, and also information for ongoing therapy input. Also, the structure for reflection and the various resources in the tool might form the basis for greater interaction between specialist practitioners and care workers, enhancing understanding of each other's roles and needs to the benefit of service users.

The environment and communication

There are two aspects of the relationship of the environment to communication which it seems important to discuss in this context:

- the effect of the physical surroundings in which an act of communication takes place
- the communicative potential or otherwise of the environment.

Concentrating first on the environment as an influence on an interpersonal interaction, there are many ways in which our surroundings can affect our ways of communicating. The very location of an interaction can carry a message about our feelings and intentions. Consider the difference between the experience of embarking on a conversation in a public context, where the presence and proximity of other people set limits on how far the conversation can go, and that of having a similar encounter in private surroundings. At all times we make choices about the physical contexts in which our interactions take place in order to influence the nature and outcomes of communication.

Then there are the many aspects of the physical surroundings which can affect the quality of communication in different ways depending on the characteristics and dispositions of the individuals involved. In terms of the external environment, the presence of buildings, traffic and noise affect the way we feel and behave, and could dispose us to completely different actions to those which feel natural in the presence of, say, hills, trees or the sea. Also, the many elements which combine to form the weather can exert a profound influence on the ways in which people behave and interact.

For indoor environments, the nature of furnishings such as chairs, tables and lighting can have significant effects on whether we feel inclined to stop and engage in communication or to keep moving. More transient variables such as the presence or absence of others, noise levels, temperature and air quality will also influence whether individuals want to spend time there and engage with one another or not. The presence of a television which is switched on can act as an inhibitor to interactions by drawing the attention of those present to it.

Different kinds of physical surroundings can have a profound effect on the ways in which people with dementia are able to express themselves, as this account from Kotai-Ewers (1999) (who has undertaken creative writing work with people with dementia in Australia) illustrates:

> After lunch we sat in the sunshine. Grant's fluency increased. He spoke of being a volunteer at the Centre. I was overcome with confusion. Could I have made a mistake? Was this really a new volunteer? For ten minutes while Grant spoke, I agonized about how I could explain my mistake to him. Suddenly his language lost cohesion. Several times during the following months I observed a similar improvement whenever we were outside. I was

intrigued as to possible causes. Was it direct sunshine? Or the freedom of open space? Or more probably a combination of these, together with the relaxing effect of nature. Some time later a sociologist assured me that researchers have found that even a picture of natural scenes can relieve tension. Presumably, for Grant at least, one of the outcomes of this release was improved verbal communication. He confirmed this preference for sunshine when I visited him at a respite home one afternoon. 'This is probably the best time. I like doing things in the warmth and things.' (Kotai-Ewers 1999)

Designing environments for people with dementia

In recent years, within the field of services for people with dementia there has developed a strong current of interest in how built environments (both external and internal) can be designed to provide maximum support, stimulation and enjoyment for people who have dementia. Marshall (see for example Judd et al. 1998, Marshall 2001, 2003) is an authority in this area, and has written about one of the principles of 'dementia-friendly design' being that the environment should 'be orientating and understandable'. This is a form of communication. Examples of particular features which fulfil this need would be signs (for example on the door of a dining room) which are easily visible and make sense. (Think of how many different kinds of notices are used to signal whether a public toilet is intended for men or women. How many of these might pose problems for someone with dementia?) The use of contrasting colours can act as ways of drawing attention to important features of the environment, such as a red toilet seat against yellow walls of a cubicle, or the edge of a step on a flight of stairs. Blending certain features in with surrounding shades (for example a white electrical socket against a white wall) acts to minimize their impact and therefore make them less likely to attract notice. The thoughtful planning of physical space to enable easy visual access and orientation is another way of enabling the environment to communicate information which supports the functioning of people with dementia and avoids adding to their disabilities. Factors such as the presence and nature of noise must also be considered, given the high levels of hearing loss present among older people. These features and others have been incorporated into the design of the Iris Murdoch Building at the University of Stirling, which has been the home of the Dementia Services Development Centre since 2002.

Alongside the potential of the physical environment to convey information to us, there is also its potential to act as a channel for us to tell others about who we are as individuals. In Marsden et al. (2001), Calkins, who has led thinking about the subject of design for people with dementia in the US, takes us back to issues which are at the core of our appreciation of the personhood of individuals with dementia.

Recognizing how the development of dementia and the changes in people's lives which come about can often undermine the potential for an environment to reinforce the individual's sense of self and communicate this to others, these authors examine how the physical environments can provide opportunities for 'personalization': the expression of one's uniqueness as a human being. Ways of adapting a person's physical surroundings to support and enhance other aspects of personhood, such as the individual's need to maintain a connection to valued roles and activities, is another major theme. The issue of privacy and the need to have a sense of control over one's environment are also explored. The following perspective from an architect, Bennett (1997), highlights the cultural dimension of concepts such as privacy:

> Privacy is not such an issue for Aboriginal people out bush where everything is settled in public. This is, however, a way of life that is not common for non-Aboriginal people and can be quite stifling for them. Aboriginal people will often draw a semicircle with a fire at its centre and spaces radiating out from this to illustrate their preferred living arrangement. This allows people to sit at the fire and share in the community, and then withdraw but still be in touch. (p. 166)

Another approach to thinking about the physical environment is provided by Craig (Craig and Killick 2001, Craig 2002), as part of a broader stream of work investigating the potential of creative activities and the arts to enhance communication. Craig (2002) highlights the many possibilities that exist, even in environments which are far from ideal in terms of their overall design, for people with dementia to be encouraged to make choices and to create features which reflect their tastes, interests and lifestyles. She highlights the real danger of feelings of alienation, disorientation and distress by the lack of stimulation inherent in situations where, for example, an individual is confined to bed and can only see white cot sides, or blank ceiling tiles for much of the day. She describes her work with one man, Jack, who was confined to bed and had not spoken for a long time. He was considered to be uncommunicative. Over a period of many weeks Craig spent time with him, giving gentle encouragement to communication through the provision of various sorts of objects and textures for him to touch and respond to. Over this time there were many changes in how Jack interacted with his surroundings and with people. He became more active and alert, spent less time asleep and became more expressive non-verbally. This in turn altered staff members' behaviour towards him, as they realized that he was making choices and expressing preferences. This is one of many examples Craig provides of people with even very severe disabilities having the capacity to respond to the approach of others, and for their apparently 'lost' personhood to become real again. We need to value these sorts of acts of communication in their own right, and allow them to challenge our assumptions about the nature of dementia as a condition.

There is a strong sensory theme in Craig's approach which builds on previous work (see a review by Ellis and Thorn 2000) exploring the potential of stimulating the senses in pleasant and meaningful ways to enhance well-being and to increase opportunities for communication and appreciating the uniqueness of individual persons with dementia. There is also an interesting overlap here with work on designing environments for people with dementia, particularly on the subject of designing gardens (Pollock 2002, Melling 2003, Cobley 2003a, 2003b)

Other work which has formed part of Killick's 'Communication Through the Arts' project, based at the Dementia Services Development Centre in Stirling University, has provided inspiration for how people's physical surroundings can become part of an inclusive and innovative approach to communication. People in a nursing home in Wales created a series of mosaic and painted murals depicting aspects of life in their town, and these were mounted in the garden of the home. A project in Devon (Wayland and Cosgrove 2002) explored the theme of 'growing things' to create a variety of different art forms, some lasting, some transient, but all of which were rooted in appreciation of both internal and external environments as a kind of 'canvas' and inspiration for creativity. Rose, a documentary filmmaker, has supported individuals with dementia in making their own short videos presenting themselves and their lives in their own ways (Rose 2001). Often these have a strong theme of the role of physical surroundings, both past and present, as a backdrop for significant experiences and as a way of continuing to project information about the self and kick-start interactions and new relationships.

Conclusion

Communication is at the heart of what makes us 'persons' in the fullest sense, and this is as true for those who have dementia as for anyone else. Indeed, in line with Kitwood's psychosocial model of dementia the maintenance and development of genuine relationships through communication has the power not only to preserve the individual's personhood, but also to alter the individual's experience and journey through the dementia, and to challenge our understanding of the nature of dementia as a condition. The socially constructed nature of personhood also means that the personhood of those surrounding the person with dementia, whether in a professional or family role, must also be recognized and nurtured.

For those coming into contact with people with dementia there is a great need for development and deepening of an understanding of what it means to communicate. In particular, a much fuller appreciation of the richness, complexity and potential of non-verbal communication is required in this context, and it is incumbent upon us all to recognize and reflect on what we bring to our encounters and relationships with people with dementia.

The influence of the physical environment, both in terms of how it affects communication and also the potential of one's surroundings to act as a channel for communication needs to be appreciated and utilized. There exists great scope for continued development in this area, particularly through the involvement of people with dementia themselves in expressing their own individuality, preferences and needs through their surroundings.

References

Allan K (2001) Communication and Consultation: exploring ways for staff to involve people with dementia in developing services. Policy Press, Bristol.

Allan K (2002a) Finding Your Way: explorations in communication. Dementia Services Development Centre, Stirling.

Allan K (2002b) Focusing, reflecting and exploring how to communicate effectively. Journal of Dementia Care 10(5): 16–17.

Baker C, Edwards P, Packer T (2003) You say you deliver person-centred care? Prove it! Journal of Dementia Care 11(4): 18–20.

Bennett K (1997) Cultural issues in designing for people with dementia. In: Marshall M (ed.) State of the Art in Dementia Care. Centre for Policy on Ageing, London.

Bowlby J (1969) Attachment and Loss, Vol 1. Hogarth Press, London.

Bradford Dementia Group (1997) Evaluating Dementia Care: the DCM method, 7th edn. Bradford Dementia Group, University of Bradford.

Brooker D (2002) Dementia Care Mapping: a look at its past, present and future. Journal of Dementia Care 10(3): 33–36.

Cobley M (2003a) A place to delight the senses and refresh the soul. Journal of Dementia Care 11(4): 2–23.

Cobley M (2003b) Designing a garden for people with dementia. Journal of Dementia Care 11(5): 22–23.

Craig C (2002) Creative Environments. Dementia Services Development Centre, Stirling.

Craig C, Killick J (2001) Transformations . . . from awakenings. Journal of Dementia Care 9(5): 10–11.

Ekman SL, Norberg A, Viitanen M, Winblad B (1991) Care of demented patients with severe communication problems. Scandinavian Journal of Caring Sciences 5(3): 163–170.

Ellis J, Thorn T (2000) Sensory stimulation: where do we go from here? Journal of Dementia Care 8(1): 33–37.

Feil N (1982) V/F Validation: The Feil Method. Edward Feil Productions, Cleveland, OH.

Gibson F (1999) Can we risk person-centred communication? Journal of Dementia Care 7(5): 20–24.

Goldsmith M (1996) Hearing the Voice of People with Dementia: opportunities and obstacles. Jessica Kingsley Publishers, London.

Judd S, Marshall M, Phippen P (1998) Design for Dementia. Dementia Services Development Centre, Stirling.

Killick J (1997) You Are Words: dementia poems. Hawker Publications, London.

Killick J, Allan K (2001) Communication and the Care of People with Dementia. Open University Press, Buckingham.

Killick J, Cordonnier C (2000) Openings: dementia poems and photographs. Hawker Publications, London.

Kitwood T (1997) Dementia Reconsidered: the person comes first. Open University Press, Buckingham.

Kotai-Ewers T (1999) Falling apart: an in-depth view of one man's progress with early onset Alzheimer's Disease. Paper given at the International Alzheimer's Conference, Johannesburg, 1999.

Lam J, Beech L (1994) 'I'm sorry to go home.' The Weekend Break Project: Consultation with Users and Their Carers. Monograph available from Department of Psychology, St Helier NHS Trust, Sutton Hospital, Cotswold Road, Sutton, Surrey, SM2 5NF.

Marsden JP, Briller SH, Calkins MP, Proffitt MA (2001) Creating Successful Dementia Care Setting: enhancing identity and sense of home. Health Professions Press, Baltimore, MD.

Marshall M (2001) Care settings and the care environment. In: Cantely C (ed.) Handbook of Dementia Care. Open University Press, Buckingham.

Marshall M (2003) Not just because we can do it. Journal of Dementia Care 11(6): 10.

Melling G (2003) A sensory garden created by, with and for residents. Journal of Dementia Care 11(5): 24–26.

Miesen B (1999) Dementia in Close-Up. Routledge, London.

Morton I (1999) Person-Centred Approaches to Dementia Care. Winslow, Bicester.

Müller-Hergl C (2003) Focus on the change agent. Journal of Dementia Care 11(6): 8–10.

Müller-Hergl C (2004) Reflection is essential. Journal of Dementia Care 12(3): 9.

Pollock A (2002) Designing Gardens for People with Dementia. Dementia Services Development Centre, Stirling.

Post SG (1995) The Moral Challenge of Alzheimer's Disease. Johns Hopkins University Press, Baltimore, MD.

Quinton A (1973) The Nature of Things. Routledge, London.

Rose S (2001) Video Portraits: acknowledging the whole person. Dementia Services Development Centre, Stirling.

Sheard D (2004) Person-centred care: the emperor's new clothes. Journal of Dementia Care 12(2): 22–24.

Sperlinger L, McAuslane D (1994) 'I don't want you to think I'm ungrateful . . . but it doesn't satisfy what I want.' Monograph available from the Department of Psychology, St Helier NHS Trust, Sutton Hospital, Cotswold Road, Sutton, Surrey, SM2 5NF.

Sutton L, Fincham F (1994) Client's perspectives: experiences of respite care. Psychologists' Special Interest Group in Elderly People Newsletter 49: 12–15.

Wayland K, Cosgrove H (2002) Light at the end of the tunnel. Journal of Dementia Care 10(6): 14.

CHAPTER 8

Speech and language therapy intervention for people with Alzheimer's disease

JACKIE KINDELL AND HELEN GRIFFITHS

This chapter is based on the accumulated clinical experience of the authors, who have worked as speech and language therapists within dementia services in the National Health Service in the UK. These services have fallen within the spectrum of mental health rather than elderly care services and have comprised a community mental health team and day hospital for people with dementia, in addition to inpatient mental health assessment and continuing care for those with severe and enduring mental health problems. People under 65 years of age with dementia have also been cared for by these services. This model of service appears to be typical of many old age psychiatry services in England, although the level of speech and language therapy provision seems to be greater than that available to many services (Ponte 2001).

This chapter outlines the contribution speech and language therapists can make in the management of individuals with Alzheimer's disease and their families and carers. This will be considered from the earliest point an individual may have contact with secondary services – that is, the point of diagnosis – and follows the person's journey through the course of the illness to the latter stages when extensive care at home or in a residential setting may be required. A series of illustrative case studies is used to demonstrate speech and language therapy input for people with dementia at different stages of the condition.

Working within a wider context

Recent years have seen a fundamental change in the conceptualization of the dementias. Dementia was considered 'a generalized impairment of intellect and memory' and the belief was that forms of dementia were indistinguishable on clinical and neuropsychological grounds. Perhaps arising from the beliefs of global intellectual impairment, a paternalistic

201

approach to the care of people with a dementia developed. Basic care was provided, but people were disadvantaged, as their communication, including language and behaviour, was seen as meaningless, negative and problematic.

That there has been a change in our conceptualization of the dementias is evident in the organization of this book. A number of chapters are organized around the notion of distinct clinical syndromes within the rubric of dementia. Although cross-cutting issues are recognized, variation in the nature of the impairments and in the evolution of the clinical syndromes is identified.

A greater understanding of the nature of dementia and the contribution of academics such as Tom Kitwood has altered the culture of care in dementia in recent years. There has been a move away from focusing solely upon the impairment, and towards reaching an understanding of the experience of the person with a dementia and the effects of the changes that the dementia brings to the family. Thus the medical model has been challenged as the guiding philosophy in dementia care. Kitwood argued that concentrating solely on the neuropathology and ignoring other important factors gave an incomplete picture of dementia, highlighting the importance of psychological and social factors in maintaining 'well-being' (Kitwood 1993). He defined an individual's dementia (D) as the result of a complex interaction between five main components: personality (P), biography (B), physical health (H), neurological impairment (NI) and social psychology (SP). He put forward the relevant factors in the following equation to explain this interaction:

$$D = P + B + H + NI + SP$$

In examining social psychology, Kitwood concentrated on the interpersonal environment of the person with a dementia and the importance of relationships in maintaining a sense of self (Morton 1999), using the term 'personhood' to capture an individual's social requirement for the maintenance of self. He suggested that this personhood required a living relationship with at least one other, where there was a bond or tie, alongside a need for some place of significance within a human grouping, 'bound together on the basis of family, friendship, occupation, religion, neighbourhood or whatever' (Kitwood 1997a). In order to maintain personhood, an individual needs not only such relationships but also to be accorded status. Personhood can be affirmed if a person feels they have been 'treated like a real person' with their feelings acknowledged and their point of view valued. However, it can be denied by being in contact with people who do not fully acknowledge a person's presence, treat or act as if they are not there or not worthy of their full attention and consideration (Morton 1999).

Within the care environment, Kitwood examined everyday interpersonal interactions involving people with dementia and found them lacking the essential ingredients of empathy, acceptance and support.

Instead, he found a range of interpersonal interactions displayed by caregivers and professionals that he regarded as damaging to personhood. This set of characteristic behaviours he termed 'malignant social psychology'. These included a range of behaviours including ignoring, disempowerment, infantilization and mockery (Kitwood 1997b). This had resonance for many working within the field and has been described as the 'old culture of dementia care', where the care and the environment could lead to a downward spiral of disability. In contrast, Kitwood outlined the need to concentrate on promoting the 'well-being' of the person with dementia. In order to achieve a state of well-being, five psychological 'needs' should be fulfilled:

- attachment
- psychological comfort
- a sense of identity
- occupation
- inclusion in groups.

Dementia makes these needs harder to attain, and the goal of Kitwood's notion of 'person-centred' dementia care can be seen as an attempt to fulfil these needs (Morton 1999). Later work concentrated on equipping caregivers with the skills, knowledge and working environments that would allow them to move from negative caregiver practices and replace these with 'positive person work' (Kitwood 1997a). Characteristics of positive practice were identified and included collaboration, validation, recognition and facilitation. These positive aspects were the hallmark of the 'new culture of dementia care' (Kitwood 1995). How to promote such values within dementia care settings is discussed in Chapter 7.

Dementia care evaluation

The tool of Dementia Care Mapping is an observational method developed by Kitwood and the Bradford Dementia Group, to evaluate the quality of care. In essence the tool evaluates both positive and negative aspects of the social psychology of a care environment (Fox 1995). Dementia Care Mapping has been widely adopted internationally to audit dementia care settings. Training in this method is delivered initially through a 3-day course, with further study for more experienced 'mappers'. Because analysis of interaction and engagement are core elements within Dementia Care Mapping, it is of interest to speech and language therapists. Attempts have been made to examine the validity of Dementia Care Mapping, with positive results (Beavis et al. 2002, Fossey et al. 2002), and inter-observer agreement has been confirmed (Fossey et al. 2002, McKee et al. 2002). However a recent study has questioned both the reliability and validity when used by routine care staff rather than professionals skilled in research, showing, for example, low levels of inter-observer agreement and difficulty in measuring well-being as a separate construct from level of dependence (Thornton et al. 2004).

Validation therapies

Another strand in the dementia care literature encompasses the analysis, understanding and response to confused speech and challenging behaviours. In response to dissatisfaction with work to orient confused older people, Feil has over a number of years developed a theory of 'validation therapy' (Feil 1993). The main aim is to listen to whatever the person with dementia is trying to communicate about his or her feelings in order to establish a dialogue and to 'validate' what is being said, rather than correcting factual errors in orientation. Validation attempts to explore the subjective inner world and reality of a person with dementia and to validate their feelings. The technique can be used in individual and group situations. Responses always facilitate and accept what is being communicated: crying and pacing behaviours may be lessened, while speech, non-verbal communication and eye contact may be improved (Feil 1992). Agitation may be lessened in individuals who are distressed by reality orientation approaches (Dietch et al. 1989) (see Chapter 11).

Stokes (2000) has taken the notion of validation further and developed the practice of 'resolution therapy'. This outlines the need to adapt Rogerian counselling skills in order to understand the person with dementia and the reasons underlying their challenging behaviour. Although dementia is a barrier to communication and contact, confused speech and behaviour should not be ignored or seen as meaningless. Instead, they should be seen as an attempt by the person with a dementia to make sense of the environment or communicate an unfulfilled need. By using techniques of reflective listening, exploration, warmth and acceptance, the caregiver can take steps to understand the hidden meaning concealed by the confusion, acknowledge the feeling that may accompany the message and – if indicated – make any practical changes to meet these needs.

It can be seen, therefore, that facilitation of communication is a core aspect of these person-centred approaches to dementia care. Speech and language therapists have a vital contribution to make to such practices, because a central philosophy within the profession is that communication is about more than just the spoken word. Speech and language therapists are skilled in the analysis of both verbal and non-verbal communication, including facial expression, gesture and intonation, and use discourse analysis techniques to examine the part played by participants in a conversation, recognizing that communication is a collaborative process (Perkins et al. 1997). An understanding of 'shared knowledge', including biography, is central to understanding discourse. Speech and language therapists look beyond the impairment and examine other factors that may impact on communication, including the environment, believing that communication is possible at some level even when severe impairment is present, and thus it is possible to maintain interpersonal relationships. Communication is multifaceted, and individuals possess a unique profile of both skills and difficulties that speech and language therapists can assess in a variety of innovative ways using a range of tools including standardized tests alongside informal and observational techniques. For this reason no one is 'beyond assessment'. The authors believe that just as other patient groups, including those with progressive diseases, have access to specialist communication assessment and advice, those with dementia should have the same opportunities.

Multidisciplinary team working

It is important that the goals of speech and language therapy are in keeping with the team's overall aims for care of the patient and carer. Liaison with the multidisciplinary team should be seen as a priority. The presence of a speech and language therapist within the multidisciplinary team allows for specific communication and swallowing needs to be included in the planning of care and incorporated in the care plan. The care plan may be defined by the team at a ward round or case conference and it is important that the speech and language therapist attends in order to be involved in these discussions (Griffiths and Baldwin 1989). Sharing of skills is also important within the multidisciplinary team; the speech and language therapist can learn a great deal by working closely with other disciplines and conversely the team benefits from increased awareness of communication problems and how to deal with them (Bryan and Maxim 2002).

Patients in England receiving a specialist psychiatric service are presently managed within the guidelines of the Care Programme Approach (Warner 2004) and have a designated care coordinator (key worker) and a detailed specific Care Programme Approach assessment and care plan. Both authors have worked within community mental health teams providing a range of communication and feeding and swallowing interventions, as well as in particular cases adopting the care coordinator role and supporting patients and carers on a longer-term basis. The ability to undertake the care coordinator role will depend on the individual therapist's experience as well as the speech and language therapist being an integral part of the team. For a review of feeding and swallowing interventions for people with dementia, see Kindell (2002).

Presentation of language and cognition

Alzheimer's disease, a progressive neurodegenerative disorder, is the commonest cause of dementia in older people and accounts for approximately one third of cases of dementia in those less than 65 years of age (Harvey et al. 1998). The disorder has characteristic clinical and pathological features. It is insidious in onset and steadily progresses over a period of years. This period may be as short as 2–3 years but is frequently considerably longer (see Chapter 4 for further information on the disease process).

The clinical syndrome of Alzheimer's disease is now outlined, with the focus on the cognitive changes that occur. It is important to recognize the nature and the range of profiles of impaired and preserved cognitive ability which may occur in Alzheimer's disease, in order to understand the impact on communication. Language processes cannot be viewed in isolation, and so in addition to understanding the changes that occur in linguistic skills, speech and language therapists need to understand the contribution that non-linguistic cognitive domains, such as memory, make to communication. This has implications for the assessment and management carried out by speech and language therapists with people who have dementia. The cognitive impairment is typically characterized by memory impairment and disturbance in one or more higher cortical cognitive functions, which impact upon occupational or social functioning and activities of daily living (APA 2000). Neuropsychiatric features may be present and may include affective disturbance, delusions and hallucinatory experiences, and behavioural disturbance (Purandare et al. 2000).

Because the clinical presentation is heterogeneous, it is likely that there is more than one form of Alzheimer's disease. A number of neuropsychological profiles have been described in Alzheimer's disease, with variation both in the presenting cognitive impairment and in the development of additional cognitive difficulties (Neary et al. 1986, Martin et al. 1986, Becker et al. 1988, Price et al. 1993). The neuropsychological impairment in Alzheimer's disease therefore varies, not only in terms of severity over the course of the illness but also in the cognitive domains involved which include memory, language, visual perception and spatial skills, praxis and executive function.

Memory impairment is often the presenting and prominent symptom in Alzheimer's disease (Bayles 2003). Patients and carers report difficulties with recent memory such as being forgetful of day-to-day events, recent conversations and appointments. Questions may be repetitively asked for information that has already been given. Personal possessions may be mislaid within the home. These memory difficulties typically represent impairment in the formation of new 'episodic' memories, that is, the memory for personally experienced, context and time specific events. Impairment in the acquisition or learning of such information leads to problems in updating memory; for example, a person may recall some details of an event but not where or when it took place. Further, events from different points in time may be recalled as though they occurred simultaneously. If the person is disorientated in time, they may talk as though past events are currently occurring, for example a retired person may speak or behave as though they are still at work. Thus the content of speech will be affected as temporal relationships become eroded and events from different points in time are juxtaposed inaccurately. However, aspects of remote memory, such as autobiographical memory for the more distant past, may be rather better retained (Greene and Hodges 1996).

The episodic memory disorder may remain a relatively isolated symptom for a number of years (Neary et al. 1986, Perry et al. 2000), this selective amnesia reflecting the relatively circumscribed distribution of pathology within the medial temporal lobe structures. Typically, however, as the disease progresses, there is involvement of the posterior association cortex and deficits emerge in other cortically represented functions in addition to memory. Therefore the episodic memory impairment is often accompanied by emerging difficulties in linguistic and visual perceptual and spatial abilities.

The development of amnesia, with emerging language disorder and difficulties in visuo-spatial skills, is probably the most common neuropsychological profile in Alzheimer's disease, with fairly consistent staging of the evolution of the neuropsychological deficits possible (Lambon-Ralph et al. 2003). However, neuropsychological profiles that differ from this typical presentation have also been described (Neary et al. 1986, Lambon-Ralph et al. 2003). For example, it has been observed clinically that some patients with Alzheimer's disease rapidly lose track, both of what is said to them and what it is they are speaking about. Some patients also lose track of what it is they are doing. Losing track may occur in the absence of significant episodic memory impairment or language disorder. Indeed, it is the relative preservation of long-term retention that permits recollection of instances of losing track and enables some patients to comment on the phenomenon. Conversation may contain interjections referring to the experience: 'what was I saying?', 'what do you want me to do?', 'it's gone'. Patients also report difficulties in joining a conversation involving a number of people, and relatives believe they adopt a 'listening' role in such a situation. Spoken output becomes fragmentary and utterances are left incomplete as the idea of what the person was speaking about becomes difficult to hold on to. One patient reported to the authors that he felt that he 'couldn't reach the conclusion of a subject' and gave the following account of losing track of a subject:

/it's very difficult to get thoughts together and communication breaks down/you think you are in a void/it's like a veil comes over and you're trying to find your way out/it's quite a terrifying situation/it's like you're going upstairs for something/you've forgotten what you've gone for/difficult because it's happening all the time/it's gone within seconds/you're desperately trying to recall/I know I'm going to make a lot of mistakes/I can't think of the word or the line/the sentence/and you feel a bit of a fool/when suddenly whilst you are talking/the memory will go/like that/(clicks fingers) frequently when I'm talking to colleagues/you can feel it's going away from you/you are losing the thread of what you were saying/it's terribly frightening that is/

The early literature on the communication disorder in Alzheimer's disease described a reduction in conversational coherence. For example, people may have problems in the use and understanding of reference over the course of a conversation and in topic management. The authors have observed that patients who lose track have these difficulties. Some studies have emphasized the important interaction between linguistic and memory systems in discourse production (Ehrlich 1994, Almor et al. 1999), but others have described the phenomena of reduced conversational coherence as a disorder of pragmatics or social skills. The relative preservation of interpersonal and social skills in many people with Alzheimer's disease leads the authors to attribute at least some of these conversational problems to impairment in memory.

Problems in holding information in temporary store may impact upon language comprehension in certain circumstances. Research suggests that some individuals with Alzheimer's disease have difficulty in 'off-line' sentence processing tasks where a verbatim record of an utterance has to be held in temporary store while an additional task is carried out (Waters et al. 1995, 1998, Croot et al. 1999). For example, the Test for the Reception of Grammar (Bishop 1989) requires a comparative judgement to be made of which out of four pictures matches a sentence 'held' in the mind. These studies suggest that such problems may be due to impairment in verbal working memory, rather than difficulties in processing syntactic structures per se.

Prominent memory deficits are, however, not a prerequisite for the diagnosis of Alzheimer's disease (Snowden et al. 1996). For example, visuo-spatial problems may be the presenting cognitive feature and overshadow any problems with memory (Ross et al. 1996, Caine and Hodges 2001). Difficulties described by patients, who often have clear insight into their visual failure, include problems in reading and writing, difficulty in reading a conventional clock face and problems in aligning objects (for example, clothes when dressing and cutlery when setting the table). They may report difficulty initially in negotiating an unfamiliar and then later a familiar environment. The visual difficulties are sometimes misinterpreted by the patient as poor eyesight, but examination reveals elementary visual functions to be intact. The difficulties reflect problems in higher-order visual processing; including visual localization, visually guided movements and the appreciation of the spatial relationships between objects. This profile of cognitive impairment suggests a pattern of atrophy within the cerebral cortex which has a more posterior distribution than is typically seen in Alzheimer's disease, which is more commonly predominantly within the parietal cortices.

Some of the consequences of impaired visuo-spatial ability on communication are evident and indeed form the basis of the person's complaints. Difficulties in the visual localization of text, tracking along a line of text and moving from one line to the next mean that reading becomes problematic (attentional alexia). Writing difficulties also occur, characterized by difficulties in letter formation and in the correct spatial localization of writing on the page, with a relative integrity of oral over written spelling. Visual localization of pictorial material is also problematic. For example, the visual localization demands of multiple picture stimuli on a single page could impair performance on comprehension tasks thus giving rise to misleading results. Other consequences of impaired visuo-spatial processing on communication are less conspicuous but nonetheless significant. Deictic terms (those that 'point') become difficult for the person to interpret. For example, the request to 'put your arm in here' and the statement 'your cup of tea is over there' have little meaning unless the visual context is shared.

Alzheimer's disease may also present with other highly circumscribed psychological disorders including language disorder. There are a number of case reports in the literature where Alzheimer's disease (confirmed by post-mortem pathological findings) presented as a language disorder and where this feature preceded the development of other cognitive symptoms by many months or even years (Pogacar and Williams 1984, Jagust et al. 1990). However, although language disorder may dominate the clinical presentation, it is typically part of a spectrum of deficits including memory and visuo-spatial impairment.

From the above review of the language and cognitive deficits it can be seen that Alzheimer's disease does not result in a unitary neuropsychological syndrome. It therefore follows that assessment and management needs to be detailed and specific to the individual.

Role of the speech and language therapist

The role of the speech and language therapist may include:

- assessment and description of skills and difficulties with regard to communication
- contribution to the process of differential diagnosis of the dementia syndrome
- ascertaining whether communication difficulties are impacting on a person's level of behavioural disturbance
- advising on feeding and swallowing
- advising and/or providing the patient with external aids to help word-finding and memory, for example, word books, diaries, calendars and clocks
- information and education for patients and carers about Alzheimer's disease and how it affects communication
- support and counselling for the patient and carer
- specific advice to carers regarding strategies to facilitate communication
- information and/or provision of external aids to communication such as life story work, reminiscence or advice on appropriate activities to encourage communication

- advising on ways to adapt the daily routine to foster communication
- analysing the impact communication problems may have on assessments carried out by other disciplines, and facilitating such assessments
- helping plan for the future, for example, with regard to legal and financial planning
- referring carers and patients on to other appropriate agencies, both statutory and voluntary for further support and advice
- liaison and advice for care providers, for example day care, domiciliary and nursing home care regarding communication
- carrying out group therapy sessions for patients and/or carers, for example activity, information and support groups (in conjunction with other disciplines)
- training caregivers regarding communication and feeding and swallowing
- facilitating patients and carers with communication problems to express their views regarding their current or future treatment or care.

The remainder of the chapter will describe the areas of work outlined above in more detail using case examples.

Referral

Within the authors' practice, referrals come from all members of the old age psychiatry team. Assessment takes place in the most appropriate location – ward, day hospital or community. Referrals from the community are always seen on a domiciliary basis as this allows for informal assessment of communication in the home situation, discussion with significant others and a more holistic assessment of the person and their current situation. It also reduces non-attendance for patients living on their own who do not have the practical or organizational resources to arrange transport or remember appointments.

Assessment

Whatever the reason for referral, assessment should always begin with the patient and carer to ascertain their views and understanding of any communication difficulty. However, it is important to remember that the needs of patients and carers are not the same, and indeed at times can be in opposition and challenge our skills of providing person-centred care. The nature and extent of the assessment by the speech and language therapist will depend on the reason for the referral. For example, an assessment undertaken to establish the nature and likely aetiology of a language disorder will be very different from that carried out when looking at the impact of communication disorder on behaviour.

Cognitive evaluation has an important contribution to make in the diagnosis and differential diagnosis of dementia. Speech and language therapists have a vital role in the assessment of individuals with language disorder. Although their focus will be on linguistic processes, the therapist should also consider the assessment of those aspects of cognitive function which may be impaired and impact on communication. The therapist may wish to undertake this wider assessment or work alongside other disciplines; for example, occupational therapy, clinical psychology or nursing. In some services the speech and language therapist is a core member of the memory clinic, undertaking neuropsychological assessment following additional training. (See Chapter 6 for more information on assessment of language in dementia.)

Intervention

The early stages – patient-focused work

In the experience of the authors, there has been a change of focus in the delivery of speech and language therapy to people with Alzheimer's disease in recent years. Increasingly, therapy involves direct work with the individual with Alzheimer's disease whereas previously intervention was generally carer-focused. A number of patients themselves are requesting advice on a range of issues, including communication. These individuals are striking in their insight and articulation, and challenge the stereotyped view of people with dementia. It is likely that the development of anticholinesterase inhibitors in the treatment of Alzheimer's disease has led to an increase in the numbers of people seeking an early medical opinion about their memory difficulties and hence the possibility of an earlier diagnosis. A number of old age psychiatry services now run 'dementia treatment clinics' identifying patients early in their illness and providing monitoring of the range of medications available (NICE 2001) alongside information and advice about the condition. Variation in the provision of speech and language therapy and service delivery issues are discussed in Chapter 12.

Innovative service developments have included time-limited support and information groups for those living with mild dementia, including Alzheimer's disease. The opportunity to have contact with others in the same situation, to share experiences and to obtain information to help guide future financial and personal care planning appears to be valued by those attending. Such forums make significant demands upon vulnerable cognitive resources and therefore support needs to be in place to help participants with the process of the meetings. In the groups run by the authors, patients and their spouses or partners, who are invited to attend together, are sent a programme outline before the meetings. Key issues are summarized on a flip chart during the meeting. The summary provides an opportunity to review and remind members what has been discussed, and an overview of each meeting is written up for group members. Participants may also require individual support during the group, and some strategies are outlined below. These strategies would also form part of the advice given when working on an individual basis with patients and their carers. The general principle underlying the strategies is to try to compensate for or reduce demands upon impaired skills. This requires an understanding of the nature of an individual's difficulties by the caregiver and behavioural change on their part. Attempts are also made to capitalize upon intact abilities.

Where episodic memory difficulties impact on communication, the conversational partner can assist in the following ways:

- Understanding that the person may inaccurately associate events from different points in time and place. This knowledge can help the carer interpret apparently confused speech. Some individuals can use external aids such as a diary to help support recent memory. Studies suggest that, for people with more severe memory difficulties, providing contextual support (autobiographical pictures and statements in the form of a memory book) can help to enhance conversation (Bourgeois 1993, Bourgeois and Mason 1996).
- Being aware that some question forms demand significant retrieval and manipulation of information from long-term memory. Questions such as 'what have you done today?' are particularly demanding.
- Writing down key pieces of information; for example, in response to repetitive questions.

When individuals have particular difficulties in keeping track, the conversational partner can assist by:

- Not presenting too much information at any one time. Difficulties in holding information in temporary store mean that the person finds it difficult to assimilate all the information presented: information needs to be presented in chunks.
- Being aware that conversations involving a number of participants may be more difficult.
- Being aware of potential problems in the use of reference and that the person may have lost track of the subject matter. Restate referents and reduce the use of pronouns and other referring terms in conversation. It may help to restate the topic of conversation if it seems that the person has lost track.
- Using a normal rate of speech. In the past there been a tendency for speech and language therapists to advise slower rate of speech to aid comprehension. However, this advice may be counterproductive if the person is losing track. A slower rate of speech is likely to increase demands on auditory verbal memory (Small et al. 1997a, b).

Where individuals have particular difficulties in word retrieval the conversational partner can assist by:

- Using cueing techniques to support word retrieval where lexical access difficulties arise in the context of relatively good day-to-day and immediate memory.

The authors have found value in identifying with the patient instances of specific difficulties with particular vocabulary. Personalized word books have then been developed for use in specific situations. Some patients have also valued the opportunity for rehearsal. Some studies have explored specific memory re-training techniques in Alzheimer's disease. For example, trials of errorless learning techniques (where clinicians present the correct information in a way that minimizes the possibility of an erroneous response, e.g. by using supportive cues and using forced choice recognition tasks) suggest that some individuals are able to improve their performance on name retrieval in face/name association tasks (Winter and Hunkin 1999, Clare et al. 2000). Errorless learning techniques are thought to be effective in Alzheimer's disease because they reduce demands on the episodic memory system.

In the experience of the authors, caregivers derive most benefit when strategies are developed in relation to a specific problem that has been identified. For example, 'difficulties in following instructions given while the carer provides assistance with dressing'. Significant visuo-spatial difficulties lead to problems in orienting items of clothing and orienting body parts to clothing, and the ability to interpret deictic and spatial terms. Thus many instructions given in such a setting, for example, 'put your arm in here, over to the right, through there' (referring to the sleeve) are meaningless when the visual context is not shared and thus impossible for the patient to follow. Understanding the limitations allows more appropriate vocabulary to be used and the carer can approach the situation from the perspective of the patient. (See Chapter 9 for detailed discussion of working with family carers of people with dementia.)

Case example

The following case example illustrates some aspects of the contribution of speech and language therapy in the management of an individual with mild Alzheimer's disease.

Case study 1

Jean (58 years of age) was initially referred to speech and language therapy for assessment. The presenting problem was one of a gradual onset of word retrieval difficulties which had developed over a period of approximately 1 year. Jean had also noted intermittent spelling difficulties. She could give examples of recent incidents of such problems. Cognitive assessment revealed problems in lexical access with good semantic specification for items she had difficulty naming. No impairment was evident on formal evaluation of memory or other cognitive functions. Other investigations, including structural imaging, did not reveal any abnormalities. It was considered that the nominal difficulties heralded the onset of a degenerative disorder which was either Alzheimer's disease or frontotemporal lobar degeneration (Snowden et al. 1996).

The care plan included repeat speech and language assessment after several months to ascertain the nature of any evolution of symptoms. This revealed slightly more difficulties in word access and increased problems in spelling, although no phonological errors were evident. Problems in carrying out mental calculation and in keeping track were emerging. Day-to-day memory remained good. An anticholinesterase inhibitor was commenced on the basis that this woman had probable Alzheimer's disease.

Jean was invited to attend the support group for patients with Alzheimer's, as described above. As a result she made some practical and financial plans for her future, including putting in place an Enduring Power of Attorney. Jean was a widow who lived independently and worked as a volunteer in a local charity shop. She adopted a very pragmatic approach to her memory and speech difficulties when at work in the shop. She told others to remind her of things that she had forgotten. If she couldn't get a word, she asked others to supply it for her and not to leave her struggling. With the speech and language therapist she developed a personal vocabulary book which included the names of flowers, people and places. She referred to this book when she was in specific difficulties and others could not assist.

Jean enjoyed ballroom dancing and regularly attended events. She was aware that she could not always remember which dance had just been announced. As she did not have a regular partner to remind her, she was finding the situation frustrating. With the speech and language therapist she compiled a short list of dance names so that when a dance was announced she could mark it giving an opportunity for rehearsal before going on the dance floor. Identifying specific problems and developing appropriate strategies appears to be more valuable than simply providing general advice that can be hard to translate into action. These strategies were important in ensuring Jean maintained her social contacts and quality of life. Jean was subsequently discharged from speech and language therapy but staff in the dementia treatment clinic who were monitoring her medication had the option to refer her back to the speech and language therapist if necessary.

The middle stages – involving significant others

As the disease progresses, approaches to therapy may involve increasing collaboration with caregivers in order to facilitate communication.

Information and support is particularly important for the family. There may be involvement of other services such as day care or paid care in the home and these care workers may also require training regarding communication issues. Difficulties with behaviour become more prevalent (Purandare et al. 2000), leading to increased stress on the carer, and problems with comprehension begin to affect everyday life. Comprehension may be affected because of linguistic or memory problems, while expressive communication may become more hesitant and fragmented alongside difficulties with reading and writing. Increasing problems with memory lead to difficulties with retaining information and in some instances to repetitive questioning. However, it must be recognized that there may be a number of reasons for repetitiveness. A sense of anxiety or being ill at ease, which may originate from the amnesia, may underlie repetitive questioning. Responding to the emotion seems a more appropriate response in this case, including any practical changes to reduce distress. The person may experience significant frustration at their communication impairment and will be aware of their difficulties; however, insight and ability to reflect on this impairment may be variable.

It is important to be aware that, even at this stage, patients may present with very different patterns of communication, memory and other cognitive impairments alongside differences in personality, pre-morbid communication style and environment, and individualized advice will still be of more benefit than general communication advice. At times advice can easily sound critical or become burdensome if it is seen as imposed rather than agreed between the person, their carer and the health worker. It is therefore essential to negotiate mutually agreeable and realistic aims and objectives with all relevant parties.

Further advice for caregivers

- **Advice for word-finding difficulties:** It is usually helpful to give the person time to think for themselves, although it is important to be aware that they may lose track and forget what they were trying to say. If they are struggling and the word is obvious, say it naturally, as you would in normal collaborative conversation. If you need to guess, try to narrow down the topic using yes/no questions. However, there may be instances when you both need to 'give in gracefully' and having an appropriate phrase for such times is useful, for example 'don't think about it now . . . it might come back to you later'.
- **Advice for confused speech and behaviour:** Be aware that confabulation at times of memory failure is not a strategy intended to deceive, and that trying to reason or argue over confused speech and behaviour at this stage is often not helpful. This is not to say that such utterances are without meaning, and so validation of feelings and emotion may be more successful than reality orientation. Exploration

of the individual's viewpoint, including past experience and lifestyle, may yield practical solutions and responses, as in resolution therapy.

- **Advice for comprehension:** Giving information in specific 'chunks' tends to reduce the load on memory, but simplify syntax too. If possible, point to or take the person to the object you are referring to. If necessary, repeat and rephrase.
- **Advice on activities to encourage communication:** Doing things together encourages a shared focus in the 'here and now' and is often easier than conversation out of context. This includes a range of practical activities, reminiscence and life story work.

Life story work has been highlighted by a number of authors (Baker 2001a, Murphy 1994) as a useful way to encourage communication, particularly in Alzheimer's disease where it can tap relatively intact remote memory and can be used to support topics for conversation. Baker (2001b) argues that life story books can be extremely beneficial in the long-term care environment, providing opportunities to share important life events and reminisce; focus conversations around a shared theme; rekindle the relationship between spouses; provide a means of carer support; provide activity-based training in communication skills for care staff; and help staff acquire detailed knowledge of people which can, in turn, be used in the planning of more person-centred care and other ward activities. Bryan and Maxim (1998) evaluated a life story initiative conducted in a residential home and involving three people with advanced dementia. The six group sessions benefited the residents and provided an effective opportunity to train two members of the care staff to use validation techniques to encourage and enhance communication with residents who have dementia. After the initiative staff reported increased interaction with residents, increased awareness of communication issues, increased knowledge of the residents which increased quality of life for residents, e.g. by staff facilitating favourite activities, and a particular value to new staff in helping them to get to know residents. If patients are to use the books themselves, particular attention needs to be paid to delivering a clear layout with simple text.

The following case study illustrates work in the middle stages.

Case study 2

May (79 years of age) lived with her husband; their children lived abroad and kept in contact by phone. She was a retired clerical officer who enjoyed ballroom dancing and holidays abroad. The specialist nurse in the dementia treatment clinic who was monitoring her response to anticholinesterase inhibitor medication referred her to speech and language therapy. The Mini-Mental State Examination was part of the assessment to monitor response to treatment, and those scoring below a certain level were judged to be unable to benefit from the medication (NICE 2001). May had scored below this level, but had become very anxious during the assessment. The nurse felt that her significant communication difficulties had compromised her performance on this task and that May's husband needed advice about his wife's communication. The speech and language therapy assessment revealed moderate to severe word-finding difficulties, leading to very hesitant speech. In contrast, May had fairly preserved comprehension at a linguistic level. However, problems with immediate memory led to losing the thread of the conversation, leading to comprehension failure. In contrast to this, her day-to-day memory was less impaired. She was, for example, able to report some recent events in her life or in the news and retained some orientation for place and time. She could indicate the correct day, month, and place she lived from a written array, although spatial problems reduced her ability to read text.

The assessment had revealed that May had some islands of preserved skills, in spite of a low score on the Mini-Mental State Examination, and that her impaired communication was indeed compromising her performance on this test. A range of more appropriate tasks was outlined to assess May's orientation, memory, language and spatial skills for the purpose of assessment and reassessment. May was prescribed the medication and these tasks were used as a baseline to measure against future change. Together with the carer's report, they provided a more appropriate way to assess and measure change in her case.

May was aware of her difficulties with word-finding and this often led to frustration. Her husband reported that he worried about how to respond when May struggled to find a word. He had some understanding of her illness, but felt he needed more information. He was increasingly taking on more tasks in the home and the therapist was worried that he was becoming tired, but he refused all offers of help. Together the therapist, May and her husband produced a life story book using photos and simple written material to illustrate her life. Pages were left blank for new events to be added (for example her imminent eightieth birthday). The book provided an excellent shared focus to encourage communication and sparked off other activities including looking through books together and listening to old records.

May had enjoyed reading magazines before her illness, but was now finding this problematic largely because of her visual localization difficulties. Advice was given regarding written material. Magazines with pictures of famous people proved less demanding and enabled her to continue her enjoyment. Alongside this work on enabling reading, discussion took place with them both to define mutually agreeable ways to help word-finding difficulties, memory and comprehension failure (see above for specific strategies). There would, however, be occasions when communication failure would occur and such strategies would be inappropriate.

In order to reduce frustration on both sides, it was important to concentrate on non-verbal information, for example the emotion inherent to the communicative context, in order to try to understand what May was saying. The agreed strategies were then incorporated into an advice sheet.

Information about Alzheimer's disease and support available was provided for them, and as a result May's husband joined the local Alzheimer's Society. Following some physical health problems he agreed to a referral to social services. This culminated in a place 2 days a week for May at a day centre. As the speech and language therapist was the team member who knew May the best, she accompanied her on her first day at the centre. May took her life story book along with her and this proved a very useful aid both for communication and to help staff get to know her. The speech and language therapist outlined to staff May's background, biography, skills and difficulties and the most productive ways to encourage her communication.

Another role for the speech and language therapist may be to enable carers and patients with communication problems to express their views regarding health and social care. Currently there is an increasing emphasis on 'service user involvement' and the National Service Framework for Older People (DH 2001) highlights this involvement as a priority. Work at Stirling University has highlighted practical ways to engage people with dementia in consultation (Allen 2003). The Alzheimer's Society is also exploring ways to involve people with dementia in the society (see *Living with Dementia*, Alzheimer's Society 2002). (See Chapter 7 for further consideration of this issue.)

The following example outlines this role.

Case study 3

Mr and Mrs Brown lived together in a first-floor flat. Mrs Brown had been diagnosed as having Alzheimer's disease 3 years ago. Her husband cared for her very well, but found the burden of care increasingly stressful. Sadly he suffered a stroke and was admitted to hospital, and then to the local stroke unit. Mrs Brown's daughter, who did not live in the area, came to stay to look after her on a temporary basis. The staff on the stroke unit soon found Mr Brown's behaviour difficult to manage; he was described by staff as 'wandering' off the unit and they felt it would be unsafe to send him home, particularly given the home situation. He was referred to the psychiatrist who, in turn, asked for further speech and language therapy assessment to determine Mr Brown's wishes regarding his future care and that of his wife. The assessment revealed severe jargon aphasia alongside difficulties in organization and planning with intact non-verbal memory. Most importantly, however, through use of verbal, non-verbal and pictorial means the speech and language therapist was able to ascertain that Mr Brown was extremely worried about his wife and wanted to go home to look after her. Closer examination of recent events revealed that his 'wandering' had actually taken him to the correct bus stop to take him home. He had been brought back to the unit but was expressing through his behaviour his resistance to this course of action. This raised a number of issues including consent to care, and practical issues regarding how both Mr and Mrs Brown would cope, should he return home. He agreed to stay in hospital for a few more days whilst assessment and additional domiciliary care could be planned.

The speech and language therapist worked with the social worker to facilitate communication with both Mr and Mrs Brown, so they could engage in this process. It quickly became clear that Mrs Brown had her own communication difficulties relating to word-finding and memory. Through slow and targeted communication the therapist facilitated discussion, stopping to rephrase, use gesture or the written word to help comprehension and clarifying when expressive difficulties occurred. The greatest challenge was to ensure that Mr and Mrs Brown could discuss this in a collaborative way as any husband and wife would wish to do. A plan was developed to enable them to return home with extra support, alongside regular monitoring visits and an action plan should a crisis occur. The speech and language therapist was able to ensure they understood the process and their views had been included in the care plan.

Another aspect to the role of the speech and language therapist may be to highlight where development of further unexpected symptoms raises questions regarding an initial diagnosis. Because the speech and language therapist has knowledge of differing disease processes, and the patterns of communication and swallowing impairment that are expected to develop with time, such a referral can aid both the initial and the re-evaluation of diagnosis. The following case example highlights this role.

Case study 4

Mr Woods, who had Alzheimer's disease, was referred because he had difficulty with swallowing. In Alzheimer's disease, problems with swallowing typically emerge late in the disease when mobility deteriorates and other physical problems emerge. However, the referral stated an unusual pattern of difficulties in that Mr Woods was described as still mobile and going out alone, yet experiencing significant swallowing difficulties. Assessment revealed difficulties with swallowing at the oral and pharyngeal stage, alongside wasting of oral musculature and other muscle groups in the body. Cognitive and behavioural problems were present, with prominent stereotyped and repetitive speech and behaviour. The speech and language therapist felt this constellation of symptoms was not consistent with Alzheimer's disease and she therefore facilitated neurological and cognitive assessment. A diagnosis of frontotemporal dementia with motor neurone disease was confirmed. As Mr Wood's physical condition was deteriorating, the team's care planning process needed to respond rapidly.

The later stages – activity, engagement and training

In the later stages of Alzheimer's disease communication and memory become significantly impaired, alongside behavioural and functional decline. Communication difficulties impact on the person's ability to understand the daily routine and interventions, such as washing and dressing, and difficulty expressing their views, choices and needs. There is some evidence that behavioural disturbance is particularly associated with difficulties with communication, and that modification of communication can reduce agitation (Hart and Wells 1997). In providing care for those at this stage it is important to optimize communication as far as possible; this is a crucial aspect to maintaining dignity and providing truly person-centred care (Kitwood 1997b). The speech and language therapist therefore has an important role to play in evaluating communication in care settings (Le Dorze et al. 2000) and in training carers to modulate their input to meet the patient's needs (Jordan et al. 2000, Maxim et al. 2001).

At this stage formal assessment may not be possible and informal assessment and observation may be more appropriate. A great deal can be learned by sitting alongside the person, engaging in simple activities together, or observing or joining in the daily routine (Tanner and Daniels 1990). In spite of severe impairment, many patients with Alzheimer's disease retain the desire to communicate and a level of 'social speech' in particular. A number of linguistic tasks including automatic speech, sentence completion and familiar songs and prayers may yield an appropriate response. Such activities alongside non-verbal aspects of communication such as eye contact, intonation and facial expression make communication, particularly in the 'here and now', possible. Response to appropriate stimulation can often reveal surprising and rewarding responses for both the patient and the caregiver. For this reason, a wide range of activities has been suggested in the literature to facilitate communication in such individuals (Powell 2000, Perrin and May 2000).

Group initiatives

Reminiscence is widely used in dementia care settings because relatively intact remote memory can be used to support meaningful and enjoyable interaction. Group sessions may involve looking at objects or pictures from the past, listening to music, or watching slides or videos. The authors have worked with occupational therapists in delivering reminiscence sessions in day hospitals and continuing care environments. These sessions were useful as a therapeutic tool, but also as a means to assess and facilitate communication and memory in an informal manner (Griffiths and Burford 1988). Because a number of patients can be assessed within the group setting, this is also an efficient use of time. Jointly delivering sessions also enables disciplines to build relationships with each other and with patients.

Dance has been used in a variety of ways to engage people with dementia. Used creatively it can facilitate a more 'failure free' means of exercise than following an exercise routine, and can encourage both verbal and non-verbal aspects of communication. A project involving one of the authors employed a dance worker. The speech and language therapist observed sessions using a checklist to analyse patients' behaviour and communication and was able to demonstrate positive results during the sessions (Kindell 2003).

Sonas aPc is a multisensory group approach that was originally developed by Threadgold (Threadgold 2002, Hamill and Connors 2004). Training in this approach is provided by the Sonas organization. This approach is popular with speech and language therapists working in old age psychiatry, and many have become trained in the method particularly to use with more impaired patients. Other speech and language therapists have facilitated training in their place of work in order for others, e.g. support workers, to carry out this type of group work. The approach uses a set format for groups, using a tape to provide music and structure.

Multisensory work is used increasingly in dementia care and a number of old age psychiatry departments have developed multisensory rooms using lighting, music, projectors and tactile stimulation. Mobile equipment of this nature can also be used in a variety of ways to provide both stimulation and relaxation and has been shown to have positive effects on mood and behaviour immediately after sessions (Baker et al. 1997).

Later-stage ethical issues

It is in the later stages of Alzheimer's disease that difficulties with swallowing emerge, and the speech and language therapist may be involved in assessment and management of such difficulties. Because such problems usually occur at a stage when the person has significant physical and communication disability formal assessment may not be possible, and structured observation at mealtimes may be more appropriate (Kindell 2002). Close working with caregivers is vital for both assessment and management. Any management decisions should take into account quality of life issues and careful exploration of ethical issues is required with regard to decisions about non-oral feeding (Gillick 2000).

The following example discusses a project and case study to demonstrate work at the later stages of Alzheimer's.

Case study 5

In 2000 the local old age psychiatry unit had two continuing care wards but no therapy input from occupational therapy, physiotherapy or speech and language therapy. The management team wanted to improve the therapeutic input to the wards but was unsure as to how best this could be achieved. A pilot project was planned and a speech and language therapist was seconded from another area to coordinate the project. Funding was secured for two part-time therapy support workers to work across all disciplines to carry out interventions. The speech and language therapist supervised the support workers with input from physiotherapy and occupational therapy delivered on a sessional basis. With regard to communication, all patients were briefly assessed individually as well as while engaged in a variety of group activities. This allowed a profile of communication to be built up, as well as awareness of those activities most appropriate to each individual, and that particularly encouraged communication. The results of these assessments were combined with those from occupational therapy and physiotherapy and an activity programme, involving both group and individual work, was then drawn up to facilitate and maintain as many of the patient's skills as possible. Physiotherapy, occupational and speech and language therapy were no longer seen as discrete spheres of activity but delivered through a holistic model of therapy. An example of this in relation to one patient (Rose) is outlined below.

Speech and language therapy assessment showed that although Rose had advanced Alzheimer's disease she still made good eye contact and enjoyed social interaction. She had very little propositional speech but she could often engage in simple social speech, for example 'oh look', 'that's nice', etc. She responded well to facial expression. Rose had severe comprehension problems exacerbated by spatial difficulties in locating sounds and speech in the environment, and ascertaining which remarks were directed to her. She was thus easily overstimulated when the environment was too noisy and this could lead to her becoming first anxious and then angry. Her spatial difficulties also affected her ability to manipulate objects, localize pictorial material and follow commands in exercise sessions. It was clear from Rose's history that she had always been a very sociable person and that talking with friends was very important to her. Therapy needed to encourage talk while minimizing other difficulties. Advice was therefore given to the therapy support workers and ward staff regarding ways to capitalize on Rose's communication skills and how best to reduce frustration.

Activities were planned which could include Rose and use her skills. For example, although she found craft activities and following exercises particularly difficult and frustrating because of her spatial difficulties, she would sit and watch most activities and make comments when prompted. She particularly enjoyed rummaging through the 'feely box' containing a variety of objects and materials of different colours and textures. She would look through simple picture books and photos, especially of children and animals. Rose loved music and was best involved in exercises when movements were more automatic such as patting a balloon, holding onto a large elastic rope or parachute, and tapping her feet. Such 'non-verbal' activities often elicited communication on a number of levels. It was important to be aware with all activities, and particularly music, that overstimulation and fatigue could be a problem. If this was not recognized, Rose could become distressed and this would lead on to difficulties in behaviour. Rose's husband was interviewed before and after the therapy programme to ascertain his views. This showed that he was realistic about what could be achieved, but that he particularly valued the stimulation his wife was receiving. Ward staff also reported an increase in the amount and quality of Rose's communication during activities.

Training

Training regarding communication and swallowing difficulties is an important role for the speech and language therapist (Maxim et al. 2001). The authors therefore work closely with the local dementia care training project which provides training to both family caregivers and staff. A regular course for relatives and carers includes a session on communication that is delivered by the speech and language therapist. Courses for staff from health, social care, private and voluntary agencies include sessions directly on communication or where communication is a central theme, for example, person-centred care and activity. Within the old age psychiatry department there is an in-service training programme for unqualified nursing and therapy support staff, and the speech and language therapist makes regular contributions to this.

For the continuing care project described above, ongoing training and supervision of the therapy support workers was vital to ensure that activity and communication aims were realistic and valued. In order for the staff to feel positive about their work it was important to foster a philosophy where positive emphasis and value was placed on the responses and engagement of patients, no matter how small. Training regarding communication difficulties was therefore provided, alongside sessions to increase awareness of one's own communicative style and ways to adapt it to meet differing individual needs on a day-to-day basis.

Maxim et al. (2001) and Bryan et al. (2002) report on the effectiveness of a 1-day training package principally aimed at care assistants in the residential sector who had received no formal training in relation to understanding communication difficulties in older people and promoting communication. The 'Communicate' training, originally designed by Speakability, was shown to be effective in terms of care workers' knowledge of communication and their perceived effectiveness in using it (see Appendix 8.1 for carer questionnaires). Analysis of a video sample of interactions with older people (the vast majority of whom had dementia) taken before and after the training showed that the training had resulted in increased use of appropriate strategies to promote communication. (Bryan et al. 2002) (see Appendix 8.2 for the schedule of basic and advanced strategies.) Maxim et al. (2001) suggest that the factors that contributed to the success of the training were:

- involvement of representatives from the local speech and language therapy service
- mixed-level groups (contrary to the trainers' expectations)
- managers and supervisors involved in the workshops
- staff having had experiences of difficulty communicating with residents and therefore valuing the opportunity to talk through actual experiences
- material which summarizes the training being available to take away
- training a large proportion of staff within a unit and including some of the least experienced staff
- linking training to a national scheme such as NVQ
- practical skill training is an essential component of a training session.

Review and discharge

As with any work involving individuals with a progressive illness, measuring the outcome of therapy can be challenging. Therapy may be very wide ranging, including direct work with the patient, work with carers, training, provision of information and advice, or practical aspects including introducing patients to day care or other community groups. For this reason we have found that a system of goal-setting is useful both to determine the aims of intervention and to judge any change on review or reassessment. We have used a modified version of the East Kent Outcome Measures Scales (Johnson 1997) because this gives the freedom to define aims around the needs of both the patient and carer, or significant others including paid carers, or the multidisciplinary team. This can also be used with the patient and/or carer to ensure expectations of therapy are realistic and areas of concern to them are specifically targeted.

Clearly defining the goals of therapy also facilitates the process of review and discharge. Working alongside and planning with the multidisciplinary team will also help here. For example, following a period of intervention, disciplines may discharge a person whilst the planned care coordinator maintains contact for support and monitoring, with a view to re-referral if needed in the future. In addition, once a relationship has been established with a patient and carer, a period of review may be agreed, with a view to the carer contacting the speech and language therapist should the situation change or deteriorate. Typically intervention peaks and troughs alongside the patient and carer's journey, with increased involvement at times of changing personal circumstances, deterioration or stress. Links with voluntary agencies such as the Alzheimer's Society are important in order for patients and carers to derive support outside statutory agencies, or when they are discharged. It is important when discharging patients that all involved understand the process of re-referral if necessary and any particular triggers that may necessitate this. In summary, reasons to plan a review and further assessment may be to:

- ascertain if advice given is actioned and maintained over time
- modify communication/swallowing advice where rapid change is occurring
- address concern about patient or carer stress and support
- address concern about the care or care environment provided.

  Reasons for discharge include:

- the episode of intervention has been satisfactorily concluded
- further speech and language therapy advice is not needed
- the carer/patient is satisfied they have access to support or further advice if needed
- other members of the team are involved and will contact the speech and language therapist if needed.

The future

The field of dementia care is a rapidly expanding and changing field. Alongside this, changes are also occurring in the wider health and social economy. The role of the speech and language therapist is therefore likely to continue to develop as a result. As the work of professionals becomes more specialized and a wider remit is devolved to support staff, it may be that there will be an increasing role for the speech and language therapist in delivering training to such individuals and in devising specific programmes for others to follow.

References

Allen K (2003) Finding Your Way: explorations in communication. Dementia Services Development Trust, Stirling.

Almor A, Kempler K, MacDonald MC et al. (1999) Why do Alzheimer patients have difficulty with pronouns? Working memory, semantics, and reference in comprehension and production in Alzheimer's disease. Brain and Language 67(3): 202–227.

Alzheimer's Society (2002) Living with Dementia. Alzheimer's Society UK, London.

APA (2000) Diagnostic and Statistical Manual of Mental Disorders, 4th edn, Text Revision. American Psychiatric Association, Washington, DC.

Baker J (2001a) Life story books for the elderly mentally ill. International Journal of Language and Communication Disorders 36: 185–187.

Baker J (2001b) How . . . I manage dementia: living in the real world. Speech and Language Therapy In Practice, Autumn, pp. 24–26.

Baker R, Dowling Z, Wareing LA et al. (1997) Snoezelen: its long-term and short-term effects on older people with dementia. British Journal of Occupational Therapy 60: 213–218.

Bayles KA (2003) Effects of working memory deficits on the communicative functioning of Alzheimer's dementia patients. Journal of Communication Disorders 36: 209–219.

Beavis D, Simpson S, Graham I (2002) A literature review of Dementia Care Mapping: methodological considerations and efficacy. Journal of Psychiatric and Mental Health Nursing 9: 725–736.

Becker JT, Huff FJ, Nebes RD et al. (1988) Neuropsychological function in Alzheimer's disease: pattern of impairment and rates of progression. Archives of Neurology 45: 263–268.

Bishop D (1989) Test for Reception of Grammar. Psychological Corporation, London.

Bourgeois MS (1993) Effects of memory aids on the dyadic conversations of individuals with dementia. Journal of Applied Behaviour Analysis 26: 77–87.

Bourgeois MS, Mason LA (1996) Memory wallet intervention in an adult day-care setting. Behavioural Interventions 11: 3–18.

Bryan K, Maxim J (1998) Enabling care staff to relate to older communication disabled people. International Journal of Language and Communication Disorders 33: 121–126.

Bryan K, Maxim J (2002) Letter to the Editor. International Journal of Language and Communication Disorders 37(2): 215–222.

Bryan K, Axelrod L, Bell L et al. (2002) Care workers and communication difficulties: an evaluation of care worker training. Ageing and Mental Health 6: 248–254.

Caine D, Hodges JR (2001) Heterogeneity of semantic and visuospatial deficits in early Alzheimer's disease. Neuropsychology 15: 155–164.

Clare L, Wilson BA, Carter G et al. (2000) Intervening with everyday memory problems in dementia of Alzheimer type: an errorless learning approach. Journal of Clinical and Experimental Neuropsychology 22: 132–146.

Croot K, Hodges JR, Patterson K (1999) Evidence for impaired sentence comprehension in early Alzheimer's disease. Journal of International Neuropsychological Society 5: 393–404.

DH (2001) National Service Framework for Older People. Department of Health. HMSO, London.

Dietch JT, Hewitt LJ, Jones S (1989) Adverse effects of reality orientation. Journal of the American Geriatrics Society 37: 974–976.

Ehrlich JS (1994) Studies in discourse production in adults with Alzheimer's disease. In: Bloom R, Obler LK, Santi S De, Ehrlich JS (eds) Discourse Analysis and Applications: studies in adult clinical populations. Lawrence Erlbaum Associates, Hillsdale, NJ, pp. 149–160.

Feil N (1992) Validation therapy with late-onset dementia populations. In: Jones GMM, Miesen BML (eds) Care-Giving in Dementia. Routledge, London, pp. 199–218.

Feil N (1993) The Validation Breakthrough. Health Professions Press, Baltimore, MD.

Fossey J, Lee L, Ballard C (2002) Dementia Care Mapping as a research tool for measuring quality of life in care settings: psychometric properties. International Journal of Geriatric Psychiatry 17: 1064–1070.

Fox L (1995) Mapping the advance of the new culture of dementia care. In: Kitwood T, Benson S (eds) The New Culture of Dementia Care. Hawker Publications, London, pp. 70–74.

Gillick MR (2000) Rethinking the role of tube feeding in patients with advanced dementia. New England Journal of Medicine 342(3): 206–210.

Greene JDW, Hodges JR (1996) The fractionation of remote memory. Evidence from a longitudinal study of dementia of Alzheimer type. Brain 119: 129–142.

Griffiths HL, Baldwin B (1989) Speech therapy for psychogeriatrics: luxury or necessity? Psychiatric Bulletin, Royal College of Psychiatrists 13: 57–59.

Griffiths HL, Burford A (1988) Thanks for the memories. Nursing Times 84(36): 55–56.

Hamill R, Connors T (2004) Sonas aPc: activating the potential for communication through multi-sensory stimulation. In: Jones G, Miesen B (eds) Care-giving in Dementia: research and applications. Routledge, London, pp. 119–137.

Hart BD, Wells DL (1997) The effects of language used by caregivers on agitation in residents with dementia. Clinical Nurse Specialist 11: 20–23.

Harvey RJ, Rosser M, Skelton M et al. (1998) Young Onset Dementia: epidemiology, clinical symptoms, family burden, support and outcome. Dementia Research Group, London.

Jagust WJ, Davies P, Tiller-Borcich JK, Reed BR (1990) Focal Alzheimer's disease. Neurology 40: 14–19.

Johnson M (1997) Outcome measurement: towards an interdisciplinary approach. British Journal of Therapy and Rehabilitation 4(9): 472–477.

Jordan L, Bell L, Bryan K et al. (2000) Communicate: evaluation of a training package for carers of older people with communication impairments. Middlesex University/University College London, London.

Kindell J (2002) Feeding and Swallowing Disorders in Dementia. Speechmark Publications, Oxford.

Kindell J (2003) Doing things differently: dance in dementia care. Journal of Dementia Care 11(2): 18–20.

Kitwood T (1993) Discover the person not the disease. Journal of Dementia Care 1(1): 16–17.

Kitwood T (1995) Cultures of care: tradition and change. In: Kitwood T, Benson S (eds) The New Culture of Dementia Care. Hawker Publications, London, pp. 7–11.

Kitwood T (1997a) The concept of personhood and its relevance for a new culture of dementia care. In: Jones G, Miesen B (eds) Care-giving in Dementia: research and applications. Routledge, London, pp. 3–13.

Kitwood T (1997b) Dementia Reconsidered: the person comes first. Open University Press, Buckingham.

Lambon-Ralph M, Patterson K, Graham N et al. (2003) Homogeneity and heterogeneity in mild cognitive impairment and Alzheimer's disease: a cross sectional and longitudinal study of 55 cases. Brain 126: 2350–2362.

Le Dorze G, Genereux MJS, Larfeuil C et al. (2000) The development of a procedure for the evaluation of communication occurring between residents in long-term care and their caregivers. Aphasiology 14: 17–51.

McKee KJ, Houston DM, Barnes S (2002) Methods for assessing quality of life and well-being in frail older people. Psychology and Health 17(6): 737–751.

Martin A, Brouwers P, Lalonde F et al. (1986) Towards a behavioural typology of Alzheimer's disease. Journal of Clinical and Experimental Neuropsychology 8: 594–610.

Maxim J, Bryan K, Axelrod L, Jordan L, Bell L (2001) Speech and language therapists as trainers: enabling care staff working with older people. International Journal of Language and Communication Disorders 36: 194–199.

Morton I (1999) Person-centred Approaches to Dementia Care. Winslow Press, Bicester, pp. 79–138.

Murphy C (1994) It Started with a Seashell. Life Story Work and People with Dementia. Dementia Services Centre, Stirling.

Neary D, Snowden JS, Bowen DM et al. (1986) Neuropsychological syndromes in presenile dementia due to cerebral atrophy. Journal of Neurology, Neurosurgery and Psychiatry 49(2): 163–174.

NICE (2001) Guidance on the use of donepezil, rivastigmine, and galantamine for the treatment of Alzheimer's disease. National Institute of Clinical Excellence, London (www.nice.org.uk).

Perkins L, Whitworth A, Lesser R (1997) Conversation Analysis Profile for People with Cognitive Impairment. Whurr, London.

Perrin T, May H (2000) Wellbeing in Dementia – an Occupational Approach for Therapists and Carers. Churchill Livingstone, London.

Perry R, Watson P, Hodges JR (2000) The nature and staging of attentional dysfunction in early Alzheimer's disease. Neuropsychologia 38: 252–271.

Pogacar S, Williams RS (1984) Alzheimer's disease presenting as slowly progressive aphasia. Rhode Island Medical Journal 67: 181–185.

Ponte N (2001) Under the survey: the elderly. RCSLT Bulletin 588: 7–9.

Powell J (2000) Communication intervention in dementia. Reviews in Clinical Gerontology 10: 161–168.

Price BH, Gurvit H, Weintraub S et al. (1993) Neuropsychological patterns and language deficits in 20 consecutive cases of autopsy confirmed Alzheimer's disease. Archives of Neurology 50: 931–937.

Purandare N, Allen NHP, Burns A (2000) Behavioural and psychological symptoms of dementia. Reviews in Clinical Gerontology 10: 245–260.

Ross SJ, Graham N, Stuart Green L et al. (1996) Progressive biparietal atrophy: an atypical presentation of Alzheimer's disease. Journal of Neurology, Neurosurgery and Psychiatry 61: 388–395.

Small JA, Anderson E, Kempler D (1997a) The effects of working memory capacity on understanding rate-altered speech. Aging Neuropsychology and Cognition 4: 126–139.

Small JA, Kemper S, Lyons K (1997b) Sentence comprehension in Alzheimer's disease: effects of grammatical complexity, speech rate and repetition. Psychology and Aging 12: 3–11.

Snowden JS, Neary D, Mann DMA (1996) Fronto-temporal Lobar Degeneration: fronto-temporal dementia, progressive aphasia, semantic dementia. Churchill Livingstone, Edinburgh.

Stokes G (2000) Challenging Behaviour in Dementia: a person centred approach. Winslow, Bicester.

Tanner B, Daniels KA (1990) An observation study of communication between carers and their relatives with dementia. Care of the Elderly 2: 247–250.

Thornton A, Hatton C, Tatham A (2004) Dementia Care Mapping reconsidered: exploring the reliability and validity of the observation tool. International Journal of Geriatric Psychiatry 19: 718–726.

Threadgold M (2002) Sonas aPc – a new lease of life for some. SIGNPOST 7(1): 35–37.

Warner L (2004) Review of the Literature on the Care Programme Approach. Sainsbury's Centre for Mental Health, London.

Waters GS, Caplan D, Rochon E (1995) Processing capacity and sentence comprehension in patients with Alzheimer's disease. Cognitive Neuropsychology 12: 1–30.

Waters GS, Rochon E, Caplan D (1998) Task demands and sentence comprehension in patients with dementia of the Alzheimer type. Brain and Language 62: 361–397.

Winter J, Hunkin NM (1999) Re-learning in Alzheimer's disease. International Journal of Geriatric Psychiatry 14: 988–990.

Appendix 8.1: Questionnaires

These questionnaires were developed as part of a Middlesex University and University College London research project to evaluate 'Communicate', a training package for carers of communicatively impaired older people (Jordan et al. 2000).

Carer questionnaires

We are carrying out some research into a training package that has been developed for people working with older people who have communication problems. The aim of the research is to find out whether this particular training is useful and effective. To help us do this, we will be using information from the following questionnaire to compare the answers of people who have received the training with those who have not.

- It is important that you try to answer all the questions.
- All your answers will be treated confidentially and will not be disclosed to anyone outside the research team.
- Please complete the following personal details to help us contact you again.
- The top page of this document will be removed on receipt so that your answers cannot be identified by name.

Name:

Contact telephone number:

Official use only:

Part 1 You and your job

If your job has changed since the last time you completed a questionnaire for this research project, please explain how it has changed:

Change of job title:

Change of organization/department:

Change in qualifications:

Change in responsibilities:

How do you rate your job currently? (please circle a number between 1 and 5):

not at all enjoyable   very enjoyable

1   2   3   4   5

Do you have face to face contact with clients?   Yes/No

What proportion of your clients have communication problems (i.e. problems talking to you or understanding what you are saying)?

None ☐   A minority ☐   About half ☐   Most ☐   All ☐

If you have answered None, please go straight to Part 2.

How long have you been working with people with communication problems?

_____

What sorts of communication problems do they have?

_____

Please give examples of any situations that you find difficult because of the communication problems of the people you care for.

_____

How do you feel when you are working with someone who has communication problems?

_____

Part 2 Training about communication

How did you get a place on the 'Communicate' workshop?

_____

Did you find the 'Communicate' workshop useful?   Yes/No

What was the most useful thing about the workshop?

_____

What was the least useful thing about the workshop?

_____

Was there anything that was not covered in the 'Communicate' training
that you think should have been included?   Yes/No
If Yes, please explain:

Have you been able to apply any aspects of the training to your work?
                                                                      Yes/No
Please explain:

Since the 'Communicate' training took place, have you received any other
training about communication and communication problems?   Yes/No

If Yes:
What did the training consist of?
When was the training?
How long was the training?
Who provided the training?

Part 3 Knowledge about communication

Please circle a number to indicate how much you feel you know about the
following, on a scale of 1 (very little) to 5 (a lot):

Normal everyday communication (talking and listening)	1	2	3	4	5
Your own talking and listening skills	1	2	3	4	5
The causes of communication problems	1	2	3	4	5
Different types of communication problems	1	2	3	4	5
Medical conditions or diseases that result in communication problems	1	2	3	4	5
Ways of changing your communication to help people understand	1	2	3	4	5
Ways of changing your communication to help people express themselves	1	2	3	4	5

How it might feel to have communication problems	1	2	3	4	5

Please indicate how competent you feel to do the following, on a scale of 1 (not at all competent) to 5 (very competent):

Notice that someone has communication problems	1	2	3	4	5
Recognize different types of communication problems	1	2	3	4	5
Change the way you communicate to help people understand you	1	2	3	4	5
Change the way you communicate to help people express themselves	1	2	3	4	5

Part 4   Attitudes towards communication problems

Please tick once only to indicate how far you agree/disagree with each of the following statements

	Strongly disagree	Disagree	Neither agree nor disagree	Agree	Strongly agree
1 Spending time talking and listening to people is an important part of my job					
2 It is frustrating trying to talk to people who have communication problems					
3 I feel confident working with people who have communication problems					
4 I feel sympathetic towards people who have communication problems					
5 It's not my problem if people can't understand me					
6 It is rewarding to work with people who have communication problems					

	Strongly disagree	Disagree	Neither agree nor disagree	Agree	Strongly agree

7   It is important to allow more
    time for people with
    communication problems

8   It is embarrassing having to talk
    to people with communication
    problems

9   My job requires good
    communication skills

10 I get annoyed when people
    don't understand me

11 It is stressful working with
    people who have
    communication problems

12 If people have communication
    problems, it's up to me to
    change the way I speak to them

13 I find it hard to cope with
    people who have
    communication problems

14 I don't have time to talk to
    people who can't communicate
    easily

15 I feel relaxed when I'm talking
    to people who have problems
    communicating

16 I don't need to talk to my
    clients to get my job done

Part 5   How to help with communication problems

Please make some suggestions about strategies you could use to communicate with people who have the following communications problems:

Someone who has difficulty hearing you:

Someone who can't understand you:

Someone who can't think of the words they want to say:

Someone who has slurred speech:

Someone who talks a lot but doesn't make much sense:

Someone who seems confused:

Someone who is reluctant to communicate:

Video sessions

Date: Test phase:

Researcher will ask the following questions and complete the form on behalf of carer on each visit. (Explanation of 5-point scale and assistance/examples to be given as necessary.)

Why are you seeing *(service user's name)* today?

Have you met *(service user's name)* before?   Yes/No

If Yes:

How long have you known *(service user's name)*?

How often do you see *(service user's name)*?

How much do you talk to *(service user's name)*?

very little				a lot
1	2	3	4	5

How easy is it to talk to *(service user's name)*?

not at all easy				very easy
1	2	3	4	5

How well does *(service user's name)* understand you?

not at all well			very well	
1	2	3	4	5

How well does *(service user's name)* communicate with you?

not at all well			very well	
1	2	3	4	5

How do you feel when you are talking to *(service user's name)*?

For carers who have received 'Communicate' training only

What have you learned about *(service user's name)* from the 'Communicate' training?

Have you changed the way you communicate with *(service user's name)* as a result of the training?

If Yes, how?

Appendix 8.2: Schedule of strategies to promote communication use by carers

Carer strategies: basic	Frequency		Comments	Carer strategies: advanced	Frequency		Comments
Appropriate positioning	Never Often Score	Sometimes Always	Too near Too far	Gains attention	Observed? Used appropriately? Required?	Y/N Y/N Y/N	Too often Too little
Uses appropriate loudness	Never Often Score	Sometimes Always	Too loud Too soft	Uses non-verbal cues (gesture)	Observed? Used appropriately? Required?	Y/N Y/N Y/N	Too often Too little
Uses appropriate level of language	Never Often Score	Sometimes Always	Too simple Too complex	Uses repetition (close)	Observed? Used appropriately? Required?	Y/N Y/N Y/N	Too often Too little
Uses appropriate rate of speech	Never Often Score	Sometimes Always	Too fast Too slow	Uses yes/no questions	Observed? Used appropriately? Required?	Y/N Y/N Y/N	Too often Too little
Allows time for comprehension	Never Often Score	Sometimes Always	Too little Too much	Uses forced alternatives	Observed? Used appropriately? Required?	Y/N Y/N Y/N	Too often Too little
Allows time to respond	Never Often Score	Sometimes Always	Too little Too much	Uses open questions	Observed? Used appropriately? Required?	Y/N Y/N Y/N	Too often Too little
Attempts to extend interaction	Never Often Score	Sometimes Always	Acknowledges Responds – to verbal – to non- verbal Elaborates Initiates repair	Uses AAC

Checks back meaning | Observed? Used appropriately? Required?

Observed? Used appropriately? Required? | Y/N Y/N Y/N

Y/N Y/N Y/N | Too often Too little

Too often Too little |

Any other strategies observed? Appropriate?

Source: Jordan et al. (2000).

CHAPTER 9

Working with family and friends as carers

COLIN BARNES

This chapter is an introduction to the importance of working with the carers of people with dementia; who they are, what they do, how to determine their needs and how to shape their expectations. It is essential to understand the carer's perspective before considering using individual or group approaches for working with them.

Communication partners and carers

Many people with dementia spend the greatest proportion of their time interacting with people not employed in the caring professions, ranging from close family members to local shop assistants to complete strangers. The quality of these interactions will be influenced by the abilities of the person with dementia and the insight, experience, skills and knowledge of their communication partner(s).

This chapter will consider the group of communication partners who typically spend the most time with, have the most historical knowledge of and are most affected by the well-being of the person with dementia – their carer.

Why work with carers?

Since carers are often the main communication partners of the person with dementia, they are most likely to influence the person's experience of communication. People with more than mild dementia have, by definition, memory impairments that are likely to render carry-over of information, habit and skill from therapy to everyday life difficult. For this reason it is important to involve carers in the aims of individual and group client therapy wherever appropriate. Lubinski (1995) suggests that even intensive therapy is less likely to have the same generalizing effect as equipping carers with the right tools to enable conversation.

The loss of meaningful interaction and conversation places increased pressure on the caring relationship (Greene et al. 1982, Gilleard et al. 1984a, 1984b, Argyle et al. 1985, O'Connor et al. 1990, Nolan et al. 2002). Gilleard et al. (1984a) found that carers of people with dementia exhibiting communication and behaviour difficulties were twice as likely to report symptoms of their own psychiatric distress as carers not experiencing these difficulties. It is therefore important that a mental health service cares for carers, who have a higher likelihood of becoming patients in their own right. Further pressure will be added to current care systems by reduction in the total number of carers in the UK. This is attributed primarily to the increased number of married women in employment (UK Census, ONS 2001). Other social trends likely to affect carer numbers are the growth in lone parenting, changes in attitude towards marriage and increased mobility among family members.

Reasons and rationale

When considering the reasons for working with carers, it is all too easy to think of carers as a resource. Nolan et al. (1994) suggest the needs of carers are often assessed in terms of providing services or training to help them continue in their caring role, rather than focusing on them as individuals in their own right who have their own needs.

It is possible to work with carers at all stages of the illness. Although evidence suggests that individual or group cognitive therapy approaches can improve communication skill and experience (Clare and Woods 2001), most of these interventions are only suitable for individuals in the mild to moderate stages of dementia.

In contrast to interventions with people who have dementia, the focus of intervention with carers is primarily directed towards:

* developing the carer's understanding, knowledge and expectations
* helping to shape the carer's behaviours in a changing world
* maintaining, enabling and maximizing existing skills and responsibilities for the client via the carer
* encouraging the carer to recognize and develop their 'expertise'
* showing some understanding of the carer's experiences.

Nolan et al. (2002) suggest that, while many authors encourage interventions designed to reduce carer stress or burden, it is equally valuable to focus on ways of increasing satisfaction and expertise in caring. Similarly, although much work has focused on the goals of reducing institutionalization and sustaining long-term caring relationships, the aim should be to enhance the quality and meaning of life for both the person with dementia and their carers.

Understanding informal carers

Between 6 and 7 million people in the UK define themselves as carers through looking after a relative, partner or friend because they are ill, disabled or frail (Victor 1997, Carers UK 2003). Of these, approximately one quarter are defined as main carers (Parker 1990) spending more than 20 hours per week caring. Of today's carers, approximately 42% are men and 58% women. The largest proportion, 54%, are aged between 35 and 59. However, older carers are more likely to be caring for someone within their own household (Marriott, 2003).

Victor (1997) describes two types of carer: co-resident (those who live with the person with dementia) and extra-resident (those who live elsewhere). Co-resident carers tend to be spouses and immediate family members; extra-resident carers are more likely to be distant relatives, friends or neighbours. Co-resident carers spend considerably more time providing care.

It is estimated that 80% of the care older people need is provided by the family (Walker 1995). Of the 750 000 people in the UK with dementia (Alzheimer's Society 2004b), the majority live in their own home or with family members, although a large minority (40%) are estimated to be living in some type of institutional care (Gordon and Spicker 1997).

Few statistics look specifically at the numbers of people caring for people with dementia. However, one study conducted in a rural area of the UK (Cumbria) suggested that 60% of people with dementia had one or more carer(s) (Gordon and Spicker 1997). The average duration of dementia from symptom onset is 8 years, and in some cases considerably longer (Alzheimer's Society 1995). Over this time period, caring for someone with dementia involves continuously increasing responsibility for the caregiver and dependence for the receiver (Samuelsson et al. 2001).

The carer's experience

The lives of carers can be very different from those of other people. For a relatively inexperienced professional, it may be helpful (if not essential) to attend a carers' meeting or group to listen to carers describe their experiences before endeavouring to advise them.

Haley et al. (1994), in a study of 170 people with dementia, found that behavioural and communication problems were rated by their carers as more stressful than daily living and self-care impairments. However, these difficulties did not necessarily worsen throughout the course of the illness, sometimes peaking early or in the middle of the illness.

In a European study by Murray et al. (1999), 280 spouse carers in 14 countries were interviewed. Carers described both passive behaviours (sleeping, withdrawal, immobility, loss of communication) and active or excessive behaviours (aggression, restlessness, aimlessness, sleep disturbance, mood swings and antisocial behaviour) in their spouses. Both patterns could be present in the same person. The most commonly expressed difficulties were:

- loss of companionship through diminished communication
- loss of reciprocity as carers experienced their partner's growing dependency
- deterioration in social behaviour.

Spouses provided increased assistance with activities of daily living while losing key elements of their marital relationship, such as companionship, emotional support, shared responsibilities and joint decision-making.

It seems possible that female carers report stress and burden more often than male carers (Bayles and Tomoeda 1996). Gilhooly (1987) found that male carers:

- adopted a more behavioural and practical approach to caring
- were more able to distance themselves from their caring duties
- found help with caregiving more socially acceptable
- found help more readily available.

All professionals therefore need to ensure that female carers are offered the help they need (Alzheimer's Society 2004a). Research suggests that those carers interviewed at point of referral to psychiatric services are more likely to present with depression, whereas those interviewed as part of an existing carer support group report a lower incidence of depression (Brodaty and Hadzi-Pavlovic 1990, Clarke and Watson 1991, Saad et al. 1995, Lubinski 1995). Brodaty and Hadzi-Pavlovic (1990) suggest that carers who are spouses are also likely to suffer greater psychological distress.

Carers of people with Lewy body dementia were significantly more likely to have a major depressive disorder associated with their relatives' increased likelihood of disturbed behaviour, when compared with carers of people with Alzheimer's disease (Lowery et al. 2000).

Extra-resident and long-distance carers

With the exception of spouses visiting residential or nursing homes, the majority of extra-resident carers are the children of the person with dementia. Some are local, though many are involved from a distance.

Extra-resident carers may have to deal with complaints from neighbours and spend time sorting out affairs and physical needs, while suffering considerable anxiety about their relative when they are not with them. Although there are often role changes for spouse carers, for children there may be additional difficulties directing their parent's behaviours or attending to their personal needs. Thompsell and Lovestone (2002) found that relatives living at a distance reported similar rates of subjective distress as nearby relatives. They suggested that those seeking to support carers may need to widen their supportive net.

Friends and neighbours

Friends may also provide care because of regular contact with each other, though friendship is more typically based on reciprocal action. Generally, it is easier to break ties with friends than with family and consequently friendship-based caring can be more vulnerable to collapse, particularly when behavioural changes manifest or family members intervene. Similarly, neighbours become involved in caring, and their relationship is both complicated, and made easier, by physical proximity. Many care out of deep friendship, though some neighbours may care out of obligation or in order to protect their own interests.

The caring career

Aneschensel et al. (1995) introduce the idea that carers have broadly three stages to their caring career:

- role acquisition (illness onset, start of care)
- role enactment (in-home care and institutional care)
- role disengagement (patient death, bereavement and social adjustment).

They propose that during each of these stages carers have a corresponding primary need for:

- education, prevention and planning
- stress management and resource enhancement
- closure and readjustment.

Aneschensel et al. (1995) add that since carers face a prolonged period of exposure to chronic stress, they may deplete or exhaust their social, personal and economic resources. Interventions over the course of caregiving therefore should reinforce these resources. They also suggest that carers' self-concept can suffer and may need building up through the successes in their role.

For carers of people with dementia, increases in disease-related burdens do not necessarily lead to increased stress; as dementia progresses care situations can deteriorate, remain the same or improve. However, carers are individuals. Some, especially perhaps the younger ones who may still be at work, struggle to accept their situation. They can become angry, but at the same time are reluctant to accept help. Others seem to almost embrace the opportunity to care or become involved in the 'caring scene'.

How carers cope

O'Brien (1999) believes that four broad factors influence carers' coping strategies in informal care settings:

- the carer's interpretation of the sufferer's condition and their own supporting role
- the quality of their relationship with the sufferer
- the coping strategies available and selected by the carer
- relationships between the carer and other sources of formal and informal support.

Murray et al. (1999) identified four positive aspects to caring:

- a sense of job satisfaction – gaining a sense of achievement from making their spouse as comfortable as possible
- reciprocity and mutual affection – making a return for care and affection shown in the past
- companionship – most likely to occur when efforts were appreciated or when their spouse could interact positively
- a sense of duty – e.g. keeping one's wedding vows.

A study by Saad et al. (1995) serves as a reminder that many carers are able to generate their own coping strategies. In their study of 109 carers, the 77 carers not experiencing depression described a number of coping strategies which included 'being firm, directing behaviour, constructing a larger sense of the illness, reducing expectations and trying to find ways of keeping your relative busy'. Nolan et al. (2002) also suggest that some carers may benefit from being taught coping thoughts, e.g. 'There are many worse off than me', as well as practical ways of coping.

Particular needs of specific care groups

There are likely to be particular care needs for specific groups of carers and persons with dementia. *Signposts to Support* (Alzheimer Scotland 2003) highlights the particular needs of different care groups in Scotland. Alzheimer Scotland surveyed approximately 28 000 carers providing for 12 000 people with severe dementia and 23 000 people with mild to moderate dementia. Even allowing for differences in geography, ethnic distribution and service provision it is worth noting that in Scotland in 2003:

- Between 800 (3%) and 5000 (18%) people under the age of 18 were involved in some way in caring for someone with dementia. They may not recognize themselves as carers, and face isolation, problems at school and conflicts with life demands and interests.
- An estimated 1605 (5%) of people with dementia are aged under 65. Their carers are more likely to be working and to have dependent children and less likely to be engaged with the benefits system before the person they care for is diagnosed.
- Between 110 (0.3%) and 690 (2%) carers are from non-white ethnic minority backgrounds. They may face problems obtaining information

and services because of communication barriers, cultural differences and inappropriate assumptions made by service providers.

- An estimated 1440 (5%) to 4930 (18%) carers of people with dementia are lesbian, gay, bisexual or transsexual. Stigma and discrimination may prevent them from accessing resources. Same-sex partnerships may also lack recognition by services.
- About 13% of the population of people with Down's syndrome have dementia. There may be about 750 households in Scotland caring for such people. Carers are often ageing parents and experience difficulty accessing suitable services.
- About 8400 (30%) carers live in rural areas and face lower earnings, lack of suitable housing, lack of flexible resources, transport problems and variable levels of community support alongside greater isolation.

Contact with carers and carer needs

Ideally, it should be part of service delivery to clearly identify and contact carers after a person with dementia has been referred to a therapy service. If the client is seen for assessment with the carer it is helpful to obtain some symptom and life history from the carer alongside examples of current difficulties and lifestyle. Professionals need to ensure that the appropriate carer is identified: this may not always be the first name that comes to the mind of the client, nor necessarily the contact name on their medical notes.

When people with dementia are first seen alone, where possible, consent should be sought to contact the carer. If the client has already been seen, it might be preferable to meet carers alone in order to give them the opportunity to be open about their feelings. Meeting carers in their home may also be preferable in order to minimize their effort and give the therapist some impression of the environment in which care and communication takes place.

The therapist may also make contact with carers in other ways, for example:

- attending carers' support groups
- leaving leaflets or posters in the hospital or local voluntary services
- attending carers' exhibitions, talks and conferences
- linking up with other services, e.g. other therapies and memory clinics
- attending day centre parties.

Carers are much more likely to respond to a telephone call or face-to-face meeting than a letter. However, their responses to an invitation to discuss communication difficulties will vary. Factors affecting initial response may include:

- understanding of what is being offered
- priorities for care

- time
- previous experience with health and social care professionals
- whether they can see benefits for themselves or the client
- whether they are thinking of their own needs or the client's
- previous communication patterns
- current stress and burden levels.

Some care should be taken in explaining the purpose of meeting with them. Ideally, the therapist should already have met the person with dementia. Therefore, they will be able to at least offer the carer an explanation of their assessment findings. They could also be offered:

- the opportunity to view a presentation on communication and memory difficulties (e.g. Barnes 2003) or discuss attending a carers' group
- advice and specific recommendations on communication and memory approaches
- the chance to borrow leaflets, books, videos or tapes
- demonstrations and examples of communication approaches
- individual therapy programmes.

Barnes (1998) looked at the effectiveness of offering advice to carers of people with dementia. He identified that carers found the idea of communication difficult to grasp, and tended not to consider the relationships between memory, communication and other activities of daily living. The study also showed that carers benefit from:

- explanation of what is communication and how memory works (their understanding of this may need to be informally tested)
- being encouraged for what they are already doing
- very specific advice

but that carers find the following difficult:

- too much advice that can be overwhelming and stressful
- very general advice that is difficult to apply
- continuously repeating what has been recommended over the long term.

Efforts are needed to ensure demands are not made of carers that they will be unable to carry out, thus creating yet more guilt and feelings of helplessness. Similarly, it is not advisable to place carers in a role that demands unsustainable or potentially harmful changes in their relationship: for example, a previously submissive partner working as therapist.

Meeting the carer

Once the meeting has been arranged, the therapist's aims may include:

- explaining the results of assessment (usually an abridged and interpreted version of the medical report)

- assessing the carer's abilities and needs
- developing an understanding of pre-morbid relationships
- assessing the nature of current interactions
- determining and shaping the carer's expectations
- identifying specific issues
- giving specific advice
- offering help through other approaches or services/professionals.

Assessment of carers

Assuming that they do agree to meet, any carer's ability to understand and apply what they learn from interventions focusing on communication and memory difficulties may depend in part on:

- their intellect and ability to think in abstract terms
- their ability to reflect and self-monitor
- their own memory or ability to use written guidelines
- other goals they are working towards
- their personal discipline
- their stress and anxiety
- support and help from other friends or members of the family
- the extent to which they are seeking to change.

Within the assessment and initial discussion with a carer, the therapist should also gain some understanding of the carer's perceptual, educational, pragmatic and social skills in order to consider how best to deliver intervention. Armstrong and Borthwick (1997) developed a specific format for assessing carers' perceptions using a questionnaire and demonstrated that this added to more objective client assessments, provided for more effective management and also prepared the carer for interventions.

Understanding pre-morbid roles and relationships

All work with people with dementia and their carers should be undertaken within the context of those individuals: who they are, what they have done, their interests, education, ambitions, roles and relationships. An understanding of these relationships should include some impression of the extent to which carer and client would normally interact and 'care for' each other. Some carers find themselves caring for someone they haven't spoken to for years; others may find themselves caring for a previously abusive partner. Where there has been strain in a relationship, it may be more difficult for the carer to attribute behaviours to the disease process. In this case carers may benefit from an explanation of the widespread effects of memory and other impairments.

Motenko (1989) suggests that a continuing sense of closeness between carer and dependant may sustain a sense of well-being in carers. Ratings of quality and closeness of pre-morbid relationships are negatively associated with carer stress (Gilleard et al. 1984a, Morris et al. 1988). Family therapists, where available, may help to at least sustain the current level of relationship (Richardson et al. 1994). Particularly in the role-acquisition stage of caring, carers may need some help in determining to what extent they are able to commit to the caring role (Aneschensel et al. 1995).

Social and cultural expectations may pressure carers to commit to caring (Murray et al. 1999). It may be appropriate in some circumstances to discourage a carer from undertaking a level of care that is well above their previous commitment. As an extension to working individually with carers, Powell et al. (1995) suggest a family conference could be held to explain the disease and its progress, to help the family prepare for the future, protect their assets and become knowledgeable about local resources.

Assessing current interactions

It is possible to gather some impression of the ways in which the carer and client interact (as well as the client's lifestyle and abilities) through less structured interviews using questions related to the person with dementia such as:

- What does s/he do during the day?
- Does s/he have any responsibilities or interests?
- Does s/he read or watch television?
- What do you talk about at mealtimes?
- What happens when people visit?
- What do you say when s/he comes home from the day centre?
- Is there anything s/he has stopped doing recently?
- What causes you the most frustration?
- What does s/he forget the most often?
- When does s/he talk the most/least?
- Does s/he have any way of helping her/his memory?
- When does conversation work best?
- Does s/he have any other ways of communicating, e.g. drawing, gesture?

Answers from these questions should give the therapist a reasonable impression of what occurs during the day – or at least what is most important to the carer.

It is also possible to assess carers by making use of audio or videotape recording, in a similar way to the SPARCC programme for carers of people with aphasia (Lock et al. 2001). Using video as both assessment and therapy tool (for feedback) has the advantage of addressing behavioural change as well as knowledge. This would involve lending the carer a video camera to record themselves interacting with the client, e.g. at mealtimes. The therapist could then meet with the carer to evaluate the tape. Bayles and Tomoeda (1996) suggest that carers most often do not realize the limitations of their relative's comprehension. This author has noted that carers can also have a tendency to over-remind their relative and may need help in prioritizing issues for reminding.

Creating expectations

The degree to which the carer feels that any intervention is beneficial or has succeeded will be influenced by the expectations they have. These may be influenced by previous contact with health professionals and by their own life values and experiences. They may underestimate or over-estimate what can be achieved. It is important that the therapist is clear about their own expectations. Goldsmith (1996) advises that a belief that successful communication is possible must exist and that without a commitment to explore this belief, we are unlikely to identify any clues to help communication.

Developing a broader understanding of what constitutes communication and interaction will help this process. It is important to be realistic about and encouraged by what can be achieved, e.g. 5 minutes' conversation or one name learned. Examples of what has been achieved with other people may be useful illustrations. However, when considering what can be achieved, it is important not to understate the likelihood of eventual deterioration.

Examining the carer's beliefs should be done in a supportive and non-judgemental way, for instance when asking why they haven't accepted more help or why they feel a day centre is inappropriate. In these examples it may be beneficial to describe in detail what is being offered and how other people benefit from it. Encouraging clients and carers to visit or try out available provision may aid decision-making.

Identifying issues for discussion and goal setting

After meeting and assessing the client and carer, the therapist and carer should have identified a number of issues influencing the perceived success of their communication. Examples of specific issues identified include:

- I'm never sure what to say to other people about him.
- Is that his memory or is he just being awkward?
- He doesn't seem able to make decisions any more.
- When he comes home from the day centre he never tells me what he's done.
- He accuses me of taking things.
- Sometimes I'm sure he doesn't recognize me.

- He doesn't do anything.
- He forgets to turn off the light at night.
- All he ever does is talk about work – he's been retired for years!
- I'm never sure how much to remind him.

For those issues that appear to warrant action, determining which of these to translate into goals will be influenced by:

- the degree to which both client and carer are motivated to change
- the extent to which the therapist feels able to influence change
- the frequency of occurrence of difficulties
- the impact change could have on client and carer
- resources available to aid change.

Barnes (2003) strongly advocates giving no more than three specific goals (or pieces of advice), ideally starting with an issue that is both commonly occurring and most likely to change. In all cases the therapist should encourage the carers for the success they are already experiencing. In some cases it may be appropriate to offer just an explanation of assessment results and services available in the future.

Bayles and Tomoeda (1993) suggest that a caregiver's conscious and unconscious beliefs about the person with dementia can have a tremendous impact on how the caregiver interacts and copes with the person. They suggest that the therapist should help shape beliefs about diagnosis, share information and provide specific practical suggestions.

Additional evidence from studies by Smith and Ventis (1990) and Bohling (1991) suggests it is advisable to intervene when carers dominate control of conversation and fail to recognize the person's attempts to initiate. It is important to be aware that carers can, with varying degrees of awareness, produce types of communication abuse ranging from direct verbal abuse to inferred abuse and ignoring or distancing (Santo Pietro 1994). Homer and Gilleard (1990) found that abuse by carers is more common in people with communication disorders.

Interventions for carers

The following sections will introduce a range of intervention approaches including leaflet, video and book loan, individualized presentations, advice or therapy, client/carer therapy programmes, counselling and fixed/open-term specific or general group meetings.

The duration of intervention

It is usually impractical for a therapist to maintain regular contact with a carer throughout their caring career. Some carers may only need to be seen once; others may benefit from a review appointment to determine progress with recommendations or to check on the effects of anticipated deterioration, for example for people with dysphagia (swallowing difficulty) or a progressive dysphasia. Although many carers' groups run indefinitely, it may be useful to run groups for a set period of time. This enables the group aims and membership to be re-evaluated.

If the therapist is expecting the carer to contact them, it is advisable to make contact as easy as possible, for example by:

- providing a leaflet or 'business card' with contact details
- suggesting examples of issues they may wish to discuss
- giving examples of how other carers have benefited from maintaining contact.

Multidisciplinary team members need to be aware that ringing up for advice on how to talk to someone may be daunting for carers.

Carer support from other agencies

It is likely that other professionals are also involved with the carer. In the UK, community psychiatric nurses, Admiral nurses (a UK specialist mental health nursing service specifically providing for the needs of carers of people with dementia), psychologists and psychiatrists, GPs, occupational therapists, counsellors, day centre workers, social workers and carer support workers (e.g. from the Alzheimer's Society) are among those who may have some contact with the carer. It may be that one person has developed a closer relationship with the carer, in which case it may be better to work with or through them. It is also important to ensure that the carer is not receiving overlapping or conflicting advice.

In a study comparing the work of the Admiral nurse service with more general support provided by a community mental health team, both were identified as equally associated with lower distress scores from carers over an 8-month period (Woods et al. 2003). Similarly, Pool (1997) outlines how occupational therapists can influence client and carer well-being through assessment, equipment and therapy to maximize functioning.

Contacts with any professionals may raise communication issues in themselves (as well as the additional burdens of remembering and attending appointments). In particular the client's (and carer's) ability to understand and consent to treatment and legal (e.g. arranging Enduring Power of Attorney) or circumstantial changes should involve some assessment of ability to comprehend and consent (Alzheimer Scotland 2003). A number of services provide more formal counselling for carers. Gallagher-Thompson (1994) and Zarit and Teri (1991) suggest that short-term counselling may reduce stress experienced by family carers.

Pusey and Richards (2001) conducted a systematic review of psychosocial interventions for carers of people. They found that individualized interventions that utilized problem solving and behaviour management approaches demonstrated the best evidence of effectiveness. Knight et al.

(1993) completed a meta-analysis of 20 studies of carer support programmes. Each used a measure of carer burden and distress and included a non-intervention control group. They concluded that group interventions have smaller effects than individual interventions such as counselling, which appeared to produce almost twice the effect size for improvement in burden and emotional dysphoria. Both interventions, however, were significantly more effective in reducing burden and distress than a respite/patient treatment control group.

Two more recent studies (Marriot et al. 2000, Charlesworth 2001) have looked specifically at the benefits of using cognitive behavioural therapy with carers of people with dementia. Both studies indicated that this approach could reduce distress and depression in these carers in comparison to non-treatment control groups. Burns et al. (2003) and Mittelman et al. (2004) showed that interventions with carers reduced stress. Two meta-analyses of caregiver interventions also concluded that caregiver interventions are effective (Schulz et al. 2002, Sorenson et al. 2002).

Using leaflets and other resources

Many organizations, such as the Alzheimer's Society, provide leaflets (printed or printable from the internet) for carers on communication and dementia. Similarly, a number of organizations have published books and videos which can be used by health professionals as well as carers for self-education. Hann (1998), Tanton (1993), Powell (2000), Koening Coste (2003) and Rau (1993) (in order of increasing complexity) are especially recommended.

However, the use of general pre-printed or recorded information assumes that the carer will be able to:

- read and follow it
- filter out what is pertinent and appropriate to their situation
- prioritize from what is usually a large selection of advice.
- implement changes in actual behaviour without help.

For these reasons all leaflets and advice should be easily understandable, succinct and given out with at least some discussion on which are the most applicable parts and how the information could be implemented in specific circumstances.

Santo Pietro (1994) reminds us that there is a difference between advice, knowledge and actual change in behaviour. She suggests that any new behaviours are best mastered with the clinician, otherwise they are unlikely to be carried over into general use.

Barnes (1998) identified key aspects of advice giving: carers found general advice difficult to put into practice, while more specific 'exactly what to do when' advice appeared to be more often remembered and successfully applied. For example, 'talk in shorter, less complex sentences' is a typical instruction on a leaflet. However, this may require of the carer a dramatic and far-reaching change in behaviour. In this example, it is better to first explain to the carer why long and complex sentences may cause difficulty. They could then be helped to think of specific situations when complex sentences or instructions are not followed. Taking one of these situations, the therapist may suggest and practise with the carer alternative ways of posing the question or instruction. An example of such a situation could be a carer who is saying to the person with dementia, 'When you go upstairs, could you shut the windows and then get dressed'. After considering the comprehension and physical agility of the person with dementia, the therapist may suggest the carer break this into two separate instructions or events, e.g. 'go upstairs and get dressed' then later 'go upstairs and close the windows'.

A list of recommended resources for use with carers is given at the end of the chapter.

Communication activity programmes for carers

Providing specific advice for carers may be enhanced by programmes of activity or therapy. This could be providing the carers with techniques to use regularly with the client or by themselves (e.g. relaxation) or with resources (e.g. pictures, videos, books, objects or worksheets). Regular daily activity can be beneficial, though it need not necessarily be varied for the client's sake. It is essential that the aims of any programme are made clear to the carer, alongside a discussion of what is realistic for them to achieve in each session.

It is unlikely that carers will be able to follow a programme indefinitely. The therapist should be sensitive to the carer's limitations and congratulate them for what they have achieved. At present all interventions in dementia care aim to slow down or minimize the impact of the inevitable progression of the illness.

Programmes can range from planning the use of just one specific response, such as what to say when they forget your name, identifying a subject to talk about, compiling or using a life story book through to using orientation or word-finding exercise sheets, for the more able client, to work through together. Carers may also want to use reflective diaries, and records of success/difficulties in communication and re-orientation to identify difficulties as they occur and help plan future goals. Typically, a programme involves providing the carer with ideas, resources and structure, accompanied by realistic expectations and beliefs that are likely to lead to an experience of success.

Carers' groups

Although individual intervention may be more timely, and gathering sufficient numbers of similar people to attend a group can take months, there are many benefits to working in groups.

Bayles and Tomoeda (1993) recommend support groups within which carers have the opportunity to receive teaching and advice and also discuss difficulties and solutions. Muir (1996) describes general carer support groups as providing an opportunity to express negative feelings, emotions and frustrations in a supportive environment.

Carers' groups typically form around statutory services such as day centres, day hospitals, nursing homes and wards or voluntary organizations. Some groups (with a tendency toward information giving) meet for a set period of time whereas others are ongoing. The latter have a tendency to have a larger membership and are representative of a wider cross-section of carers.

A study by Gordon and Spicker (1997) shows that carers participating in support groups or in contact with mental health professionals had greater knowledge than people yet to be in contact with the service. However, knowledge does not necessarily predict behavioural adherence (Chadwick et al. 2002). Brodaty and Gresham (1989) compared the value of a carer education group with a patient memory training group and found that the carer education group resulted in significantly less psychological stress for carers at a 12-month follow-up, and at 30 months significantly fewer admissions to long-term care.

Worthy of special mention is the 'Alzheimer's café' concept (Miesen and Blom 2000), which provides a social event and meeting place for people with dementia with their carers. It has three goals:

- to provide information about dementia and caring
- to encourage speaking openly about difficulties
- to promote the emancipation of people with dementia and their families.

Groups for communication difficulties

A small number of studies have looked more specifically at the value of communication-based (fixed-term) training groups for carers. These are described below.

Danielle Ripich (1996) carried out the FOCUSED Program with 19 carers, before and after which they were asked to complete questionnaires assessing changes in knowledge, attitudes, stress and burden. The results showed improve satisfaction with communication and decreased problems relating to communication breakdown for caregivers of persons with Alzheimer's disease (see Chapter 11 for full details of the FOCUSED Program).

Schulman and Mandel (1988) provided three 2-hour workshops on communication for families of elderly people in nursing homes including (though not exclusively) people with dementia. The results of a questionnaire suggest that 86% of family members believed their visits with residents had improved in one or more respect, while 76% reported a greater understanding and knowledge of communication problems and more awareness of appropriate strategies required to manage communication.

Brodaty and Peters (1991) invited carers (and clients) to a 10-day residential training course shortly after diagnosis of dementia. This included discussion and training on reality orientation, reminiscence, behaviour modification and therapeutic activities. At a 12-month follow-up the group attendees were found to have had significantly fewer admissions to institutions and decreased psychiatric morbidity compared to a control group. At 39 months, 53% of the trained carer group patients were still at home compared with only 13% of the control group. In addition, only 20% of the trained carer group patients had died compared with 41% of the non-trained. They argued that carer training had brought about reduced admission to institutions and, as a direct result of avoiding institutionalization, fewer deaths. They also calculated a cost saving on state-provided care of US$6000 per patient. Thus they conclude that carer training can also be cost effective.

McCallion et al. (1999) provided a Family Visit Educational Program (FVEP) for 32 randomly assigned carers who were compared to 32 non-attending control carers. The study was conducted in five nursing homes. The FVEP included four 1.5-hour group sessions and three 1-hour family conferences. It covered topics of verbal and non-verbal communication and effective structuring of family visits. They found that the FVEP was effective for reducing residents' problem behaviours and for decreasing their symptoms of depression and irritability. FVEP also improved the way family members and visitors communicated with residents, though had little if any impact on the way nursing staff interacted.

Done and Thomas (2001) compared the effectiveness of providing carers with workshop training against reading a booklet. Thirty carers were randomly assigned to the workshop whereas 15 read the booklet. After 6 weeks both groups reported reduced communication and behaviour problems at home, although the workshop participants demonstrated a significantly higher awareness of communication strategies when evaluating video-clips of actor interactions. Hopper (2001) provided a summary of interventions with carers to facilitate communication in dementia.

Working individually with carers

Bayles and Tomoeda (1996) recommend working individually with carers on communication difficulties in dementia. The Chatter Matters presentation and approach was developed for working individually with carers (Barnes 2003). Carers are visited at home and initially interviewed informally about their concerns and impressions of the client's difficulties, which are added to those already identified from the client's assessment.

Carers are then invited to view the Chatter Matters presentation. This contains a total of 40 presentation pages each covering a different topic (with a planning sheet), though a small number of pages are used for an individual carer according to the issues and difficulties identified so that a presentation of approximately 15 minutes takes place. After this the carer is invited to identify any issues most relevant to their situation and needs or interests. The therapist then helps the client to identify no more than three specific ideas that may help enable or maintain communication. Within the discussion there is also some element of encouragement for what the carer is already doing. After the discussion recommendations are written down, the therapist negotiates with the client the amount of support required to implement each of the issues suggested. This may range from weekly contact to 3-monthly reviews.

The Chatter Matters presentation covers:

- understanding communication and the effects of dementia
- keeping the quality and content of communication balanced
- understanding why memory loss affects communication
- what helps communication
- using objects to enable communication
- using internal and external memory aids
- using correction and reality orientation
- using distraction and reminiscence
- allowing the person to succeed using validation techniques
- going along with confused ideas
- when to use which approaches
- word-finding and difficulty with expression
- comprehension and difficulty with understanding
- decision-making
- watching television
- coping with repetition
- planning for visitors and visiting
- using life history as a conversation aid
- reacting to difficult behaviour
- what to do and expect when conversation is very difficult.

Future developments and research

A firmer commitment from therapy services to working with carers is advocated. This should be fuelled by more research evidence showing how working with carers can change their behaviour as well as their knowledge and ultimately benefit the client. Despite the development of some approaches, there is still scope for identifying the most effective means of carer training. Would-be researchers are advised to consider contemporary approaches to research in this area suggested by Nolan et al. (2002) and an ethical framework devised by Vaas et al. (2003).

There is considerably less evidence for helping us determine which carers are likely to benefit from particular types of approaches. Further research should also be carried out to determine what 'successful' carers and communicators do, think and feel alongside innovative ways of sharing and developing these ideas with others. Standards of practice and service provision need to incorporate specific provision for carers (see Chapters 3 and 8).

Summary

In summary:

- A large proportion of care and communication experienced by people with dementia comes from informal family and friend carers.
- Carers of people with dementia are likely to experience increased stress and burden over a period of years. The loss of meaningful interaction can increase this pressure.
- Carers may be able to make modifications to the communication environment and style, though initially this may be a difficult concept for them to consider.
- When contacting carers, take care to explain what is meant by communication difficulties and communication interventions.
- As well as assessing the person with dementia, try to gain some understanding of the carer's lifestyle, situation, relationships, abilities, beliefs and expectations as well as the stage in their caring career.
- When working with carers, avoid treating them as resources. Encourage them to value their own expertise while forming realistic expectations about what can be done now and what will happen in the future.
- Try to work with carers individually to develop their understanding, knowledge, expectations and behaviours in order to reduce or share their burden and help maintain, enable and develop communication between them and the person they care for.
- Encourage carers, to join carers' groups to gain further information and understanding alongside the social support and the unique empathy and problem-solving potential that can come from their fellow carers.
- Use leaflets, books, videos and other resources by guiding the carer through that which is most appropriate to their situation.
- Avoid offering too much advice; rather, base advice and goals on what is most important to carers as well as what is most amenable to change.
- Enable the carer to access ongoing support by providing contact details and ensuring that they understand how further support may be beneficial.

References

Alzheimer Scotland (2003) Signposts to Support: understanding the special needs of carers of people with dementia. Alzheimer Scotland, Edinburgh.

Alzheimer's Society (1995) Right from the Start: primary heath care and dementia. Alzheimer's Society UK, London.

Alzheimer's Society (2004a) Policy Position Paper on Carer Support. Alzheimer's Society UK, London.

Alzheimer's Society (2004b) Policy Position Paper on Demography. Alzheimer's Society UK, London.

Aneschensel CS, Pearlin LI, Mullan JT et al. (1995) Profiles in Caregiving. The Unexpected Career. Academic Press, San Diego, CA.

Argyle N, Jestice S, Brook CPB (1985) Psychogeriatric patients: their supporters' problems. Age and Ageing 14: 355–360.

Armstrong L, Borthwick S (1997) The power of carer perceptions. Human Communication February/March, pp. 6–8.

Barnes CJ (1998) An investigation into the value of providing communication advice and training for carers of individuals with dementia. Unpublished MA dissertation. University of Portsmouth.

Barnes CJ (2003) Chatter Matters. A presentation for carers of people with communication and memory difficulties. Colin Barnes Publications, Portsmouth (*http://chattermatters.mysite.freeserve.com*).

Bayles K, Tomoeda C (1993) The ABCs of Dementia. Canyonlands Publishing, Tucson, AZ.

Bayles K, Tomoeda C (1996) Understanding and Caring for Dementia Patients: caregiver training audiotape. Canyonlands Publishing, Tucson, AZ.

Bohling HR (1991) Communication with Alzheimer's patients: an analysis of caregiver listening patterns. International Journal of Ageing and Human Development 33(4): 249–267.

Brodaty H, Gresham M (1989) Effects of a training programme to reduce stress in carers of patients with dementia. BMJ 299: 1375–1379.

Brodaty H, Hadzi-Pavlovic D (1990) Psychosocial effects on carers of living with persons with dementia. BMJ 299: 1375–1379.

Brodaty H, Peters KE (1991) Cost effectiveness of a training program for dementia carers. International Psychogeriatrics 3(1): 11–21.

Burns R, Nichols LO, Martindale-Adams J et al. (2003) Primary care interventions for dementia caregivers: 2-year outcomes from the REACH study. Gerontologist 43: 547–555.

Carers UK (2003) Stretched to the Limit. Annual Review 2002–2003. Carers UK, London.

Chadwick DD, Joliffe J, Goldbart J (2002) Carer knowledge of dysphagia strategies. International Journal of Language and Communication Disorders 37(2): 345–359.

Charlesworth G (2001) Can cognitive therapy reduce depression in depressed carers of people with dementia? Research Fellowship Report, Alzheimer's Society UK, London.

Clare L, Woods RT (2001) Cognitive rehabilitation in dementia. In: Clare L, Woods RT (eds) Neuropsychological Rehabilitation Special Issue 11(3/4). Psychology Press, Hove, pp. 193–517.

Clarke C, Watson D (1991) Informal carers of the dementing elderly: a study of relationships. Nursing Practice 4(4): 17–21.

Done DJ, Thomas JA (2001) Training in communication skills for informal carers of people suffering from dementia. International Journal of Geriatric Psychiatry 16: 816–821.

Gallagher-Thompson D (1994) Direct services and interventions for caregivers. A review of extant programs and a look to the future. In: Cantor MH (ed) Family Caregiving; Agenda for the Future. American Society For Aging, San Francisco, CA, pp. 102–122.

Gilhooly MLM (1987) Senile dementia and the family. In: Orford J (ed) Coping with Disorder in the Family. Croom Helm, Beckenham, pp. 138–168.

Gilleard CJ, Belford H, Gilleard E et al. (1984a) Emotional distress among the supporters of the elderly mentally infirm. British Journal of Psychiatry 145: 172–177.

Gilleard CJ, Gilleard E, Gledhill K, Whittick J (1984b) Caring for the elderly mentally infirm at home: a survey of the supporters. Journal of Epidemiology and Community Health 38: 319–325.

Goldsmith M (1996) Hearing the Voice of People with Dementia. Jessica Kingsley Publishers, London.

Gordon D, Spicker P (1997) Demography, needs and planning: the challenge of a changing population. In: Hunter S (ed) Dementia Challenges and New Directions. Research Highlights in Social Work Series, No 31. Jessica Kingsley Publishers, London.

Greene JG, Smith R, Gardiner M, Timbury GC (1982) Measuring behavioural disturbance of elderly demented patients in the community and its effects on relatives: a factor analytic study. Age and Ageing 11: 121–126.

Haley WE, Wadley VG, West CAC, Vetzel LL (1994) How care-giving stressors change with severity of dementia. Seminars in Speech and Language 15(3): 195–205.

Homer AC, Gilleard C (1990) Abuse of elderly people by their carers. BMJ 301: 1359–1362.

Hopper T (2001) Indirect interventions to facilitate communication in Alzheimer's disease. Seminars in Speech and Language 22: 305–315.

Knight BG, Lutzky SM, Macofsky-Urban F (1993) A meta-analytic review of interventions for caregiver distress: recommendations for future research. Gerontologist 33(20): 240–248.

Lock S, Wilkinson R, Bryan K (2001) Supporting Partners of People with Aphasia in Relationships and Conversations (SPPARC). Winslow, Oxford.

Lowery K, Mynt P, Aisbett J et al. (2000) Depression in the carers of dementia sufferers: a comparison of the carers of patients suffering from dementia with Lewy bodies and the carers of patients with Alzheimer's disease. Journal of Affective Disorders 59(1): 61–65.

Lubinski R (1995) Dementia and Communication. Singular Publishing, San Diego, CA.

McCallion P, Toseland RW, Freeman K (1999) An evaluation of a family visit education program. Journal of the American Geriatrics Society 4(7): 203–214.

Marriot A, Donaldson C, Tarrier N, Burns A (2000) Effectiveness of cognitive-behavioural family interventions in reducing the burden of care in carers of patients with Alzheimer's disease. British Journal of Psychiatry 176: 557–562.

Marriott H (2003) The Selfish Pig's Guide to Caring. Polperro Heritage Press, Clifton upon Teme, Worcestershire.

Miesen B, Blom M (2000) The Alzheimer Café. A guideline manual for setting one up. Translated by G Jones. Dutch Alzheimer's Society.

Mittelman MS, Roth DL, Haley WE, Zarit SH (2004) Effects of a caregiver intervention on negative caregiver appraisals of behaviour problems in patients with Alzheimer's disease: results of a randomised control study. Journal of Gerontology Psychological Sciences and Social Sciences 59B: 27–34.

Morris LW, Morris RG, Briton PG (1988) The relationship between marital intimacy, perceived strain and depression in spouse caregivers of dementia sufferers. British Journal of Medical Psychology 62: 173–179.

Motenko AK (1989) The frustrations, gratifications and well-being of dementia caregivers. Gerontologist 29: 166–172.

Muir N (1996) Management approaches involving carers. In: Bryan K, Maxim J (eds) Communication Disability and the Psychiatry of Old Age. Whurr, London.

Murray J, Schneider J, Banerjee S, Mann A (1999) Eurocare: a cross-national study of co-resident spouse carers for people with Alzheimer's disease: II – A qualitative analysis of the experience of caregiving. International Journal of Geriatric Psychiatry 14: 662–667.

Nolan M, Grant G, Caldock K, Keady J (1994) A framework for assessing the needs of family carers: a multi-disciplinary guide. BASE Publications, Guildford.

Nolan M, Ingram P, Watson R (2002) Working with family carers of people with dementia. Dementia 1(1): 75–93.

O'Brien V (1999) Dementia care in South Lakeland. Challenges and Potentials. South Lakeland Alzheimer's Society, Kendal, Cumbria.

O'Connor DW, Pollitt PA, Roth M et al. (1990) Problems reported by relatives in a community study of dementia. British Journal of Psychiatry 156: 835–841.

ONS (2001) Census 2001. Office for National Statistics. The Stationery Office, London.

Parker G (1990) With Due Care and Attention, 2nd edn. Family Studies Policy Centre, London.

Pool J (1997) Helping carers change their role. Journal of Dementia Care 5(3): 24–25.

Powell JA, Hale MA, Bayer AJ (1995) Symptoms of communication breakdown in dementia: carers' perceptions. European Journal of Disorders of Communication 30: 65–75.

Pusey H, Richards D (2001) A systematic review of the effectiveness of psychosocial interventions for carers of people with dementia. Aging and Mental Health 5(2): 107–119.

Richardson CA, Gilleard CJ, Lieberman S, Peeler R (1994) Working with older adults and their families – a review. Journal of Family Therapy 16: 225–240.

Ripich D (1996) Alzheimer's Disease Communication Code: the FOCUSED program for caregivers. Psychological Corporation, Austin, TX.

Saad K, Hartman J, Ballard C et al. (1995) Coping by the carers of dementia sufferers. Age and Ageing 24: 495–498.

Samuelsson AM, Annerstedt L, Elmstahl S, Samuelsson S, Gratstrom M (2001) Burden of responsibility experienced by family caregivers of elderly dementia sufferers. Scandinavian Journal of Caring Sciences 15(1): 25–33.

Santo Pietro MJ (1994) Assessing the communicative styles of caregivers of patients with Alzheimer's disease. Seminars in Speech and Language 15(3): 236–254.

Schulman MD, Mandel E (1988) Communication training of relatives and friends of institutionalised elderly persons. Gerontologist 28(6): 797–799.

Schulz R, O'Brien A, Czaja S et al. (2002) Dementia caregiver intervention research: in search of clinical significance. Gerontologist 42: 589–602.

Smith C, Ventis D (1990) Cooperative and supportive behaviour of female Alzheimer's patients. Paper presented at the annual meeting of the Gerontological Society of America, Boston.

Sorenson S, Pinquart M, Duberstein P (2002) How effective are interventions with caregivers? An updated meta-analysis. Gerontologist 42: 356–372.

Thompsell A, Lovestone S (2002) Out of sight out of mind? Support and information given to distant and near relatives of those with dementia. International Journal of Geriatric Psychiatry 17(9): 804–807.

Vaas AA, Minardi HA, Ward R et al. (2003) Research into communication patterns and consequences for effective care of people with Alzheimer's and their carers. Dementia 2(1): 21–48.

Victor CR (1997) Community Care and Older People. Stanley Thornes, Cheltenham.

Walker A (1995) Integrating the family in the mixed economy of care. In: Allen I, Perkins E (eds) The Future of Family Care for Older People. HMSO, London.

Woods RT, Wills W, Higginson IJ, Hobbins J, Whitby M (2003) Support in the community for people with dementia and their carers: a comparative outcome study of specialist mental health service interventions. International Journal of Geriatric Psychiatry 18: 298–307.

Zarit SH, Teri L (1991) Interventions and services for family caregivers. Annual Review of Gerontology and Geriatrics 11: 287–310.

Recommended resources for carers

Clare L, Wilson BA (1997) Coping with Memory Problems. Psychological Corporation, Bury St Edmunds.

Hann L (1998) The Milk's in the Oven. A booklet explaining dementia to children. Mental Health Foundation (*www.mentalhealth.org.uk*).

Koening Coste J (2003) Learning to Speak Alzheimer's. The new approach to living positively with Alzheimer's disease. Vermillion, London.

Marriott H (2003) The Selfish Pig's Guide to Caring. Polperro Heritage Press, Clifton upon Teme, Worcestershire.

Martyn C, Gale C (1999) The BMA Family Doctor Guide to Forgetfulness and Dementia. Dorling Kindersley, London.

Powell J (2000) Care to Communicate. Helping the Older Person with Dementia. Hawker Publication, London.

Rau MT (1993) Coping with Communication Challenges in Alzheimer's Disease. Singular Publishing, San Diego, CA.

Tanton M (1993) Helping Communication in the Person with Dementia. Published by the author. Available from M. Tanton, 38 The Marsh, Pudsey, W Yorks LS28 7NY.

CHAPTER 10

Developing speech and language therapy services in older age mental health

VICTORIA RAMSEY, MARY HERITAGE AND KAREN BRYAN

The role of the speech and language therapist (SLT) within older people's mental health (OPMH) services is relatively new and is therefore undergoing significant change and development. Currently in the UK the SLT is only partially recognized as a core member of the mental health team, and SLT provision is very variable. A number of key documents have recently supported the need for SLT provision to mental health as a specialist intervention (see Chapter 1).

Because of the lack of services nationally, SLTs need to influence the commissioning of new services and develop existing services to meet required standards. When developing such services, it is important to ensure that all components of the service are planned and that there is a clear understanding of the local population and need. Those planning new SLT services should seek to form good links with other professionals and agencies and promote the service in a clear and confident manner. Any new developments should be considered in the broader context of the current changes elsewhere in older people's services (e.g. in intermediate care, reform of social services and the single assessment).

This chapter will briefly review the history of services for older people with mental health needs and consider the development of new and existing services.

Speech and language therapy services in older age mental health

The provision of SLTs to mental health services is a relatively recent development for the profession. Historically, the SLT's involvement with this client group has developed from mainstream adult services where SLT has treated communication and swallowing disorders, primarily with people with dysphasia. Older people with mental health problems were seen on acute wards following a crisis or because of an acute admission, perhaps for a hip fracture or a chest infection. Management of long-term mental health problems, originally situated in psychiatric institutions and latterly provided in community settings, has rarely attracted dedicated SLT provision, although notable centres of excellence have emerged.

However, changes in the ethos of patient care, from a medical model toward a more social or therapeutic model, have led to rehabilitation being considered as an important component of the care process in dementia (Clare and Woods 2001). Professions such as occupational therapy and psychology have found their place within the OPMH multidisciplinary team, and understanding of the importance of SLT input to this client group is increasing. Social models of disability focus on the individual person and how that individual experiences their condition. Factors such as the person's environment, life experience, culture and beliefs are taken into consideration, and an understanding of these factors and how they affect the person is considered to be as important as the clinical diagnosis. Compared to 'medical' approaches, the 'person-centred' approach can be seen as less fatalistic towards the individual. It supposes that each person will respond to having a disease in a unique way and as a consequence each will have different needs and strengths which can be met or optimized through therapy. The person-centred, individualized approach opens up opportunities for therapeutic intervention to be successful, whereas a purely medical model may consider such interventions as futile, given the inevitability of some types of disease progression. Therapeutic intervention maximizes strengths and gives alternative strategies where the person or their carer encounters difficulties.

Given this context, a wider understanding has emerged of what SLTs can offer OPMH services. A patient's environment can be adapted to maximize communication opportunities, families can be supported to avoid communication breakdown and to increase insight into their relative's condition. Training can enable carers to develop strategies for functional communication. (See Chapter 1 for a review of the emerging evidence for the effectiveness of SLT with people with mental health problems, and Chapter 9 for a discussion of working with carers.)

The provision of SLT in OPMH services has developed in an ad hoc way. Bryan and Maxim (1998) referred to a service which is 'fragmented and variable owing to reliance upon local initiatives and resources'. Services that exist in the UK have little national consistency and this has led to a number of challenges which are described below.

Current provision of speech and language therapy within OPMH services

The provision of SLT services within mental health services varies widely across the country. The range includes specialist services providing training and student supervision, to those providing some SLT input via the generic adult service.

A national survey of SLT managers and clinicians was conducted in 2000 to get a picture of service provision to OPMH across the country (Stevens et al. 2000, Ponte 2000). The survey showed that although 67% of respondents reported providing a service to OPMH, only 30% of those services were provided by specialist SLTs. In addition, 52% of respondents indicated that no full-time OPMH clinicians were involved in the service, and in 39% of cases an ad hoc service was the only SLT provision to mental health clients.

Ponte outlines the significant changes that have occurred in the NHS in the period between the 1990 and 2000 surveys. A shift has occurred from the internal market of the 1980s and 1990s to the integrated care system, promoted and underpinned by the National Service Frameworks. Despite this shift in patient care focus, Ponte found that little in fact had changed in terms of the number of services providing SLT to mental health of the elderly (MHE) services. Although the total number of SLTs working in specialist MHE posts increased in between 1990 and 2000, there was only a net increase of 5.5% of services providing SLT to OPMH. Ponte (2000) suggests that

> The Government's pledge to abolish the current 'unfairness between different parts of the country' in terms of service provision, means that each area's Health Improvement Programme should include a designated speech and language therapy service to the MHE client group, including specific and nationally consistent service standards for referral, assessment, intervention and discharge. (p. 13)

To date, this has not happened.

The experience of many who work in the field is that once a service is established, it is possible to be successful in bidding for extra sessions or posts, but initiating a new service is very difficult. The research of Stevens et al. (2000) appears to support this view.

However, the development of SLT services needs to be viewed within the context of the more general development of older age mental health services. Old age psychiatry is a relatively new branch of medicine with a significant increase in services over the last decade where the value of multidisciplinary assessment has been clearly demonstrated (Dening 1992). In 1998, the Geriatric Psychiatry section of the World Psychiatric Association and the WHO, with the collaboration of the International Psychogeriatric Association, issued a consensus statement on the organization of care in old age psychiatry (Graham et al. 1998). A survey of service arrangements in old age psychiatry in England sent to 438 old age psychiatrists (Challis et al. 2002) showed substantial variation in the three domains of comparison for the 73% who responded. Only 12% of services reported that the majority of their initial assessments were multidisciplinary, with 11% of services reporting zero multidisciplinary assessments. Only 30% of assessments were multidisciplinary and, when these were carried out, over 90% were undertaken by consultants and nurses. The involvement of social workers (78%), occupational therapists (74%) and psychologists (52%) was less likely. Only 31% of teams were integrated for case management, although 61% were integrated for policies and 58% for access routes. For community orientation, 60% or more services undertook the majority of initial assessments in people's own homes, and 53% had at least two specific links with residential and nursing homes. Linkage with social services was variable with only 8% of services reporting joint management and governance arrangements, but higher percentages for joint training (54%) and team membership (59%). Although 84% of the services reported linkage with primary care, outreach clinics and consultant time spent in primary care were less common (12% and 14% respectively). The survey indicates that service variability continues to exist and many services are not yet fully compliant with the standards in the National Service Framework for Older People (DH 2001).

Draper (2000) undertook a meta-analysis of studies investigating the effectiveness of old age psychiatry services. The evidence base to support the effectiveness of components of such services is becoming evident. However, there is a need to evaluate the role of specific disciplines such as speech and language therapy within old age psychiatry services and to examine the extent to which professional roles can be shared via models of working such as cross-disciplinary skill mix and consultancy models.

The current trend in health and social care is towards a more integrated way of working. Becoming more focused as a profession in this field will not only help SLT with its profile, but also ensure that patients fully benefit from knowledge and expertise. In order to do this, SLTs need to consider their 'niche market' and to focus resources on those areas, providing solid evidence for the effectiveness of our practice.

Developing a new service

Understanding the local mental health service

In order to ensure that any new SLT provision fits in with the structure, it is important to understand how the mental health service is configured in terms of staffing, teams and management accountability.

At the time of writing many mental health services are currently organized as mental health trusts. It is good practice for mental health trusts to have strong working links with both primary care trusts (PCTs) and social services departments, because both organizations are likely to have some responsibility for aspects of care for the person with mental health problems.

Mental health trusts are often large organizations which span a number of geographical, social service and PCT borders. One mental health trust may manage patients from several PCTs and local authorities. The creation of these large trusts has come about from the merger of existing services, which may have led to a variety of service provision within one trust. One example of this historical inheritance is a trust where one region has a well-established OPMH service and the other area a well-established service for younger adults. Problems of equity of service arise in such a case and ideally would be addressed by raising the level of both types of services to offer established provision across both areas within the trust. However, if services are required to offer parity to their patients across the board without extra resources, established services may be diluted.

Issues of accountability and structure need to be clarified before a new service is developed. Issues such as the following should be explored:

- Would the new SLT service be managed within the mental health service or would it be managed by the local PCT and have a service level agreement with the mental health trust?
- Who is directly responsible for line management, service development and resources?
- To whom are the SLTs accountable for day-to-day operational issues, and for professional and clinical issues?

If SLT services are to be 'bought in' from another organization, there must be clear links with those making decisions about the direction of these services and speech and language therapy needs to be included as part of that planning process.

Understanding the way that other existing therapy services such as dietetics or physiotherapy function within the mental health service can give vital clues about how best (or not) to set up the SLT service.

Whether the service to mental health will be managed by the SLT service or whether it will be directly resourced and managed by the mental health service has to be a local decision and one that takes into account local factors. There are several models of service provision:

- A SLT service can be employed by the same organization (e.g. a mental health trust) that provides specialist care. A SLT or team is more likely to be included in service reviews and strategic planning under this model. It also helps in terms of service accountability where aspects of clinical governance, including outcome measures, are shared within the context of a specialist organization.
- A SLT can be provided by a 'host' organization to the specialist organization, usually under the terms of a contract or service level agreement. If the SLT specialist service is provided by a small team, or a single practitioner, this may be a more robust model. SLTs can represent a more significant staff group if they are employed by one umbrella organization providing smaller and more specialist services to other partner organizations. Maintaining continuous professional development and providing flexible career paths is easier within a large uniprofessional service. However, speech and language therapy staff need to identify

on a day-by-day basis with the integrated team in their specialist area. Provision of student placements and succession planning for the future workforce are facilitated by this model. It may also facilitate consultation between SLTs working in mental health settings and those specializing in other related areas such as neurology, community rehabilitation, acute medicine and ENT.

It is worth considering some issues that arise from both situations. Where the SLT service is provided from a uniprofessional department (usually part of a PCT, but it could be part of an acute trust) there may be problems about who is responsible for managing the SLT service. Service level agreements between the managing department and the trust need to be clear, detailed and regularly reviewed and may consider the following:

- who provides what
- who funds training
- where stationery comes from
- responsibility for secretarial support
- responsibility for technical provision and support (e.g. computers).

Good relationships which may exist between managers who draw up initial contracts are not always permanent and when staff change, service issues are hard to negotiate if the contract is not clear and detailed. Therefore, it is important to think about every aspect of the running of a department, and to ensure that responsibility is clearly specified. In terms of reviewing service level agreements, it is vital that these are undertaken within the framework of the annual planning cycle. This avoids the SLT service being isolated and also means that any new resources assigned to the service will filter down to speech and language therapy.

SLTs often feel positive about being part of a speech and language therapy department with the advantages of professional supervision and support, access to training and career development. Speech and language therapy in mental health is a relatively new discipline and is often challenging in terms of recruitment. If there are good links with the speech and language therapy department and career structures and progressions are available, then this can make posts attractive. If the service is to have newly qualified therapists, they will require close supervision and that provision is more easily provided from a big department. Being part of such a department can also avoid clinical isolation, which is sometimes experienced by therapists working in mental health posts outside such departments. However, the current direction of service provision in the NHS is toward integrated team working and away from uniprofessional 'silo' working. There are advantages to being part of an interdisciplinary team, including ease of communication, joint and shared goal setting and joint care planning which can facilitate more holistic care for the patient.

It is also vital to understand how mainstream SLT services manage people with mental health problems. Many older people with mental health problems are not known to specialist services but are managed within primary care, acute medical and surgical services or other services appropriate for their individual health needs. SLTs with specialist experience and skills in mental health need to be able to outreach and advise their colleagues working in other areas to enhance management of communication difficulties related to mental health issues. The wider team that provides care to any older person needs to be able to draw on specialist staff to provide an individualized care package that meets the person's needs.

Staffing

The variety of structures in the configuration of staff groups within different trusts often emerge because of local resource decisions or because of a special clinical interest among staff. Many services in the NHS have not been set up as part of a 'strategic plan' but have arisen in a more ad hoc way, so again it is important to understand how local relationships work before deciding how the SLT service should be provided. Not only must staff groups and management structures be understood, but also the inter-relationships between agencies such as volunteer groups, nursing and residential homes and other statutory organizations.

Management structures in the UK are devolved and therefore there is considerable local variation. Three possible management structures are shown in Figure 10.1.

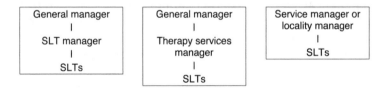

Figure 10.1 Possible management structure for SLT services.

There are positive and negative aspects of each model shown in Figure 10.1, and whether or not structures work depends upon factors such as:

- effectiveness of management structures
- efficiency and speed of decision-making within transparent systems
- flexibility within the structure
- communication channels
- adequacy of funding
- clarity and ownership of service goals
- numbers and grading of staff.

Staffing configurations will depend upon the agreed remit of the service. Staff could have a generic remit, e.g. all adults with communication or eating, drinking and swallowing disorders including those with mental health problems, or a more specialist remit with all or a significant part of the time allocated to OPMH. Ideally there would also be an appropriately graded trust or regional specialist and probably a remit within a specialist OPMH service or team. There is potential for such posts to develop into therapist posts, embracing the wider roles for allied health professionals published by the Department of Health (DH 2000b).

Appropriate skill mix should also be considered. SLT assistants can be a valuable asset to a SLT team and, given the correct direction and support, can boost the therapy time offered to patients. With the right training, SLT assistants can run groups and carry out individual programmes that have been set by the SLT.

As well as management support, any SLT working in OPMH will need adequate professional support. This could be provided by:

- **Peer support:** Other SLTs who have a similar caseload will be able to share information, resources and best practice. A network of colleagues in the same or in other organizations will ensure that individuals do not become professionally isolated (RCSLT 1996). Regular supervision should be provided according to the standards of the employing organization and should provide opportunities for reflective practice and information sharing. Those who are exposed to particularly challenging or emotionally demanding situations within their work should have access to local specialist supervision to enable them to manage such cases, and such supervision should be available from an experienced person at short notice. Peer support can be provided by regional or national networks such as special interest groups which provide continuing professional development opportunities.
- **Senior support:** SLTs will need support from an experienced colleague within the same organization to ensure that workload capacity matches demand, and that clinicians have the knowledge and skills to manage the cases referred to them. There should be referral routes to other specialists who can undertake joint assessments, especially where there is a dual diagnosis, e.g. Alzheimer's disease and depression.
- **Specialist mental health support:** SLTs with general or specialist adult caseloads that include people with mental health problems need to be able to access support and training from/alongside other professionals who work with similar clients: psychiatrists, mental health nurses, occupational therapists, psychologists. These individuals need to know how to access one another and what the skills and knowledge bases of their colleagues are. Such information would ideally emerge from regular meetings of the multidisciplinary team who share a base, but can be provided by looser networks that provide opportunities to maintain effective working relationships. Local interest groups, interdisciplinary projects (research, policy or care pathway development, audit and standard setting) are also useful in this respect, as a focus for team building.

Understanding the population needs

There are many mental health services where speech and language therapy does not exist (Ponte 2000). Within these services there will be older people who have communication and eating/drinking needs, and it is important to understand how these needs may be managed in a service without speech and language therapy. Generally, it is fair to presume that these needs are not being met but identifying and documenting unmet needs can provide a baseline from which to measure the effectiveness of a newly established service, as well as providing a platform from which to request further resources. Information on unmet need should be presented using appropriate statistical data, linked in to current national and local plans. By making use of such information, the need for a speech and language therapy service is demonstrated in clinical terms, as well as in terms of the organizations' strategy.

Local demographics will also influence the type of service that is required. Factors such as:

- the percentage of the population with mental health problems
- the percentage of older people (which will inevitably correlate to the numbers of people with dementia)
- incidence of key conditions

will affect the provision of a service that should respond to the volume of need. But other social factors will also influence the decision to assign resources (e.g. unemployment rates, presence of ethnic minority groups, housing, and transport). The range of services already provided to older people in that area will influence development of new SLT services. In some areas, there are well-organized and integrated community services which provide physical and social support and which dovetail with mental health services. In other areas, services to the older population are fragmented, with professionals providing their clinical speciality independently of other services. It is important to understand existing service provision and how the speech and language therapy service will relate to other services for older people. Key professionals providing community support include GPs, district nurses, social workers and home care workers, occupational therapists, physiotherapists and podiatrists. It would be beneficial to meet with representatives from these groups to discuss the vision for the new speech and language therapy service and how it can be accessed. Such discussions should include commissioning representatives from the PCT with responsibility for mental health services to ensure that providers and commissioners share the same vision. Groups of staff with a common clinical interest working across disciplines and even organizations, forming clinical networks which cut across hierarchical organizational hierarchies, are a common model for the development of clinical services. SLTs should seek out these networks in order to influence prioritization of new developments and investment.

Stakeholders

Where possible, it is beneficial to get the views of stakeholders. This may refer to senior managers, other professionals who will refer into your service, or patients/service users, carers and the voluntary sector. Views of stakeholders can be gained by using questionnaires, by running consultation groups or by gaining views via other forums such as managers' meetings. Patients and families, carers or staff will have valuable opinions about the way in which SLT intervention should be most appropriately targeted. Representative groups from the voluntary sector can provide the 'user voice'. Find out who are the appropriate people in the organization to whom findings should be presented, and set a time to discuss the proposals. It is now a legal responsibility for health and social care organizations to involve service users in the planning and evaluation of all services. Service users with communication disabilities are vulnerable to exclusion from these consultations unless specialist advice on communication strategies is available.

Risk assessment

Measuring the effect of a lack of speech and language therapy service on patients with eating and drinking problems is relatively straightforward. Dysphagia, if not managed, results in malnutrition (Hudson et al. 2000) and dehydration, and is a causal factor in repeated chest infections and choking risk. Studies that look at the incidence of swallowing difficulty in dementia show a high rate of dysphagia: 68% of those in one residential home had such a difficulty (Steele et al. 1997). The onset of feeding dependence correlates with the onset of dysphagia in dementia. It is therefore essential that staff and relatives caring for the person with dysphagia are aware of ways in which they can assist and prompt without reducing the person's ability to self-feed (Siebens et al. 1986). The outcome of inappropriate management of eating and drinking difficulties may be a higher incidence of death from chest infection. Managers and commissioners are responsible for addressing such risk issues and may be able to find funding to address local risk around nutrition and morbidity in older people through the provision of speech and language therapy. Demonstrating the need for communication therapy may be more difficult. However, there is now stronger evidence to support the benefits of speech and language therapy to both patients and carers (see Chapter 1).

Defining the service

The proposed service should have clear aims. These might include providing:

- assessment and intervention to enable individuals to achieve optimal functional communication and to enable teams to provide effective care
- assessment and management of eating, drinking and swallowing difficulties

- information, advice and appropriate interventions to support both family and professional carers and to prevent communication breakdown
- training and coaching based on assessment which enables teams to manage or prevent challenging behaviours
- appropriate advocacy to clients who are unable to communicate their own needs and wishes effectively
- education and support to other members of the multidisciplinary team relating to communication and dysphagia
- consultation, training and advice to SLTs and other professionals working outside of this specialist area
- audit and research.

It is then vital that agreed aims are reflected in the service level agreements. One way of ensuring that the speech and language therapy service is recognized is to set objectives and service developments in conjunction with the organization's targets. If it can be demonstrated that speech and language therapy provision contributes to the achievement of annual trust targets, managers and commissioners will recognize the benefits of service development. There should also be agreed standards for dealing with referrals within timescales, completion of assessments and reporting back to the team, therapy plans and documentation of outcomes. There should also be a protocol for discharge that would include:

- recording of progress and any ongoing needs
- any review or follow-up
- how to access the service and when this would be appropriate
- referral to appropriate agencies or organizations
- protocol for circulation of discharge information.

Best practice guidelines

The Royal College of Speech and Language Therapists (www.rcslt.org.uk) provides clinical guidelines, clinical standards and a position paper (RCSLT 2005) on standards for speech and language therapy services for older people with dementia. Information and guidelines on speech and language therapy involvement in the care of people with dementia can also be found on the websites for professional associations in the USA, Canada and Australia (www.asha.org, www.caslpa.ca, www.speechaustralia.org). These are useful tools for clinicians and managers who are developing new services and/or setting standards and procedures for existing services. Where feasible, new services should adhere to best practice guidelines.

Commissioning

Again arrangements will vary, but service level agreements may provide:

- blocks of service for an estimated number of clients, client contacts or successful outcomes

- specific defined (or restricted) services, e.g. assessment and advice only
- case by case purchase to an agreed remit
- an agreed number of therapist sessions per year
- purchased as above but from another provider.

Not all of these arrangements are equally desirable. Best practice dictates that the SLT prioritizes workload within defined parameters and in consultation with local management. Therefore, the most flexible provision may be the purchase of an agreed number of sessions per year, commensurate with local population needs.

Sites of provision

Again the exact remit of a new service will depend upon the local service configurations in OPMH. The aim should be to provide a seamless service for the client wherever they may be situated. This may include:

- specialist acute wards/units (usually hospital based)
- generic secondary care provision such as wards/units for older people
- memory clinics or dementia clinics
- community hospital or intermediate care provision
- day hospital/unit or day centre provision, including that provided by voluntary agencies
- residential and nursing home settings (mainly in the private sector)
- domiciliary provision.

Where a service does not have the resources to extend to all of these settings, information on unmet need should be collated and used to make a case for future service planning.

Identifying resources

The term 'resources' refers not only to finance, but also to people, equipment and time. In an ideal world, therapy services would be set up according to patient need and be flexible and responsive to that need. However, services are bound by resources and the ability to recruit staff into posts. It is therefore imperative to have a clear understanding of the resources that are available before embarking on designing the service. Being realistic and transparent about what can be offered and how best to use the time will support the delivery of a good quality service which can then be built on and expanded. If the service tries to provide comprehensive care with too few resources, the staff in post will be overburdened with work, and the patients will not achieve the best outcomes. In such a context it is easy to lose sight of the benefits that the service can offer.

Types of SLT intervention for OPMH

The range of disorders seen and the type of interventions offered should be made clear in the service or care protocols, reflecting multidisciplinary team aims and trust priorities. Ideally the service would cater for clients with all types of mental health problems, which may include:

- the dementias (although there may be other specialist services for some groups, such as younger people with dementia and people with Down's syndrome (see Chapter 4)
- depression and other affective disorders
- schizophrenia.

Local protocols for acceptance and acknowledgement of referrals are needed. Referral patterns also need to be monitored, so that changes in referral patterns or numbers can be used in any future contract negotiations. Given demographic changes (see Chapter 1), an increase in referrals over the next 10–15 years would be expected as the older population increases in size. The following components need to be defined within any service.

Assessment

- communication and/or eating and swallowing problems
- observation of abilities and difficulties
- contribution to differential diagnosis/care planning
- as a baseline for intervention.

(For more information see Chapter 6.)

Intervention

- Providing advice for the multidisciplinary team after assessment on the patient's functional communication ability and providing a baseline for monitoring progression of the person's condition. In some cases to help make an accurate diagnosis.
- Advice to the patient and their carers based on the information that assessment provides.
- Interventions aimed at assisting the carer to promote communication (see Chapter 9).
- Individual or group intervention to work directly on improving or enhancing communication. This might include initiatives such as life story work (Bryan and Maxim 1998). The process of putting together the life story resource is a speech and language therapy intervention in its own right, as the person is required to reminisce or comment on pictures or memorabilia provided by family and friends. The life story resource that is produced can be used as an 'anchor' for conversation and encourages meaningful interactions between the person and their carers or visitors. Later on, the books can be used by those around the

patient (particularly in the care setting) as a way of gaining information about the patient to shape the patient's care and environment. These stories are, in a sense, the patient's communication when most other methods of communication are no longer available.

* Provision of strategies to assist with communication and/or eating and drinking (see Kindell 2002).
* Modification of the environment to enhance communication.
* Re-assessment and evaluation of outcomes.

(See Chapters 5, 8 and 11 for more information on intervention.)

Group work

Group activities are a regular part of life in most OPMH settings. They are often run by occupational therapists, nursing staff, psychologists and assistants. The therapeutic goals of groups vary. Some of the generic goals are to:

* increase social contact and enhance social communication
* heighten memory and awareness skills
* encourage activities such as art or exercise
* provide support through the sharing of experience.

Groups may be for people with a variety of diagnoses or disease specific (e.g. for people with Parkinson's disease).

Groups might also use specific techniques, such as:

* validation
* reminiscence
* reality orientation
* life story work

(See Chapters 1 and 8 for more information.)

Underpinning all of these techniques is communication, and therefore many of the tasks chosen to facilitate the group will use speech, language and communication skills. The role of the SLT in group work varies depending upon the needs of the service and SLT provision. It may be advisory, in terms of both suitability of activities and how to successfully incorporate individuals with specific speech, language and communication difficulties into a group. Involvement in groups can also be used as a means of training others by co-working or facilitation, through modelling effective communication strategies. SLTs may decide to run their own groups, but these would usually target specific language tasks such as word-finding and naming, or individuals who are finding it difficult to cope with more generic group provision because of specific communication difficulties. When working with people with dementia, it is extremely important that the task does not emphasize a patient's disabilities and a way of ensuring that a patient's problems are not highlighted is to ensure that the group is run in an informal way and individuals are not pressured to respond, but that there is an open invitation to answer questions. The clinician needs to be particularly aware of any patient who appears to find the activity stressful and change the course of the group as appropriate.

Wherever possible, it is best to run a group in a day hospital or ward setting with a care nurse/assistant. In doing this collaboratively, the SLT gains a member of staff who has regular contact with the patients and the member of staff benefits from observing speech and language therapy techniques, ideally implementing those techniques in their working practice. If regular groups are run, care assistants can attend on a rotation basis, which will function as communication training.

Working with other members of the multidisciplinary team is also very positive and helps to work towards joint goal sharing and setting. Shortage of time often prevents this joint work occurring but even if regular joint groups are not possible, staff may be able to run groups together on a more ad hoc basis or around a particular issue or patient group.

Groups may also be organized by the voluntary sector (such as the local Alzheimer's Society) and the SLT may decide to approach them to offer some sessions on managing communication issues. The advantage of this approach is that these groups are linked into the support of the Alzheimer's Society and help to build networks across the community. Involvement in groups run by outside agencies or fellow professionals has the added benefit for the SLT of raising the profile of what is offered to the older person with mental health problems.

It may be advantageous to run groups with some sort of review and/or break mechanism in place to avoid long-term groups that can become stagnant. It is important to keep in mind clear objectives for the group which are also linked in to individual patient goals. The aims and objectives for each member of the group should be set and measured and those goals be made clear through the activities that are chosen for the group.

Training and enabling other colleagues and students

This may include:

- other professionals informally or as part of a multidisciplinary programme
- student SLTs and others
- volunteers
- assistant qualification programmes

(see Chapter 6).

Measuring outcomes

How we measure success in a deteriorating condition can be problematic. Goal setting can be useful (DH 1997) and can include functionally meaningful goals such reading/discussing newspapers or other notable effects such as increased confidence or more interest in cognitive activities while undergoing the activities. Care Aims is a model that helps define the SLT's practice in terms of goal setting (Malcomess 2001).The Care Aims model is a way of describing what a SLT does via eight categories of care which outline types of intervention that a SLT may provide. The SLT uses a flow chart as a way of deciding when intervention is indicated and what type of intervention is most appropriate. The patient/user/carer/ staff then works in collaboration to develop and work toward goals and monitor progress. The eight categories of care outlined in Care Aims are as follows:

- assessment (needs analysis)
- rehabilitation (improving)
- curative (resolving)
- enabling (facilitating)
- supportive (supporting)
- maintenance (sustaining)
- anticipatory (preventing)
- palliative (relief).

The advantage of using a model such as Care Aims is that it enables the SLT to describe a range of interventions which captures the scope of the SLT's work.

Measurement outcomes may also come from patient and carer questionnaires, which capture the perceptions of changes to a patient's functioning after interventions.

Promoting the service

Part of setting up and developing a good service is establishing relationships with colleagues and managers and ensuring that they are part of the process. Even when good relationships have been established, the arrival of a SLT or two, where none had worked previously, may not be noticed. Other team members have very busy schedules and may not automatically communicate the new speech and language therapy service to their teams or colleagues in the community as a matter of course. Communicating a presence must therefore be seen to be part of the setting up process and will pave the way for good communication and more appropriate referrals later on. In order to do this, it may be necessary to contact all professionals involved with a patient which could include the immediate staff within the community mental health team (CMHT) and the wards, GPs, local community staff, the local speech and language therapy service, the acute hospital, day centres, residential and nursing homes and social services staff (i.e. the older people service teams). It is vital that senior managers are aware of the new service and what it sets out to do. It is worth producing information that includes a summary of the case for the service (audit), identified areas of need and evidence from published research of the benefits of the service to support the case for SLT intervention.

Look out for opportunities to promote the service. Multidisciplinary teams have regular meetings and journal clubs and are often looking for speakers. It may be appropriate to visit some teams and give a brief talk, explaining the nature and purpose of the service, while others (e.g. GPs) may benefit from written information in the form of a leaflet or an email. It is important to send information to outside agencies such as the Alzheimer's Society and social service colleagues. However the service is provided, ensure that the information is a clear explanation of the referral process, with relevant and accurate contact details.

Developing existing services

Established speech and language therapy services need to be developed for two reasons:

- The variance between services that currently exists needs to be addressed partly by new services and partly by developing existing ones.
- There needs to be flexibility within a service to adequately meet the changing needs of patients and their carers, both in terms of local demographics and in new evidence on intervention. An example of this latter need for change is the dramatic developments in the drug treatment in dementia. Those working in speech and language therapy services when these drugs were introduced found themselves responding to greater need for pre- and post-treatment assessment and advice to families. As therapeutic approaches are developed, it may be appropriate to bring them into speech and language therapy intervention. The service should be dynamic, with developments providing an effective service.

This sense of development must be balanced against resource issues such as time and staff. If a service is too responsive, in terms of quality or range, it will require the SLTs working in it to take on inappropriate work. When new developments require integration into a service, the service manager needs to consider what existing areas of activity could cease or change in order to take on this new role. Unless these questions are resolved, the service will become unmanageable. New local initiatives (e.g. a new service for patients with early-onset dementia) can provide opportunities for SLTs, where successful bids for new resources are possible.

A further tension for a developing service is the question of stability: a service that is constantly changing does not have adequate time to become established and staff may feel that they do not have enough time to gain experience and confidence in delivering their interventions. If there are areas of good service, then those should be maintained. Much of what has been said in the earlier section of this chapter on developing new services is relevant to the development of existing services. However, a number of issues particularly relevant to improving existing services are discussed below.

Auditing current service provision

If the service is to be developed, the speech and language therapy team needs to be able to assess its current way of providing services. This means auditing some or all of the following information:

- the number of patients
- the rate of referral
- the type of disorder that is managed
- the number of one-to-one contacts, groups and other types of intervention
- the amount of time spent doing other things, e.g. training and administrative tasks.

This service review as a group can be conducted by the speech and language therapy service or by the multidisciplinary team and can be a very helpful exercise to prevent a service becoming tired.

It may also be helpful to audit other staff groups' perceptions of the service. The perception from inside the service about how well the service is performing can be quite different from the outside view. The perspectives of other members of staff, patients, and carers about the service and changes which they might like to see, given an opportunity for new developments, are valuable. When soliciting other people's views, there must be balance between wanting to know what others think and what the service is able to provide, so that expectations of change are realistic.

The effectiveness of multidisciplinary team working can also be audited. Working within the multidisciplinary team is the most effective and appropriate way for the SLT to practice. During the planning phase of a service issues should be clarified to ensure that the multidisciplinary team's work runs smoothly. Issues such as the following may need further consideration:

- line management
- team management
- liaison processes
- representation at meetings.

Benchmarking

Benchmarking is a form of audit and is a method of comparing a service against similar local services or national standards. Benchmarking will indicate where a service is successful and where it is not meeting required standards. It can be compared with national standards such as the

National Service Framework for Older People in the UK (DH 2001) and the Royal College of Physicians Sentinel Stroke Audit (RCP 2002) (which includes many common aspects of services to adults with complex acquired disorders). Managers may also use their own networks and the professional body's resources to identify best practice and the geographical location of well-developed speech and language therapy services in the field. It is possible to informally benchmark a particular service against its local counterparts for factors such as:

- size of population (including demographic information relating to proportion of older people, or ethnicity)
- overall size of service
- number of specialist sessions funded and ring-fenced
- grade of specialist sessions
- number of non-specialist sessions where this client group is represented on the caseload
- skill mix of non-specialist sessions
- non-case-based activity: research, education, policy development
- case-based-activity: involvement in diagnostic clinics; assessment, intervention options available (group work, carer support, etc).

Where a service exists but is not comprehensive, SLTs and local managers have a duty to provide adequate information so that the prioritization of funding for competing services reflects the real needs of service users rather than existing patterns of provision. Where there is no service and therefore no local 'champion' to inform commissioners, initiatives such as the RCSLT (2005) position paper may be useful and, indeed, are designed to assist in such circumstances.

Risk assessment

Risk assessment is another facet of benchmarking, but here the risks associated with not providing a comprehensive service are demonstrated. By the very nature of communication disability, the following risks may be evident for the local population:

- lack of diagnosis or incorrect diagnosis
- social isolation or exclusion
- depression which may be associated with mental health problems and communication disability
- negative impact on relationships and carers.

Social isolation is a known risk factor for suicide, 16% of all suicides in England, Wales and Northern Ireland in 1998 being people aged 65 or over. Suicide in older people is strongly associated with depression, physical pain or illness, living alone and feelings of hopelessness and guilt (Health Survey for England, DH 2000a). Older people are also more likely to complete suicide (Bird and Faulkner 2000). The National Suicide Prevention Strategy for England (DH 2003) sets out actions to be taken to address the particular needs of older people, especially those who are judged to be vulnerable and those with a physical illness and depression. Enabling older people to access the services that they need, particularly in relation to depression, social isolation and physical illness, is therefore important. SLTs should be aware of the risk factors for suicide and should know what steps to take if they suspect that a person is at risk.

Clinical governance

Managers have responsibilities within the NHS for clinical governance, which is the system through which NHS organizations are accountable for continuously improving the quality of their services and safeguarding high standards of care. The following issues should be considered:

- Are duty of care considerations fully met?
- Are SLTs who provide a service to people with mental health problems and their carers sufficiently trained and supported?
- Are staff up to date with the current evidence base and best practice?
- Are staff able to access specialist supervision or networks?
- Do staff have access to other professionals working in specialist mental health services (psychiatrists, nurses, psychologists, occupational therapists)?
- Where is a second opinion service available from?
- Where do non-specialist services fall short of the standards set by the trust, by the profession and by the government? What are the risks involved in this shortfall?
- Are the clinical network or the clinical governance leads in the trust with responsibility for mental health provision aware of any risks and able to express these to commissioners?

Effective caseload management

Managing a caseload efficiently is a fundamental skill for all SLTs, but there are some particular issues in managing a caseload of OPMH patients that are worth highlighting in the context of a developing or new service.

The nature of mental health problems is that a high proportion tend to be chronic. Indeed, patients with dementia have a progressive condition that will deteriorate. Many types of speech and language therapy intervention will require reviewing and monitoring over a course of time and change will be implemented as appropriate. Once a clinician engages in some type of intervention with a patient, they embark on a duty of care. It is likely that once involved with a patient, the clinician will become aware that the patient has other speech and language therapy needs.

Because management often requires assessment and review of the patient's changing needs and abilities, the SLT may have an increasing caseload of patients needing review who have to be prioritized against causing unnecessary stress on the therapist. In order to avoid this problem, a framework for managing patients should be agreed amongst the team of SLTs before a service starts. Effective risk assessment and prioritization is essential. Risk assessment must be based on clinical evidence and experience using an appropriate risk assessment tool. The team should agree a prioritization strategy that ensures that those patients who will benefit from the speech and language therapy service receive input at the right time. The patient's context is vital in considering timing of intervention. A patient who is coping well at home and attending a day hospital may not be a priority for a language assessment compared to another patient who is experiencing early symptoms of dementia which are affecting communication with their spouse.

The use of a suitable framework for caseload management enables the therapist to ensure that they are providing appropriate care for their patients (e.g. Care Aims; see p. 276). Viewing intervention as episodes of care that are time limited and having a review mechanism helps to avoid an increasingly large review list regardless of clinical need.

Accessing support

Linking with other SLTs who work in mental health through specific interest groups and study days provides a valuable source of support and idea sharing which can give SLTs innovative ways of practising. Such groups are usually made up of SLTs with very different skills and interests, and may provide a way of learning about very different approaches to intervention. In terms of evidence-based practice, developing the service or perhaps planning audit or research and development, the team should be encouraged to have regular time to update their knowledge using journals, books and the internet. This knowledge can then be used to steer the team towards a service that makes best use of current research. Similarly, taking part in in-service training or journal clubs with other disciplines is a way of information sharing and ensuring that everyone in the team keeps up to date.

Developing protocols and pathways

The need for a service to work to agreed protocols is discussed above. Stevens et al.'s survey (2000) showed that only 22% of existing services worked to such protocols. Development of a care pathway or protocol for the service should use best practice guidelines. Many services that are poorly resourced are likely to struggle to meet such guidelines, but they can be used as a baseline against which to audit service provision, demonstrating what is being provided and enabling the development of bids to expand that provision.

Competencies

Pre-registration curricula for speech and language therapy education include awareness of the full range of adult disorders and service areas, but such knowledge needs to be expanded by continuing professional development. On graduation SLTs need to be able to recognize language difficulties and symptoms that suggest a degree of cognitive impairment. Training around lifespan development may include the ageing process and the social, physiological, psychological and communicative changes that are associated with normal ageing, compared to those pathologies that are common among older people. Where training establishments do not have suitably trained staff to provide the training outlined above, specialists from speech and language therapy and psychiatry or psychology should be used to deliver elements of the programme. It would also be very helpful to consider the impact of involving older people/carers to describe real-life scenarios. Placements involving work in OPMH are needed in order to encourage students to become interested in this field. All services should try to encompass some aspect of student training and training, and education establishments need to be flexible on issues such as caseloads and assessment formats to facilitate such placements.

SLTs working with a general adult caseload may also need to increase their knowledge of OPMH issues, given the demographic shift that is occurring, and the move away from age-defined services. In relation to continuing professional development, the following areas may need greater provision:

- underlying pathologies and risk factors: neurology, presentation, incidence
- changing philosophy of care
- intervention approaches: pharmacological, psychological, behavioural
- social impact on patient and carers
- impact on communication and swallowing
- role of speech and language therapy within the multidisciplinary context
- application of speech and language therapy interventions within the care group
- models of service provision and relationship of speech and language therapy within each.

Sharing the skills of speech and language therapy is one of the key things that we can offer the multidisciplinary team. Good communication can ease a difficult situation, prevent frustrations and tensions from building up; and being able to facilitate someone's communication can make the difference between a person getting their message across or failing. Looking after people with chronic mental health difficulties is challenging and demanding, but is made easier if those caring are armed with good communication styles and a knowledge of some basic strategies that will facilitate communication. SLTs are often asked to provide training on eating and drinking issues, but are less often asked for communication training. Opportunities must therefore be sought and taken whenever possible, and a training session on eating and drinking issues can incorporate aspects of good communication style. After all, helping someone to eat and drink at lunchtime is a regular and important communication opportunity.

Developing services in an environment of change

Given the current picture of speech and language therapy services in OPMH that was discussed in the introductory section of this chapter, there is no doubt that service development across the UK is needed. Indeed Ponte (2000) found that out of the 33% of departments that offered no service to OPMH, 18% of those had plans to develop services. The structure of health and social services is undergoing significant change at present, and any service developments in speech and language therapy must be considered within this context.

The general picture of future services to older people is one of integrated working (and all care groups in the future) where the person is at the centre of the assessment and intervention process. Services will be organized in such a way that duplication will be eradicated: professionals are encouraged to think about their core skills and those things that they currently do that could be done by someone else. This means letting go of some of the more traditional roles that, for example, a SLT may consider to be part of her job, and facilitating a team approach where joint practice is commonplace.

At the heart of this change is a desire to put the patient first and to organize services in a streamlined and efficient way. This often causes discomfort among staff who are concerned about the way that some of the proposed changes will affect their jobs. However, there are benefits to SLTs. As communication is central to most people's lives, communication problems impact on all those around and working with that person. Working more closely with other professionals enables us to provide communication therapy that can be adopted by all those around the patient. We are able to adopt skills and practices from other professional groups and share our skills. Responsibility and goal setting are likewise shared, and the individual clinician receives support from her team colleagues. Most importantly the patient benefits. Better communication and a holistic approach to care mean that repetition is reduced and a range of professionals are focused on providing a group of goals that are shared and agreed with the patient.

It is certainly a time for professions to look seriously at what they do and how they deliver it. But if we do that promptly and efficiently, then we will develop services that are modern and efficient and based on the best evidence. It is vital that SLTs have a role in the change process. In order to do this the profession must be well informed and engaged with debate. In terms of the OPMH service there are many opportunities which should be grasped by SLTs as the service modernizes to provide a better quality of care to its patients.

References

Bird L, Faulkner A (2000) Suicide and Self-harm. Mental Health Foundation, London (*www.mentalhealth.org.uk/*).

Bryan K, Maxim J (1998) Enabling care staff to relate to older communication disabled people. International Journal of Language and Communication Disorders 33: 121–126.

Challis D, Reilly S, Hughes J et al. (2002) Policy, organisation and practice of specialist old age psychiatry in England. International Journal of Geriatric Psychiatry 17: 1018–1026.

Clare L, Woods R (2001) Cognitive rehabilitation in dementia. Neuropsychological Rehabilitation special issue 11(3): 193–517.

Dening T (1992) Community psychiatry of old age: a UK perspective. International Journal of Geriatric Psychiatry 7: 757–766.

DH (1997) Rehabilitation – a guide. Department of Health, London.

DH (2000a) The Health Survey for England. Department of Health, London.

DH (2000b) Government's New Strategy for Therapists and Allied Health Professions Sets Out Key Role in Delivering NHS Plan. Department of Health, London.

DH (2001) National Service Framework for Older People. Department of Health, London.

DH (2003) National Strategy for Prevention of Suicide for England. Department of Health, London.

Draper B (2000) The effectiveness of old age psychiatry services. International Journal of Geriatric Psychiatry 15: 687–703.

Graham N, Diener O, Dyfey A-F et al. (1998) Organisation of care in psychiatry of the elderly – a technical consensus statement. Ageing and Mental Health 2: 246–252.

Hudson HM, Daubert CR, Mills RH (2000) The interdependency of protein-energy malnutrition, aging and dysphagia. Dysphagia 15: 31–38.

Kindell J (2002) Feeding and Swallowing Disorders in Dementia. Speechmark Publications, Oxford.

Malcomess K (2001) The reason for care. RCSLT Bulletin 595, November: 12.

Ponte N (2000) A survey of speech and language therapy provision to the mental health elderly population. MSc project, University College London.

RCP (2002) Concise Report on the National Sentinel Stroke Audit 2001/02. Prepared on behalf of the Intercollegiate Stroke Working Party by the Clinical Effectiveness and Evaluation Unit, Royal College of Physicians, London.

RCSLT (1996) Communication Quality Two. Royal College of Speech and Language Therapists, London.

RCSLT (2005) Speech and Language Therapy Provision for People with Dementia. Royal College of Speech and Language Therapists, London.

Siebens H, Trupe E, Siebens A et al. (1986) Correlates and consequences of eating dependency in institutionalised elderly. Journal of the American Geriatric Society 34: 192–198.

Steele CM, Greenwood C, Ens I et al. (1997) Mealtime difficulties in a home for aged: not just dysphagia. Dysphagia 12(1): 43–50.

Stevens S, Maxim J, Binder J, Ponte N (2000) A survey of speech and language therapy provision to the mental health elderly population. Report commissioned by RCSLT and SIG Old Age Mental Health.

CHAPTER 11

A survey of services for cognitively impaired elderly in the USA

DANIELLE RIPICH AND JENNIFER HORNER

The White House Conference on Ageing convenes approximately once every 10 years. The first meeting, held in 1961, resulted in the passage of the Older Americans Act as well as adoption of health-care programmes known as Medicare and Medicaid, and establishment of the National Institute on Ageing. The fourth conference, held in 1995, placed a high priority on Alzheimer's disease (AD), ranking it fifth on the list of 75 resolutions of the conference. Delegates to the White House Conference on Ageing will meet again in 2005 to develop policy recommendations to the President and Congress of the United States. Although a list of resolutions has not yet been developed, the Fifth White House Conference on Ageing will seek, once again, to promote 'the dignity, health, independence, and economic security of current and future generations of older persons' (AoA 2004a).

The purposes of this chapter are:

- to explain the demographics of dementia in the USA and the costs associated with providing health care to elderly individuals with dementia
- to survey the range of services that provide a continuum of care for elderly people, as well as the numerous governmental and private organizations that support research, education and service on behalf of the elderly
- to describe federal laws that support the provision of services for the elderly, including Medicare, Medicaid and Administration on Ageing programmes, and to highlight the research and educational programmes provided under the auspices of the Health Resources and Services Administration
- to summarize the major disability rights laws in the USA
- to review advances in the provision of speech and language treatment to people with dementia.

Dementia: demographics and costs

Dementia has many aetiologies, for example vascular dementia, Lewy body dementia, Parkinson's disease, Creutzfeldt–Jakob disease, frontal lobe dementia, progressive supranuclear palsy, and AD. AD 'is considered the most common form of dementia worldwide, accounting for approximately two-thirds of cases in epidemiological studies' (Leifer 2003, p. S281; US GAO 1998). Horner et al. (2004) have reviewed current taxonomies of dementia, Norman et al. (2004) surveyed diagnostic and treatment approaches from the perspective of the speech-language pathologist, and the Academy of Neurologic Communication Disorders and Sciences (ANCDS) has recently completed a comprehensive technical report on the state-of-the-art of evidence-based practice (Bayles et al. 2004). (See Chapter 2 for information on types of dementia and presenting symptoms and Chapter 4 for more information on language breakdown in dementia.)

Demographics

The life expectancy of Americans increased dramatically in the twentieth century. By 2050, about 80 million people will be 65 or older, and they will represent close to 20% of the population (US Census Bureau 1995). The incidence of dementia in the USA, per 1000 individuals, is as follows (Fitzpatrick et al. 2004, p. 199):

• white women, 34.7
• white men, 35.3
• African American women, 58.8
• African American men, 53.0.

The incidence of AD versus vascular dementia is 19.2 versus 14.6 for Caucasians, as compared to 34.7 versus 27.2 for African Americans (Fitzpatrick et al. 2004, pp. 201–202). African Americans not only have a higher incidence of dementia, but also have more dementia-related behaviours than whites (for example, hallucinations and combativeness) (Sink et al. 2004, p. 1280). These demographic statistics inform policy-makers and the health professions about educational and service needs.

As life expectancy increases, the prevalence of dementing illnesses will also increase. At present, the prevalence of AD in the USA for individuals aged 65 or older is estimated to be 6–10% (Leifer 2003). Prevalence increases with age:

> The prevalence rate for AD doubles approximately every 5 years, from 1% to 2% in the 65- to 74-year range to 25% and over for those aged 85 and older. (Cummings and Cole 2002, in Leifer 2003, p. 281)

Currently, the estimated number of Americans affected by AD ranges from almost 2.5 to 4 million, and is expected to be 7.5–14.3 million by the year 2050 (US GAO 1998, p. 7, Leifer 2003, p. 281).

Costs

In the USA, health-care costs account for approximately 15% of the gross domestic product, which represents $US 1.6 trillion in annual expenditures (from private and public sources combined) (Levit et al. 2004, p. 147). Almost 20% ($US 320 billion) of the total cost results from the provision of health care to individuals older than 65 through the federally funded Medicare programme (Levit et al. 2004, pp. 148–149).

This section briefly reports total health-care costs in the USA, the costs for providing health care to elderly people, the costs for long-term care (in nursing homes and in the community), and, finally, costs associated specifically for care provided to individuals with dementia. Further details of two major health-care programmes, Medicare and Medicaid, are provided later in the chapter.

Long-term care requires substantial funding. An estimated 6 million elderly and 3.5 million non-elderly required long-term care services in 2000 (Kaiser 2004, p. 1).

> In 2002, a total of $139 billion was spent on long-term care in the U.S. for people of all ages, with $103.2 billion spent on nursing home care and $US 36.1 billion spent on care in the community. (O'Brien and Elias 2004, p. 2)

Medicaid paid 43% of all long-term care, and 50% of long-term care provided in nursing homes. Not unexpectedly, 70% of nursing home residents have dementia and about 50% are 85 years and older (O'Brien and Elias 2004, pp. 3–4).

The cost of health care for individuals with dementia of all types is estimated to be $US 50–100 billion annually (Leifer 2003, p. S287), or as much as one third of the total costs associated with caring for all elderly Americans. These figures do not include research and educational programmes funded by the National Institutes of Health, private foundations, the States, or service demonstration projects funded by the Administration on Ageing or other federal or State agencies.

Resources for elderly individuals

An important case was heard by the US Supreme Court in 1999. In *Olmstead* v. *LC*, the Court stated: 'Unjustified isolation, we hold, is properly regarded as discrimination based on disability' (p. 12), and segregating people with cognitive or psychiatric disabilities is a violation of the Americans with Disabilities Act (p. 15; see also O'Brien and Elias 2004, p. 15). In response to this decision, President Bush issued an Executive Order from which the following is an extract:

> The Federal Government must assist States and localities to implement swiftly the Olmstead decision, so as to help ensure that all Americans have the opportunity to live close to their families and friends, to live more

independently, to engage in productive employment, and to participate in community life. (Bush 2001)

The basic ideas expressed by the US Supreme Court Justices – opportunity, independence and participation – are the driving forces behind current policies that fund various levels of health care, as well as many of the initiatives on behalf of elderly individuals by both governmental agencies and professional organizations (O'Brien and Elias 2004).

Levels of care

A wide range of services is available for older Americans with dementia or other disabling conditions. These services address emergency medical needs, acute medical or surgical needs, inpatient or outpatient rehabilitation, home health care either before or after hospitalization, assisted living (or 'continuing care') retirement communities, extended care nursing facilities, home health services and other non-residential services, and hospice care, provided either at home or in residential facilities during the final months of life. The US Department of Commerce provides standard industry definitions for these various levels of care (see box).

North American Industry Classification System (NAICS) definitions

- **Freestanding ambulatory surgical and emergency centres:** 'This U.S. industry comprises establishments with physicians and other medical staff primarily engaged in (1) providing surgical services (e.g., orthoscopic and cataract surgery) on an outpatient basis or (2) providing emergency care services . . . on an outpatient basis. Outpatient surgical establishments have specialized facilities, such as operating and recovery rooms, and specialized equipment, such as anesthetic or X-ray equipment.'
- **General medical and surgical hospitals (except government):** 'Nongovernment establishments, known and licensed as general medical and surgical hospitals, primarily engaged in providing diagnostic and therapeutic inpatient services. These establishments also provide continuous nursing services and typically provide a variety of ancillary services, such as outpatient, laboratory, operating room, and pharmacy services. These establishments have an organized medical staff, inpatient beds, and equipment and facilities to provide complete health care.'
- **Specialty (except psychiatric and substance abuse) hospitals:** 'This industry consists of establishments known and licensed as specialty hospitals primarily engaged in providing diagnostic and medical treatment to inpatients with a specific type of disease or medical condition (except psychiatric or substance abuse). Hospitals providing long-term care for the chronically ill and hospitals providing rehabilitation, restorative, and adjustive services to physically challenged or

disabled people are included in this industry . . . . These hospitals may provide other services, such as outpatient services, diagnostic X-ray services, clinical laboratory services, operating room services, physical therapy [occupational therapy, and speech-language pathology] services, educational and vocational services, and psychological and social work services.'

- **Home health care services:** 'This industry comprises establishments primarily engaged in providing skilled nursing services in the home, along with a range of the following: personal care services; home-maker and companion services; physical therapy; medical social services; medications; medical equipment and supplies; counseling; 24-hour home care; occupation and vocational therapy; dietary and nutritional services; speech therapy; audiology; and high-tech care, such as intravenous therapy.'
- **Continuing care retirement communities:** 'This U.S. industry comprises establishments primarily engaged in providing a range of residential and personal care services with on-site nursing care facilities for (1) the elderly and other persons who are unable to fully care for themselves and/or (2) the elderly and other persons who do not desire to live independently. Individuals live in a variety of residential settings with meals, housekeeping, social, leisure, and other services available to assist residents in daily living. Assisted-living facilities with on-site nursing care facilities are included in this industry.'
- **Nursing care facilities:** 'This industry comprises establishments primarily engaged in providing inpatient nursing and rehabilitative services. The care is generally provided for an extended period of time to individuals requiring nursing care. These establishments have a permanent core staff of registered or licensed practical nurses who, along with other staff, provide nursing and continuous personal care services.'
- **Home health care services:** 'This industry comprises establishments primarily engaged in providing skilled nursing services in the home, along with a range of the following: personal care services; home-maker and companion services; physical therapy; medical social services; medications; medical equipment and supplies; counseling; 24-hour home care; occupation and vocational therapy; dietary and nutritional services; speech therapy; audiology; and high-tech care, such as intravenous therapy.'
- **Services for the elderly and persons with disabilities:** 'This industry comprises establishments primarily engaged in providing nonresidential social assistance services to improve the quality of life for the elderly, persons diagnosed with mental retardation, or persons with disabilities. These establishments provide for the welfare of these individuals in such areas as day care, nonmedical home care or homemaker services, social activities, group support, and companionship.'

Source: US Census Bureau (2002)

Agencies and organizations

The federal government and numerous private organizations provide many resources for individuals with dementia and their families, as well as for the health professionals who care for them. Several major agencies and organizations are listed at the end of the chapter. Most States have corresponding departments of health, departments of social services, and legal services that are specially designed to serve the needs of elderly people with cognitive impairments.

The National Institute on Ageing (NIA) is one of 27 institutes and centres comprising the National Institutes of Health (NIH) which oversees research, education, and information dissemination pertaining to the biological, behavioural, and social aspects of ageing and dementia. The Alzheimer's Disease Education and Referral Centre (ADEAR) is a service of the NIA. The Agency for Healthcare Research Quality (AHRQ) is charged with initiating and disseminating research regarding evidence-based clinical practices, clinical outcomes, and practice guidelines. The Food and Drug Administration (FDA) oversees all experimental pharmaceutical and gene therapy research, as well as the labelling and marketing of approved drugs and devices in the USA.

The US Department of Health and Human Services (DHHS) oversees a wide range of programmes that have been authorized by Congress. These include the Administration on Ageing (AoA), the Centers for Disease Control and Prevention (CDC), the Centers for Medicare and Medicaid Services (CMS) and the Indian Health Services (IHS), which serves native Americans. CMS's Health Care Financing Administration (HCFA) with DHHS reimburses physicians and other health professionals for all reasonable and necessary medical and rehabilitative services that they provide to older Americans under the Medicare and Medicaid programmes. The Veterans Health Administration (VHA) is a special branch of government that provides a range of health services to all veterans of foreign wars, including special services for AD and other types of dementia.

In addition to governmental organizations, there are a number of professional and private organizations that concern themselves with the health and well-being of older Americans, including those with dementia. These include the Alzheimer's Association, the American Medical Association, the Academy of Neurology, the American Psychiatric Association, the American Geriatrics Society, and the Gerontological Society of America. The Academy of Neurology, for example, makes publicly available several practice guidelines pertaining to diagnosis of dementia, mild cognitive impairment, the risk of driving by patients with Alzheimer's dementia, and management of dementia. Finally, the Commission on Law and Ageing of the American Bar Association, one of the largest groups of legal professionals in the world, establishes policy directives pertaining to enforcement of the legal rights of elderly people, including their right to live in safe environments that are free of physical, emotional, and financial neglect or abuse.

The programmes and organizations mentioned in this chapter embrace the obligation of society to provide for individuals who are ageing, especially those who are ill, or who have cognitive impairments. These organizations each have their individual missions, but are similar with regard to their service to elderly Americans: they advocate for the elderly, disseminate research findings, fund demonstration or research projects, and both educate and support patients, caregivers and professionals.

Federal laws and programmes

The US Public Health Service (PHS) is the umbrella federal agency for many services, including those pertaining to elderly people who are cognitively impaired. The PHS, governed by statutes passed by the US Congress, oversees the administration of laws that help to assure the health, safety and welfare of citizens. These laws include a range of entitlement programmes, most of which are administered in collaboration with the 50 States. For the purposes of this chapter, the most important are the Medicare and Medicaid statutes, and the Older Americans Act (all of which were signed into law by President Lyndon Johnson in 1965).

The Medicare insurance programme is governed by Title XVIII of the Social Security Act; the Medicaid programme, by Title XVIX of the Social Security Act. The Older Americans Act (OAA) established the Administration on Ageing (AoA), and is articulated in Chapter 35 in Title 42 of The Public Health and Welfare laws (Programs for Older Americans 2003). In addition, DHHS's Health Resources and Services Administration (HRSA) oversees the education and training of health professions. Specifically, HRSA's Geriatric Education Centers collaborate with universities to assure that health professionals are adequate in number and expertise to serve the needs of elderly individuals.

Medicare

Individuals who are 65 and older, have specified disabilities, or who have permanent kidney failure are entitled to health insurance benefits under the Medicare programme (Mold et al. 2004, Kaiser 2004b). For individuals aged 65 and older, Medicare is available to those who meet an employment criterion, namely those who have worked at least 40 quarters, and have contributed the appropriate level of their earnings to the Social Security Fund (Mold et al. 2004, p. 601). Approximately 41 million Americans are insured through one or more of the Medicare programmes (see box), some of which require beneficiaries to pay premiums and co-payments. According to the Kaiser Foundation, Medicare benefits 35 million older Americans and an additional 6 million who are not elderly but have qualifying disabilities (Kaiser 2004b).

Medicare: the federal insurance programme for Americans age 65 and older

Parts A, B and C include qualified speech-language pathology services.

- Part A. Inpatient hospital care, skilled nursing facility, hospice, and home health care.
- Part B. Physical [including occupational therapy, and speech-language pathology] and outpatient hospital care, lab tests, medical supplies, and home health.
- Part C. Primary and tertiary care provided through managed care plans, now called the 'Medicare Advantage' programme.
- Part D. Prescription drug benefit to be implemented in 2006 (Medicare Prescription Drug, Improvement, and Modernization Act of 2003).

Source: US Department of Health and Human Services (2004a)

In 2002, Medicare benefit payments for the elderly amounted to $US 295 billion (19% of total spending for personal health care in the USA). These payments were distributed as follows: inpatient hospital care, 39%; physical and clinical services, 26%; managed care, 14%; skilled nursing facilities, hospital outpatient services, and other outpatient benefits, each 5%; hospice care, 2% (Kaiser 2004b).

As a result of an important regulatory change in 2001, Medicare now reimburses for qualified rehabilitation services provided to individuals with dementia. Before that date, reimbursement for services such as speech and language treatment or physical therapy was denied, because most dementias are recognized to be progressive, and, therefore, therapy services were presumed to lack effectiveness in preventing, delaying, or ameliorating the effects of dementing illness. In 2001, the Centers for Medicare and Medicaid Services (CMS) of the DHHS revised this policy, and wrote a memorandum to contractors that stated:

> Contractors may not use [reimbursement] codes for dementia alone as a basis for determining whether a Medicare covered benefit was reasonable and necessary because these codes do not define the extent of a beneficiary's cognitive impairment. For example, a claim submitted with only a diagnosis of Alzheimer's Disease . . . may entitle a beneficiary to evaluation and management visits and therapies if the contractor determines that these therapies are reasonable and necessary when reviewed in the context of a beneficiary's overall medical condition. (US Department of Health and Human Services 2001)

Medicaid

Individuals who do not meet the requirements for Medicare may be eligible for Medicaid, which is funded through a partnership between the federal and State governments (see box).

Medicaid: the State–federal programme for some low-income elderly patients and families

Eligibility: The federal government sets basic criteria based on special needs; each State has the option of expanding eligibility based on category of need, or medical need.

Income: Income at defined levels relative to the Federal Poverty Level (FPL) is one determinant of federal and/or State eligibility; Medicaid is means-tested and is not insurance.

Matching funds: If the State programme meets basic eligibility requirements set by the federal government, the federal government will match the funds spent by the State.

'Categorically needy' persons (at the option of each State), e.g.:
* institutionalized individuals at defined income levels
* non-institutionalized individuals receiving care under home and community-based waivers
* certain low-income aged, blind or disabled adults.

'Medically needy' persons (at the option of each State), e.g.:
* certain low-income individuals with special medical needs
* other individuals who must reduce ('spend down') their income to the State's medically-needy income level by incurring medical expenses.

Mandatory State Medicaid services, e.g.:
* inpatient hospital services
* physician services
* nursing facility services for persons aged 21 or older
* rural health clinic services
* home health care for persons eligible for skilled nursing services
* laboratory and X-ray services.

Optional State Medicaid services, e.g.:
* diagnostic services
* clinic services
* prescribed drugs and prosthetic devices
* optometrist services and eyeglasses
* transportation services
* rehabilitation and physical therapy services
* home and community-based care to certain persons with chronic impairments.

Sources: US Department of Health and Human Services (2004b),
O'Brien and Elias (2004)

The Medicaid programme is designed to meet the health-care needs of many (but not all) individuals who are poor; Medicaid is means tested and is not an insurance programme. The federal guidelines stipulate basic eligibility requirements and services (if the State wishes to receive matching funds); thereafter, each State has the leeway to further define additional eligibility criteria and benefits relative to the income, age and health of the beneficiaries. Other individuals who meet Supplemental Security Income (SSI) requirements may also be eligible for Medicaid, i.e. individuals who are older, blind, or disabled (Mold et al. 2004, p. 602; Kaiser 2004a).

Approximately 50 million Americans receive health and long-term care benefits from the Medicaid fund. In 2002, Medicaid accounted for $250 billion in health-care spending in the USA (17% of all spending for personal health care); of this, the federal government financed 57%, while the States funded the remainder (Kaiser 2004a). Medicaid benefit payments were distributed as follows: inpatient hospital care, 31%; physicians and clinical services, 21%; nursing home care, 13%; home health care, 32%; prescription drugs, 2% (Kaiser 2004b). Notably, each year, shared State and federal Medicaid monies 'pay for nearly half of all nursing home care' (Kaiser 2004a). Elders accounted for 9% of Medicaid enrollees, and 27% of all expenditures; other disabled people accounted for 16% of enrollees, and 43% of all expenditures (Kaiser 2004a).

Despite the range of statutory 'safety nets' for health care for medically needy elderly people under federal and state law, a large number of Americans either are not eligible or do not enrol in either the Medicare or Medicaid programmes. Although they represent a small percentage (1.1%), the number of citizens affected is substantial. The result is that approximately 350 000 people aged 65 and older in the USA are uninsured (Mold et al. 2004, p. 603).

Administration on Ageing

Programs for Older Americans are enabled by the Older Americans Act, and are administered by the Administration on Ageing (AoA 2002, Programs for Older Americans 2003). As articulated in AoA's 2002 Annual Report, its priorities are to develop 'a more balanced, consumer-oriented long term care system,' to promote 'disease prevention and health promotion interventions,' to support caregivers, and to prevent 'elder abuse, neglect, and exploitation' (AoA 2002, p. 7). To achieve these goals, the AoA provides printed and web-based information and assistance, initiates research, offers grants to the States, and provides a host of meaningful services to elderly Americans (see box).

Programs for Older Americans (2003): Congressional declaration of objectives

'The Congress hereby finds and declares that, in keeping with the traditional American concept of the inherent dignity of the individual in our democratic society, the older people of our Nation are entitled to, and it is the joint and several duty and responsibility of the governments of the United States, of the several States and their political subdivisions, and of Indian tribes to assist our older people to secure equal opportunity to the full and free enjoyment of the following objectives:

1 An adequate income in retirement . . . .
2 The best possible physical and mental health which science can make available without regard to economic status.
3 Obtaining and maintaining suitable housing . . . .
4 Full restoration services for those who require institutional care, and a comprehensive array of community-based long-term care services . . . .
5 Opportunity for employment with no discriminatory personnel practices because of age.
6 Retirement in health, honor, dignity – after years of contribution to the economy.
7 Participating in and contributing to meaningful activity within the widest range of civic, cultural, education and training and recreational opportunities.
8 Efficient community services, including access to low-cost transportation . . . .
9 Immediate benefit from proven research knowledge which can sustain and improve health and happiness.
10 Freedom, independence, and the free exercise of individual initiative in planning and managing their own lives . . . .'

All of the programs offered through the AoA are available to cognitively impaired individuals. For example, over its 30 year history, the AoA's Elderly Nutrition Program (ENP) has delivered 6 billion meals to elderly individuals living at home through a programme known as 'Meals-On-Wheels' (AoA 2002, p. 12). It provides assistance to caregivers of elderly individuals through its National Family Caregiver Support Program (NFCSP), estimated to be 22 million people who assist family members, neighbours and friends. Since the programme was established in 2000, the NFCSP has served 325 000 caregivers (AoA 2002, p. 16). The AoA's Senior Legal Services programme provides over 1 million hours of legal assistance to elderly Americans each year (AoA 2002, p. 21), and funds State and local elder protective services through its National Center on Elder Abuse (AoA 2002, p. 22).

In addition, the AoA also administers the Alzheimer's Disease Demonstration Grants to States Program (ADDGS), which is designed to

expand the availability of diagnostic and community-based support services for persons with AD, their families, and their caregivers, as well as to improve the responsiveness of the home and community-based care system to persons with dementia. (AoA 2002, p. 26)

The recipients of these programmes are elderly (almost 80% are 75 and older), and represent both white and non-white Americans (about 50% each). About two-thirds have household incomes of less than $US 15 000, about half live in rural communities, and most require assistance with four or more activities of daily living (AoA 2002, p. 28).

In 2004, the ADDGS awarded demonstration grants to 38 State government agencies (AoA 2004b). The AoA will give almost $US 7 million in 2004 for the development of innovative programs (AoA 2004c). A few illustrations will demonstrate the diversity and innovativeness of the types of services offered to individuals with AD. These diverse projects, among other goals, intend to expand culturally and linguistically appropriate services to dementia patients, provide home and community services, train ethnically diverse health professionals, provide screenings for memory loss, expand adult day care, provide hospice referrals and caregiver support, establish 'empowerment groups' for individuals with early AD, provide services to under-served individuals representing minorities, facilitate the development of Alzheimer's programs in long-term care facilities, and expand professionals' education about Alzheimer's dementia (AoA 2004c).

Health Resources and Services Administration

The HRSA, within the DHHS, provides grants to individuals and States pertaining to the education of health professionals, and facilitates community–university partnerships in the provision of services. HRSA conducts workforce analyses, identifies health professional shortage areas, and facilitates rural educational and clinical programmes through Area Health Education Centers. HRSA's current funding opportunities emphasize 'increasing the diversity of the health-care workforce and preparing health-care providers to serve diverse populations and to practice in the nation's 3000 medically underserved communities' (US Department of Health and Human Services 2004a).

In 1983, HRSA's Bureau of Health Professions initiated support for a nationwide network of Geriatric Education Centres (GECs). The GECs provide funds to accredited schools of allied health to foster the education of health professionals regarding health promotion, disease prevention, and rehabilitation services for elderly individuals. According to HRSA's website, GECs have provided training to 375 000 health professionals since 1985. Through partnerships with universities, GECs train both students and faculty, provide continuing education to clinicians, and fund traineeships. In addition, GECs provide 'clinical geriatrics training in nursing homes, chronic and acute care hospitals, ambulatory care centers and senior centers' (Bureau of Health Professions 2004a). In addition, it has developed a white paper entitled *A National Agenda for Geriatric Education*. The recommendations pertaining to the allied health professions call for collaboration between schools of allied health and GECs to assure that the health professionals, including dentists, nurses, physician assistants, physical therapists, occupational therapists, and speech-language pathologists, among others, are adequate in number and expertise to provide care to elderly individuals (Bureau of Health Professions, 2004b).

Civil rights laws protecting the rights of cognitively-impaired elderly

Table 11.1 summarizes the major disability rights laws in the USA. These laws protect individuals of all ages, with or without cognitive impairments. These laws are enforced by the US Department of Justice (US DOJ).

Table 11.1 Civil rights laws that protect the rights of disabled Americans, including those with cognitive and communication impairments

Air Carrier Access Act of 1986	49 U.S.C. s 41705
Americans with Disabilities Act of 1990	42 U.S.C. ss 12101 et seq.
Architectural Barriers Act of 1968	42 U.S.C. ss 4151 et seq.
Civil Rights of Institutionalized Persons Act	42 U.S.C. ss 1997 et seq.
Fair Housing Amendments Act of 1988	42 U.S.C. ss 3601 et seq.
National Voter Registration Act of 1993	42 U.S.C. ss 1973gg et seq.
Section 504 of the Rehabilitation Act of 1973	29 U.S.C. s 794
Telecommunications Act of 1996	47 U.S.C. ss 255, 251(a)
Voting Accessibility for the Elderly and Handicapped Act of 1984	42 U.S.C. ss 1973 et seq.

For example, Title III of the Americans with Disabilities Act (ADA) covers both public and private entities that own and operate, for example, restaurants, stores, hotels, theatres, schools, transportation depots, doctors' offices, and day care centres. The law stipulates that no 'public accommodation' may discriminate by excluding, segregating or otherwise treating disabled people differently from others:

> [Public accommodations] also must comply with specific requirements related to architectural standards for new and altered buildings; reasonable modifications to policies, practices, and procedures; effective communication with people with hearing, vision, or speech disabilities; and other access requirements (US Department of Justice 2001, p. 5).

Section 504 of the Rehabilitation Act (which governs agencies or programmes funded by the federal government), like the ADA, requires ease of access, reasonable modifications to programmes, and access to communication devices for those with hearing or vision difficulties (US Department of Justice 2001, p. 17).

Title IV of the ADA requires telephone companies to provide 'telephone and television access for people with hearing and speech disabilities' through the use of telecommunications relay services and communications assistants (US Department of Justice 2001, p. 7). In addition, the Telecommunications Act assures that disabled people will have access to 'a broad range of products and services such as telephones, cell phones, pagers, call-waiting, and operator services' (US Department of Justice 2001, p. 8).

The Fair Housing Act protects disabled people by preventing landlords and sellers from discriminating against them (US Department of Justice 2001, p. 9), and the Air Carrier Access Act helps assure that public airlines will accommodate them (US Department of Justice 2001, p. 11). The Voting Accessibility for the Elderly and Handicapped Act 'requires states to make available registration and voting aids for disabled and elderly voters,' including the provision of telecommunications devices (US Department of Justice 2001, p. 12). Finally, the Civil Rights of Institutionalized Persons Act gives the US Attorney General authority to investigate nursing homes and other institutions to assure not only that residents are safe, but also that administrators and health professionals preserve and protect the legal rights of all institutionalized residents. These safeguards are particularly important for elderly cognitively impaired people (US Department of Justice 2001, p. 14).

In addition to the broad range of social and health-care programmes in the USA, and the panoply of civil rights laws designed to protect the safety, health and welfare of cognitively impaired elders, intervention and treatment programmes frequently used by speech and language pathologists who care for cognitively impaired elderly people are available. There are also a number of cognitively focused programmes, but these will not be included in the following review.

Treatment and intervention for people with dementia

As a result of the degenerative nature of AD, people with the disease are initially cared for by family and eventually need institutionalization for long-term care. Primary caregivers maintain that communication is the single most distressing problem they face, and they experience a gradual erosion of sociability. Therefore, the goal of quality caregiving should be to prolong and promote communication between these patients and primary caregivers for as long as possible and on as high a level as possible. Researchers report that family caregivers are sensitive to the communication problems and can identify the progression of the symptoms (Bayles and Tomoeda 1991, Orange, 1991). However, these caregivers need adequate training to communicate effectively with this increasing patient population. (See Chapter 9 for a discussion of working with family and friends as carers.) Developing the communication skills of professionals such as nurses, social workers and physicians as well as direct caregivers can enhance the quality of life for the person with dementia (Ripich et al. 1995, 1999a, McCallion et al. 1999a, 1999b) (see Chapter 8 for further information).

A considerable need exists for speech and language pathologists (SLPs) and other health-care professionals to shift from a more traditional medical model based on assessing pathology and restoring function to a more holistic model based on maintaining function (Clark 1995). The American Speech–Language–Hearing Association stresses the need for improving the quality of life and quality of care, which are rights of every individual including those who suffer from dementing disease, in the assessment and management of people with AD and related disorders. The components of quality of life include physical, mental, and spiritual health; cognitive ability; family and social relations; work and hobby activities; economic success and subjective well-being (Whitehouse and Rabins 1992). Since social interaction and interpersonal relations are a component of quality of life (Larson 1978, Mendola and Pelligrini 1979, Ishi-Kuntz 1990), ASHA encourages SLPs to provide programmes to maintain functional communication for as long as possible. An innovative and flexible treatment programme designed for people with dementia will address these quality of life issues. These treatment programmes can be implemented by direct intervention, which entails working with the patient, and/or indirect intervention, which is intended for caregivers of people with dementia. The Academy of Neurological Communication Disorders and Sciences in conjunction with ASHA have completed a technical report on the practice guidelines for cognitive-linguistic disorders associated with Alzheimer's dementia. This report reviews all current research on intervention in this area.

Direct intervention

With direct intervention, the communication specialist works with people with dementia on the goals of maintaining residual functional communication (Clark 1995). In this section, we briefly review direct approaches that have been used in treating people with dementia in both group and individual sessions. Many of the group treatment strategies can be taught to caregivers to use with the person with AD in other settings. Likewise, many of the individual treatments can be adapted for small group settings.

Group treatment

Group treatment even at more advanced stages of dementia provides opportunities to interact socially in a structured and supportive environment. Consisting of simple, informative sessions that review previous life experiences, group treatment has been successful for people in the moderate stages of AD (Hughston and Merriam 1982). Group sessions can include basic cognitive or sensory activities structured for success such as identifying textures and scents, and word, object and melody recognition tasks.

SLPs treating people with AD in groups need to assess baseline communicative abilities and determine outcomes (e.g. initiation, verbal and non-verbal responses, total words, total utterances, content, generalization, affect, interaction with other residents, interaction with staff, etc.), which can be measured through discourse analysis. These outcomes should be used to establish goals that are realistic, functional, tailored to the cognitive level of the group participant, and focused on optimal functioning and maintenance of communicative skills. In order to be reimbursable by Medicare and medical or private insurance, goals must be designed to achieve measurably functional gains within a reasonable period of time. Additionally, facilitators, other than SLPs, need to be familiar with the communication level of participants to engage group members in the activity, cue appropriately, and promote interaction. The clinical interventions for groups are summarized in Table 11.2.

Reality orientation

Reality orientation (RO) (Folsom and Folsom 1974) consists of two approaches:

* the one-to-one basic approach, in which awareness of barriers in the environment, correction for sensory deficits, attention to non-verbal communication, and structuring communicative exchanges by the caregiver are addressed with each encounter
* formal RO classes in small groups, in which signs and information boards are recommended with activities that are structured for success (Stephens 1969).

This approach has been studied and has shown positive outcomes (Baldelli et al. 1993, Metitieri et al. 2001, Zanetti et al. 1995). Although sometimes criticized through the years, it has been frequently taught, and some techniques are still used.

RO can be multifaceted and adapted to many settings and individuals while respecting the individuality and dignity of the person with dementia. Respectfully calling the person's attention to upcoming holidays and events can promote activity and interest (Miller and Morris 1993). As in any treatment method the attitudes, values and principles of the caregivers will determine how effective the approach is in a client-centred environment.

Validation therapy

As a response to the negative reaction to RO, Feil (1992) developed validation therapy with the goals of stimulating verbal and non-verbal communication, restoring dignity and well-being, and resolving meaning in life for the person with dementia, particularly for those in later stages

Table 11.2 Direct clinical interventions for groups

Intervention	Authors	Goals	Measures/Data	Results	Advantages/Limitations
Reality orientation	Folsom and Folsom (1974), Baldelli et al. (1993)	To reinforce awareness by calling attention to upcoming events or current environment	Measures verbal orientation, affect, functional behaviour	Numerous studies report: Increase in verbal orientation Improved affect Decreased mood No functional behaviour changes noted	Easily implemented Easily adapted to events and settings Criticized as having little theoretical basis and not impacting functional behaviour
Validation therapy	Feil (1992)	To help validate the feelings To identify four stages of conflict To intervene appropriately at each stage	No quantitative measures or data	Anecdotal reports show: Improved affect Positive behaviours during group sessions	Used in over 500 institutions in US May be best used with late stage patients
Reminiscence therapy	Harris, (1997, 1998), Nomura (2002)	To improve communication and discourse skills To improve memory To recall personal events To maintain cognitive stimulation	Varies depending on the goal of therapy	Improved MMSE score for people with dementia in day care setting participating in reminiscence groups	Reminiscence therapy can be conducted in a naturalistic environment Activities can be tailored to meet the needs of individuals or groups Culturally and linguistically appropriate Recall of unpleasant events is a possible risk

(Feil 1992). Rather than confront or correct people with dementia, the SLP empathically 'validates' or confirms a person's emotional states and helps resolve past conflicts. Additional studies of validation therapy effectiveness have shown a generally positive impact (Brack 1997, Toseland et al. 1997, Touzinsky 1998).

Reminiscence therapy

Reminiscence is a naturally occurring process that entails the review of life events. As a therapeutic approach it may be particularly appealing for people with dementia as an opportunity to communicate with others since it focuses on long-term memory (Harris 1997, 1998, Zgola and Coulter 1988, Harris and Norman 2002). Reminiscence can be encouraged informally by requesting advice, looking at family photographs, looking at old news magazines, discussing hobbies, military experiences, and past jobs. Discussions of traditional foods and celebrations, hobbies, school experiences, songs, and pets and artefacts such as tools and household objects borrowed from a local museum have been used in a group to provide sensory stimulation and to recall competencies and achievements from the past (Zgola and Coulter 1988). Triggers such as music, food, poems, faces, colours, objects and smells can be useful for recall. Reminiscence activities are adaptable to meet the needs of the participants by selecting tasks that are both culturally and linguistically appropriate.

In a group, reminiscence has many benefits such as developing relationships, entertaining peers, enhancing status of participants, assisting with identity formation, facilitating resolution, reorganization and reintegration of life, and establishing a sense of personal continuity (Anderson 1983). Furthermore, reminiscence has been associated with improved self-esteem in nursing home residents (Osborne 1989). Ziol et al. (1996) developed a group programme with a variety of communication activities that incorporate aspects of RO and reminiscence for those at mild and moderate stages, with suggested variations in the activities for those at later stages.

Individual treatment

Individual treatment allows the clinician to develop personalized activities designed to enhance communication for as long as possible. The person with dementia is taught strategies to compensate for deficits in memory, such as orientation, word-finding, naming, and recall. Compensatory strategies are also provided to assist with new learning. Although caregivers are not trained in the strategies, they can be present during individual sessions to observe the strategies the person with dementia is learning. Their presence at some sessions may be beneficial because it provides a mutual understanding of the communication goals established and the strategies developed to achieve them. Table 11.3 summarizes a number of individual treatments for dementia.

Table 11.3 Direct clinical interventions for individuals

Intervention	Authors	Goals	Measures/Data	Results	Advantages/Limitations
Memory compensations: notebooks, wallets, notes and look books	Bourgeois (1992) Bourgeois et al. (1997)	To create wallets containing relevant pictures and written information To train patients to self-prompt To improve conversational content using familiar persons, places and events To improve the use of factual information	Seven discourse measures scored for: Baseline conversations Training conversations Maintenance phase conversation	Some showed: Decline in non-productive statements Maintenance of performance levels Novel utterances were similar to baseline levels	Used to improve factual information in conversations with little systematic training Patients required minimal training Patients responded to prompts to look at or read their wallets May not be useful in later stage of dementia
Montessori-based activities	Judge et al. (2000)	To provide successful skills performance that involves multi-sensory experiential activities	Constructive engagement in daily activities, passive behaviour and disruptive behaviours assess change resulting from Montessori-based tasks	Improvements in constructive engagement Decreases in passivity and disruptive behaviours	Activities: Work well in the daily routine Help maintain current abilities Provide opportunities for interaction between persons with dementia and caregivers Help maintain the quality of life Can be adapted to group exercises

Table 11.3 continued

Intervention	Authors	Goals	Measures/Data	Results	Advantages/Limitations
Spaced retrieval	Brush and Camp (1998)	Persons with dementia and MMSE scores of 9–25 are given strategies Goals: To assist new learning To retain information or motor tasks by recalling information or motor tasks over increasingly longer intervals	Training sessions are designed around daily living tasks Information is designed to provide repetitive success If the patient fails to recall the trainer drops back to the previous success interval level and moves ahead more slowly	Variable results reported with subjects across early, middle and late stages	Easily modified to fit the individual's functional living needs Can be used even in late stages to help recall caregiver's name or one-step motor task May require significant time from the trainer to establish the recall information or motor task Family caregivers can be trained in this method Persons with dementia may learn a limited number of associations Previously learned information may interfere with severe episodic memory impairments
Errorless learning with quizzes	Arkin (1991)	To maximize success in answering quiz questions	Successful recall of information	Narratives and quizzes were more successful than the repetition Middle- and late- stage patients showed improvements	Shows greater success than spaced retrieval Can be used by family members

Memory/communication compensations

Training in memory and communication strategies and compensations is appropriate particularly in early stages when people with dementia are more aware of communication breakdown. During this stage the SLP can reassure and train the client to ask for repetition or review and compensate with circumlocution, gesture, and associated words for semantic deficits. A memory notebook with autobiographical information, calendar, and sections for things to do, maps, and daily logs (Sohlberg and Mateer 1989) can draw upon more intact procedural memory abilities to compensate for short-term memory failure. Bourgeois (1992) demonstrated the use of developing memory wallets with pictures and sentences about familiar people, places, and events. The use of external strategies such as written 'Post-it' notes, alarms, daily pill organizers, or audio- and videotapes can help to maintain independent function for as long as possible.

Engaging people with dementia with collections of pictures of familiar categories (flowers, boating, fishing, golfing, home decorating, local landmarks, etc.) can decrease agitated behaviour and increase interaction (Maureen Denis, personal communication, 16 August 1996). These 'look books', strategically placed within the environment, can be used informally either to distract or to serve as a focus for reminiscence in a group setting.

Montessori-based activities

Montessori methods are structured to provide successful skills performance involving multisensory experiences of daily activities for people with dementia and help them maintain current abilities (Judge et al. 2000). They provide opportunities for interaction between people with dementia and caregivers, and maintain the quality of life. Improvements in constructive engagement and decreases in passivity and disruptive behaviours have been reported (Judge et al. 2000).

Spaced retrieval

In spaced retrieval, people with dementia with Mini-Mental State Examination (MMSE) scores between 9 and 25 are given strategies to assist new learning and retention by recalling information or motor tasks over increasingly longer intervals. Training sessions, which provided repetitive success, are designed around daily living tasks (Brush and Camp 1998). If the patient is unable to recall, the trainer returns to the previous success interval level and moves ahead more slowly. The approach is easily modified to fit the individual's functional living needs and can be used even in late stages to facilitate recall of a caregiver's name or performance of one-step motor tasks.

Errorless learning with quizzes

In errorless learning, taped narratives with questions are structured to maximize success in answering quiz questions (Arkin 1991). The tape always provides the correct answer after a pause, to verify successful recall of information.

Indirect intervention

With indirect intervention, caregivers of people with dementia are trained to apply strategies to improve communication interaction. Communication breakdown is consistently listed among the top stressors in caregiver surveys of stress, strain and burden (Rabins 1982, Zarit 1982, Kinney and Stephens 1989). It appears that caregiver training in facilitating strategies could provide useful tools to the caregiver communication partner. Care of people with AD could be improved significantly by enhancing the communication skills of caregivers. The ability of caregivers to draw on strategies and techniques for dealing with communication problems in these people would reduce their own stress and frustration, and improve their competence in delivering quality care. In addition, the caregivers would be better able to promote the use of residual functional communication abilities, to provide appropriate social communication opportunities, and possibly to keep family members at home longer. Nurses and nursing assistants could also benefit from improved communication with their patients with AD. Several caregiver training programmes will be discussed in the remainder of the chapter.

Caregiver training programmes

Communication training for caregivers can increase knowledge, improve communication satisfaction, and decrease hassles related to communication breakdown. Education in specific communication strategies can alter attitudes toward people with AD. Providing adequate training to caregivers is essential to quality of life issues. Additional benefits may be caregivers' greater satisfaction and sense of accomplishment in their critical day-to-day activities. Caregivers can benefit from training in communication strategies and this training may improve the quality of life for people with AD. After briefly reviewing a training programme developed by Clark and Witte (1989), the FOCUSED Program (Ripich 1993) is discussed in detail.

Making family visits count

Clark and Witte (1989) developed this communication training programme for family members to improve quality and satisfaction in visits to relatives in nursing homes. In small practice groups, family members view prepared videotapes, taking note of facilitative communicative techniques and learning how to individualize strategies. In a communication stress management program for caregivers, Clark (1991) teaches family members to understand the nature and progression of language changes in AD, and to increase and apply problem-solving skills to reduce caregiver stress and burden. Caregivers learn appropriate expectations and the importance of maintaining the person with dementia in communicative situations.

The FOCUSED Program

To improve communication with people with dementia, Ripich and Wykle (1990a, 1990b) developed the *Alzheimer's Disease Communication Guide: The FOCUSED Program for Caregivers* (Ripich 2004a, 2004b, 2004c). The acronym FOCUSED organized strategies based on the seven major elements for communication maintenance for easy recall: Face-to-face, Orient, Continue, Unstick, Structure, Exchange and Direct. This programme consists of didactic materials to better prepare family and professional caregivers to communicate with people with AD. It was based on an interactive discourse model of conversational exchanges (Terrell and Ripich 1989), and supported by additional discourse studies (Ripich et al. 1997a, 1997b, 2000a, 2000b, 2002, Ripich and Pope 2005). The key points of the programme are indicated in Table 11.4.

The training programme is divided into five 2-hour modules for family or professional caregivers, with an optional module for professional caregivers on cultural differences:

- **Module 1:** AD and the associated communication and language decline. This module discusses characteristics, pathology, and incidence of AD. The components and processes of language are presented. Participants learn how physicians make a diagnosis of probable AD and how language in aphasia and AD differ.
- **Module 2:** The differences between memory decline in normal ageing and Alzheimer's disease, and the effects of depression on the person with AD. In this module, the caregiver is taught to understand changes in memory in the normal elderly, to recognize symptoms of depression, and to differentiate these symptoms from those of dementia. This module also discusses how depression can exacerbate the communication difficulties of the person with AD.
- **Module 3:** Interpersonal skills and the value of effective communication skills in the care of people with AD. The critical importance of social communication to keep the person with AD engaged in communication to prevent excessive functional decline and maintain abilities is discussed. Participants learn verbal and non-verbal approaches to good communication. A discussion of empathy provides a foundation for promoting sensitive interpersonal exchanges, thereby demonstrating respect for the person with dementia and supporting the self-esteem of both the caregiver and the person with AD.

Table 11.4 FOCUSED communication strategies

F   *Face-to-face communication*
        Face the person with Alzheimer's disease directly
        Call their name
        Touch the person
        Gain and maintain eye contact

O   *Orient to topic of conversation*
        Orient the person with Alzheimer's disease to the topic by repeating key
        words several times
        Repeat and rephrase sentences
        Use nouns and specific names

C   *Continue topic of conversation*
        Continue the same topic of conversation for as long as possible
        Restate the topic throughout the conversation
        Indicate to the person with Alzheimer's disease that you are introducing a
        new topic

U   *Unstick communication blocks*
        Help the person with Alzheimer's disease become 'unstuck' when they use a
        work incorrectly by suggesting the intended word
        Repeat the sentence the person said using the correct word
        Ask, 'Do you mean . . .?'

S   *Structure with yes/no and choice questions*
        Structure your questions so that the person with Alzheimer's disease will be
        able to recognize and repeat a response
        Provide two simple choices at a time
        Use yes/no questions

E   *Exchange conversation*
        Keep up the normal exchanges of ideas we use in everyday conversation
        Keep the conversations going with comments such as, 'Oh, how nice,' or
        'That's great'
        Do **not** ask 'test' questions
        Give the person with Alzheimer's disease clues as to how to answer your
        questions

D   *Direct, short, simple sentences*
        Keep sentences short, simple and direct
        Put the subject of the sentence first
        Use and repeat nouns (names of persons or things) rather than pronouns
        (he, she, it, their, etc.)
        Use hand signals, pictures and facial expressions

- **Module 4:** The FOCUSED strategies to promote effective communication with people with AD. This is a critical module which outlines the seven-point programme. The programme incorporates numerous strategies into a framework that is easy to recall and apply. A series of role-play exercises and videotaped vignettes are used to demonstrate the seven points of the programme.

- **Module 5:** The stages of AD and concurrent communication characteristics including how to assess and recognize the person with AD at each stage and maximize their communication. Though fully aware of the heterogeneity of the progress of AD and the fact that dividing the progression into stages is an arbitrary device, the literature repeatedly reports three main levels of language deterioration designated as mild, moderate and severe. In Module 5 these stages are described, the seven points of the FOCUSED programme are reviewed, and the implementation of strategies and communication goals at each stage are discussed.

- **Optional Module for Professional Caregivers:** Cultural considerations are extremely important issues in helping the professional caregiver care for the person with AD. The conflicts that arise in a caregiving situation may be further complicated by the differences in cultural and socioeconomic backgrounds of extended-care residents and nursing assistant staff. The resultant disparity in values and interpersonal dynamics accentuates the communication difficulties that are characteristic of people with AD. Therefore, didactic and experiential content that enhances caregivers' understanding of cultural considerations affecting that interpersonal communication process is presented. A number of investigations have been completed that examine the efficacy of the FOCUSED programme, and the results indicate a number of positive outcomes.

FOCUSED caregiving communication training studies

Investigation of the FOCUSED training programme has shown it to be an effective tool for caregivers to improve communication with AD patients. A series of studies examined the effects of the FOCUSED training on various caregivers. One of these studies was an investigation with 16 nursing assistants in a long-term care facility. Post-intervention analysis showed significant improvements in attitude toward AD patients, knowledge of AD and increased knowledge of communication strategies in comparisons of pre- and post-training assessments (Ripich et al. 1995).

In another study, the impact of FOCUSED was studied to determine if training effects were different in family caregivers who were African American than white family member caregivers of people with AD. African American and white caregivers completed pre- and post-training self-report measures of positive and negative affect, depression, hassles, physical health, knowledge of AD, and communication satisfaction. Results showed communication training increased knowledge of AD and communication satisfaction. African American caregivers showed greater positive effect than did white caregivers. In addition, African American caregivers showed significant declines in perceived daily hassles after communication training, whereas white caregivers did not (Ripich et al. 1998).

Additionally, the longitudinal effects of FOCUSED training were studied on self-report measures from 19 caregivers of people with AD compared to those of a control group (n=18) at entry, post-training, 6 months, and 12 months after training. These self-reports measured affect (positive and negative), depression, health, general hassles, communication hassles, and knowledge of AD. When effects of training on these measures were examined over time, the training group showed decreased communication hassles and increased knowledge of AD. No significant changes were found in the control group (Ripich et al. 1998).

Another study of 54 caregivers of people with AD was conducted to investigate the effects of caregiver FOCUSED training on question and answer exchanges. The questioning patterns of the two groups of FOCUSED training caregivers planning a menu with their family member with AD were compared to a control group of 22 caregivers. Data were collected over three visits (entry, 6 months and 12 months). Analysis revealed that for all caregivers, open-ended questions, when compared with yes/no and choice questions, resulted in more failed responses by people with AD. Following training at 6 months, FOCUSED caregivers asked fewer open-ended questions compared to the control group. This suggests that communication partners of people with AD can be trained to structure questions that result in more successful communication (Ripich et al. 1999b).

These studies show the feasibility of FOCUSED as an effective behavioural intervention for caregivers that improves communication with people with AD. Post-training caregivers showed improved attitudes, knowledge, and knowledge of communication. African American caregivers demonstrated greater positive effect and declines in perceived communication hassles after training. Communication of trained caregivers and people with AD showed more successful question-and-answer exchanges and fewer failed exchanges than those of controls. In combination, these studies present a strong case for caregiver intervention as a way to improve and maintain communication.

How effective are interventions?

Direct intervention

RO has been criticized for having little theoretical basis (Hussian 1981), for having no value (Reisberg 1981), for showing no generalization to other areas of behaviour, and being too rigid, boring and unstimulating (MacDonald and Settin 1978). Reports of validation therapy show inconsistent results of improved affect or positive effects (Peoples 1982, Fritz 1986, Dietch et al. 1989) when measuring communicative interaction in a group setting (Morton and Bleathman 1991). Baines and colleagues (1987) reported attendance at reminiscence sessions to be higher than at RO sessions. For the individual strategies, people with dementia improved conversational content, with some subjects demonstrating improvements for up to 30 months following intervention using memory wallets (Bourgeois 1992). Also, using errorless learning with quizzes was more successful in improving memory on training tasks for middle- and late-stage subjects than the repetition task or spaced retrieval (Arkin 1991).

Indirect intervention

The series of studies that examined the effects of the FOCUSED training on various caregivers suggests significant improvements in attitude toward AD patients, knowledge of AD and increased knowledge of communication strategies in comparisons of pre- and post-training assessments (Ripich et al. 1999b). The comparison of caregivers of people with AD revealed that African American caregivers showed greater positive effect and significant declines in perceived daily hassles after communication training, whereas white caregivers did not (Ripich et al. 1998). Follow-up evaluations at 6 and 12 months after training showed decreased communication hassles and increased knowledge of AD in caregivers and no significant changes in the control group (Ripich et al. 1998). Overall, these studies show the feasibility of FOCUSED as an effective behavioural intervention for caregivers that improves communication with people with AD.

Continual reassessment during intervention

Continual reassessment is an important part of the intervention process in this highly variable and heterogeneous symptom complex. Evaluation at 6-monthly intervals provides information regarding change and/or maintenance of competencies. Results of minimal or no change can be a very encouraging factor for many people with dementia and their families. Identification of further decline in an area can focus and structure case management. Furthermore, the intervention process must ideally be multidisciplinary to address the scope of problems arising from this disorder. A collaborative perspective on the person with dementia, caregiver and family counselling, education and communication treatment provide the optimal opportunity for comprehensive support of all aspects of direct and indirect intervention.

Pharmacologic treatment of AD

The American Academy of Neurology (Doody et al. 2001) developed recommended management practices for pharmacologic and non-pharmacologic treatments. The following recommendations were reported:

- Cholinesterase inhibitors should be considered in patients with mild to moderate AD.
- Vitamin E (1000 I.U. by mouth twice daily) should be considered in an attempt to slow progression of AD (Guideline).
- There is insufficient evidence to support the use of other antioxidants, anti-inflammatory agents, or other agents specifically to treat AD because of the risk of significant side effects in the absence of demonstrated benefits.

- Oestrogen should not be prescribed to treat AD (Standard).
- Some patients with unspecified dementia may benefit from ginkgo biloba, but evidence-based efficacy data are lacking.
- There are no adequately controlled trials demonstrating pharmacologic efficacy for any agent in ischemic vascular (multi-infarct) dementia.
- Antipsychotics should be used to treat agitation or psychosis in patients with dementia.
- Selected tricyclics, MAO-B inhibitors, and SSRIs should be considered in the treatment of depression.

Use of drug interventions is discussed further in Chapter 2.

In summary, a broad array of interventions is available to SLPs who treat communication-impaired dementia patients in collaboration with other health professionals. Both direct and indirect approaches aim to maintain, facilitate and support communication by the individual with dementia from the early to the late stages of the disease. Concern for the quality of life of individuals with dementia has led to the development of innovative techniques, such as validation therapy, reminiscence therapy, and caregiver training. The FOCUSED Program, for example, educates family members and professional caregivers about AD, explains the impact of memory deterioration, trains participants in the use of verbal and non-verbal approaches, and uses role-play exercises and videotaped vignettes to assure empathic and culturally sensitive communication.

Conclusion

The US government, in partnership with individual State governments and private and professional organizations, is contributing substantially to the health care and related needs of elderly individuals with cognitive impairments, including the needs of caregivers. This chapter described the structure of current service delivery in the USA, and reviewed commonly used intervention and management practices for dementia.

With advances in our knowledge about health and health care, individuals are living to older ages; in turn, the prevalence of dementia is increasing. In response, governments throughout the international community are responding to the needs of individuals with cognitive impairment – by distributing greater social resources to health care, and by creating innovative public–private partnerships. This chapter has reviewed initiatives in the USA: the levels of care, the costs of care, the sources of governmental and private support, the laws that protect disabled elderly, and the innovative behavioural treatments that are showing great promise.

Specifically, this chapter has reviewed the substantial advances in knowledge regarding speech and language pathology treatments that have been realized in the recent past. This is an age when 'evidence-based practice' is highly valued; despite the progressive nature of dementing illness, the evidence proves that individuals with cognitive impairment can learn, and can benefit from our interventions.

There is additional work to be done in all phases of health-care services for elderly individuals with cognitive impairment. However, the progress made in the last few decades demonstrates the commitment in the USA to meet the needs of individuals who are affected by old age, and especially those who are affected by cognitive decline. Speech and language pathologists play a vital role in this effort.

References

Anderson JR (1983) A spreading activation theory of memory. Journal of Verbal Learning and Verbal Behavior 22: 261–295.

AoA (2002) Annual Report: What We Do Makes a Difference. Administration on Ageing, US Department of Health and Human Services (*www.aoa.gov*).

AoA (2004a) HHS Names Executive Director of White House Conference on Ageing. Administration on Ageing, US Department of Health and Human Services (*www.hhs.gov/news*).

AoA (2004b) Alzheimer's Demonstration Program, Fact Sheet. Administration on Ageing, US Department of Health and Human Services (*www.aoa.gov/alz/public/alzabout/aoa_fact_sheet.asp*).

AoA (2004c) Alzheimer's Demonstration Program, FY04 Project Summaries and Activities. Administration on Ageing, US Department of Health and Human Services (*www.aoa.gov/alz/public/alzabout/demo_projects/2004.asp*).

Arkin S (1991) Memory training in early Alzheimer's disease: an optimistic look at the field. American Journal of Alzheimer's Care and Related Disorders and Research 7(4): 17–25.

Baines S, Saxby P, Ehlert K (1987) Reality orientation and reminiscence therapy: A controlled cross-over study of confused elderly people. British Journal of Psychiatry 151: 222–231.

Baldelli MV, Pirani A, Motta M et al. (1993) Effects of reality orientation therapy on elderly patients in the community. Archives of Gerontology and Geriatrics 17: 211–218.

Bayles KA, Tomoeda CK (1991) Caregiver report of prevalence and appearance order of linguistic symptoms in Alzheimer's patients. Gerontologist 31: 210–216.

Bayles KA, Kim E, Mahendra N et al. (2004) Technical Report, Practice Guidelines for Cognitive-Linguistic Disorders Associated with Alzheimer's Dementia. Academy of Neurologic Communication Disorders and Sciences, Minneapolis, MN.

Bourgeois MS (1992) Evaluating memory wallets in conversations with persons with dementia. Journal of Speech and Hearing Research 35: 1344–1357.

Bourgeois MS, Burgio LD, Schuls R, Beach S, Palmer B (1997) Modifying repetitive verbalisations of community dwelling patients with AD. The Gerontologist 37: 30–39.

Brack H (1997) Validation therapy with disoriented very old persons: impact of group interventions on activities of daily living, on aspects of behavior, cognition and general well-being. Unpublished doctoral dissertation, University of Montreal.

Brush JA, Camp CJ (1998) Using spaced retrieval as an intervention during speech-language therapy. Clinical Gerontologist 19(1): 51–64.

Bureau of Health Professions, Health Research and Services Administration (2004a) Geriatric Education Centres (*http://bhpr.hrsa.gov/interdisciplinary/gec.html*).

Bureau of Health Professions, Health Research and Services Administration (2004b) A National Agenda for Geriatric Education: White Papers Recommendation, Allied and Associate Health Recommendations (*http://bhpr.hrsa.gov/interdisciplinary/gecrec/gecrecallhlth.html*).

Bush GW (2001) Community-based Alternatives for Individuals with Disabilities. Executive Order of US President George W. Bush, 19 June (*www.whitehouse.gov/news/releases/2001/06/20010619.html*).

Clark LW (1991) Caregiver stress and communication management in Alzheimer's disease. In: Ripich D (ed.) Handbook of Geriatric Communication Disorders. Pro-Ed, Austin, TX.

Clark LW (1995) Interventions for persons with Alzheimer's disease: strategies for maintaining and enhancing communicative success. Language Disorders 15: 47–65.

Clark LW, Witte K (1989) Dealing with dementia in long-term care. Mini-seminar presentation for Annual Convention on New York State Speech, Language, and Hearing Association, Kiamesha Lake, NY.

Dietch JT, Hewett LJ, Jones S (1989) Adverse effects of reality orientation. Journal of the American Geriatrics Society 37: 974–976.

Doody RS, Stevens JC, Beck C et al. (2001) Practice parameter: management of dementia (an evidence-based review). Neurology 56: 1–16.

Feil N (1992) Validation therapy. Geriatric Nursing 13: 129–133.

Fitzpatrick AL, Kuller LH, Ives DG et al. (2004) Incidence and prevalence of dementia in the cardiovascular health study. Journal of the American Geriatrics Society 52: 195–204.

Folsom JC, Folsom GS (1974) The real world. MH 58(3): 29–33. National Association for Mental Health, Inc.

Fritz A (1986) The language of resolution among the old-old: the effect of validation therapy on two levels of cognitive confusion. Unpublished paper, Chicago.

Harris JL (1997) Reminiscence: a culturally and developmentally appropriate language intervention for older adults. American Journal of Speech Language Pathology 6(3): 19–26.

Harris JL (1998) The Source for Reminiscence Therapy. LinguiSystems, East Moline, IL.

Harris JL, Norman ML (2002) Reframing reminiscence as a cognitive-linguistic phenomenon. In: Webster JD, Haight B (eds) Critical Advances in Reminiscence: from theory to application. Springer, New York, pp. 95–105.

Horner J, Norman ML, Ripich DN (2004) Dementia: diagnostic approaches and current taxonomies. In: Johnson AF, Jacobsohn BH (eds) Medical Speech-Language Pathology: a practitioner's guide. Thieme Verlag, New York.

Hughston GA, Merriam SB (1982) Reminiscence: a non-formal technique for improving cognitive functioning in the aged. International Journal on Ageing and Human Development 15: 139–149.

Hussian RA (1981) Geriatric Psychology: a behavioral perspective. Van Nostrand Reinhold, New York.

Ishi-Kuntz M (1990) Social interaction and social well-being: comparison across stages of adulthood. Ageing and Human Development 30: 15–35.

Judge KS, Camp CJ, Orsulic-Jeras S (2000) Use of Montessori-based activities for clients with dementia in adult day care: effects on engagement. American Journal of Alzheimer's Disease 15(1): 42–46.

Kaiser (2004) The Medicaid Program at a Glance. Henry J. Kaiser Family Foundation, Washington DC (*www.kff.org*).

Kaiser (2004b) Medicare at a Glance. Henry J. Kaiser Family Foundation, Washington, DC (*www.kff.org*).

Kinney JM, Stephens MAP (1989) Caregiving Hassles Scale: assessing the daily hassles of caring for a family member with dementia. Gerontologist 29: 328–332.

Larson R (1978) Thirty years of research on the subjective well-being of older Americans. Journal of Gerontology 33: 109–125.

Leifer BP (2003) Early diagnosis of Alzheimer's disease: clinical and economic benefit. Journal of the American Geriatrics Society 51: S281–S288.

Levit K, Smith C, Cowan C et al. and the Health Accounts Team (2004) Health spending rebound continues in 2002. Health Affairs 23: 147–159.

McCallion P, Toseland RW, Freeman K (1999a) An evaluation of a family visit education program. Journal of the American Geriatrics Society 47: 203–214.

McCallion P, Toseland RW, Lacey D, Banks S (1999b) Educating nursing assistants to communicate more effectively with nursing home residents with dementia. Gerontologist 39: 546–558.

MacDonald MIL, Settin JM (1978) Reality orientation vs. sheltered workshops as treatment for the institutionalized ageing. Journal of Gerontology 33: 416–421.

Mendola WF, Pelligrini RV (1979) Quality of life and coronary artery bypass surgery patients. Social Science Medicine 13: 457–461.

Metitieri T, Zanetti O, Geroldi C et al. (2001) Reality orientation therapy to delay outcomes of progression in patients with dementia: a retrospective study. Clinical Rehabilitation 15: 471–478.

Miller E, Morris R (1993) Management of dementia. In: Miller E, Morris R (eds) The Psychology of Dementia. John Wiley & Sons, Chichester, pp. 110–132.

Mold JW, Fryer GE, Thomas CH (2004) Who are the uninsured elderly in the United States? Journal of the American Geriatrics Society 52(4): 601–606.

Morton I and Bleathman C (1991) The effectiveness of validation therapy in dementia – a pilot study. International Journal of Geniatic Psychiatry 6, 327–330.

Nomura T (2002) Evaluative research on reminisence groups for people with dementia. In Webster JD and Haight BK (eds) Critical Advances in Reminischence Work from Theory to Application. Springer Publishing Co. New York, pp. 289–299.

Norman ML, Horner J, Ripich DN (2004) Dementia, communication and management. In: Johnson AF, Jacobson BH (eds) Medical Speech-Language Pathology: a practitioner's guide.Thieme Verlag, New York.

O'Brien E, Elias R (2004) Medicaid and Long-Term Care. Kaiser Commission on Medicaid and the Uninsured. Henry J. Kaiser Family Foundation, Washington, DC.

Olmstead v LC (98–536) 527 US 581 (1999) (*http://supct.law.cornell.edu/supct/html/98-536.ZS.html*).

Orange JB (1991) Perspectives of family members regarding communication changes. In: Lubinski R (ed) Dementia and Communication. Mosby-Year Book, St Louis, MO, pp. 168–187.

Osborne C (1989) Reminiscence: when the past eases the present. Journal of Gerontological Nursing 15: 6–12.

Peoples N (1982) Validation therapy versus reality orientation as treatment for disoriented institutionalized elderly. Unpublished Master's Thesis, University of Akron, Akron, OH.

Programs for Older Americans (2003) 42 United States Code s 3001, 7 January (www.access.gpo.gov).

Rabins P (1982) Management of irreversible dementia. Psychosometics 22: 591–597.

Reisberg B (1981) Brain Failure: an introduction to current concepts of senility. Free Press/Macmillan, New York.

Ripich DN (1993) A communication strategies program for caregivers and Alzheimer's disease patients. In: Clark L (ed) Communicating with the Elderly: a practitioner's guide. Print Media Production Co., New York, pp. 61–72.

Ripich DN (2004a) Communicating with Persons with Alzheimer's Disease: revised FOCUSED trainer's manual. The FOCUSED Program for Caregivers.

Ripich DN (2004b) Communicating with Persons with Alzheimer's Disease: revised FOCUSED caregiver's guide.The FOCUSED Program for Caregivers.

Ripich DN (2004c) Communicating with Persons with Alzheimer's Disease: FOCUSED training tapes of five modules. The FOCUSED Program for Caregivers.

Ripich DN, Pope C (2005) Speak to me, listen to me: conversations in Alzheimer's disease. In: Davis BH (ed) Alzheimer Talk, Text and Context. Palgrave, Basingstoke.

Ripich DN, Wykle M (1990a) A program for nursing assistants, with Alzheimer's patients. Paper Presented at the American Gerontology in Higher Education Conference, Kansas City, MO.

Ripich DN, Wykle M (1990b) Developing healthcare professionals' communication skills with Alzheimer's disease patients. Paper presented at the Annual Meeting of the American Society on Ageing, San Francisco, CA.

Ripich DN, Wykle M, Niles S (1995) Alzheimer's disease caregivers: the FOCUSED Program. Geriatric Nursing 16(1): 15–19.

Ripich DN, Carpenter B, Ziol E (1997a) Procedural discourse in men and women with Alzheimer's disease: a longitudinal study with clinical implications. American Journal of Alzheimer's Disease 12(6): 258–271.

Ripich DN, Carpenter B, Ziol E (1997b) Comparison of African-American and white persons with Alzheimer's disease on language measures. Neurology 48: 781–783.

Ripich DN, Ziol E, Lee M (1998) Longitudinal effects of communication training on caregivers of persons with Alzheimer's disease. Clinical Gerontologist 19: 37–55.

Ripich DN, Ziol E, Durand EJ, Fritsch T (1999a) Training Alzheimer's disease caregivers for successful communication. Clinical Gerontologist 21(1): 37–57.

Ripich DN, Kercher K, Wykle M, Sloan D, Ziol E (1999b) Effects of communication training on African-American and white caregivers of persons with Alzheimer's disease. Journal of Ageing and Ethnicity 1(3): 1–16.

Ripich DN, Carpenter B, Ziol E (2000a) Conversational cohesion in men and women with Alzheimer's disease: a longitudinal study. International Journal of Language and Communication Disorders 35(1): 49–65.

Ripich DN, Fritsch T, Ziol E, Durand E (2000b) Compensatory strategies in picture description across severity levels in Alzheimer's disease: a longitudinal study. American Journal of Alzheimer's Disease 15(4): 217–229.

Ripich DN, Fritsch T, Ziol E (2002) Everyday problem solving in African- and European-Americans: an exploratory study. International Psychogeriatrics 14(1): 83–95.

Sink KM, Covinsky KE, Newcomer R, Yaffe K (2004) Ethnic differences in the prevalence and pattern of dementia-related behaviors. Journal of the American Geriatrics Society 52: 1277–1283.

Sohlberg MM, Mateer CA (1989) Introduction to Cognitive Rehabilitation: theory and practice. Guilford Press, New York.

Stephens L (ed.) (1969) Reality Orientation: a technique to rehabilitate elderly and brain-damaged patients with a moderate to severe degree of disorientation. American Psychiatric Association, Washington, DC.

Terrell B, Ripich D (1989) Discourse competence as a variable in intervention. Seminars in Speech and Language Disorders 24: 77–92.

Toseland RW, Diehl M, Freeman K et al. (1997) The impact of validation group therapy on nursing home residents with dementia. Journal of Applied Gerontology 16: 31–50.

Touzinsky L (1998) Validation therapy: restoring communication between persons with Alzheimer's disease and their families. American Journal of Alzheimer's Disease 13(2): 96–101.

US Census Bureau (1995) Sixty-five plus in the United States. Economics and Statistics Administration, US Department of Commerce (*www.census.gov/ population/socdemo/statbriefs/agebrief.html*).

US Census Bureau (2002) Definitions, North American Industry Classification System (NAICS). US Department of Commerce (*www.census.gov/epcd/www/ naics.html*).

US Department of Health and Human Services (2001) Centres for Medicare and Medicaid Services (25 September). Program Memorandum: Medical Review of Services for Patients with Dementia (Transmittal AB-01–135). US Department of Health and Human Services.

US Department of Health and Human Services (2004a) Medicare Information Resource. Centers for Medicare and Medicaid (*www.cms.hhs.gov/medicare/ default.asp*).

US Department of Health and Human Services (2004b) Medicaid: a brief summary. Centers for Medicare and Medicaid (*www.cms.hhs.gov/publications/ overview-medicare-medicaid/default4.asp*).

US Department of Justice (2001) Civil Rights Division, Disability Rights Section. (*www.usdoj.gov/crt/ada/adahom1.htm*).

US GAO (1998) Alzheimer's Disease: estimates of prevalence in the United States. Report to the Secretary of Health and Human Services (# GAO/HEHS-98-16), US Government Accounting Office, Washington, DC, p. 7.

Whitehouse PJ, Rabins PV (1992) Quality of life and dementia. Alzheimer Disease and Associated Disorders 6: 135–137.

Zanetti O, Frisoni GB, Leo D De et al. (1995) Reality orientation therapy in Alzheimer disease: useful or not? A controlled study. Alzheimer Disease and Associated Disorders 9(3): 132–138.

Zarit JM (1982) Predictors of burden and stress for caregivers of senile dementia patients. Unpublished Doctoral Dissertation. University of Southern California, San Diego, CA.

Zgola JM, Coulter LG (1988) I can tell you about that: a therapeutic group program for cognitively impaired persons. American Journal of Alzheimer's Care and Related Disorders 3(4): 17–22.

Ziol E, Dobres R, White L (1996) Communicative Interaction: group activities for cognitively impaired elderly. Imaginart International, Bisbee, AZ.

Governmental and professional dementia resources in the United States

Academy of Neurology (*www.aan.com/professionals*)
Administration on Ageing (*www.aoa.gov*)
Agency for Healthcare Research Quality (*www.ahrq.gov*)
Alzheimer's Association (*www.alz.org*)
Alzheimer's Disease Education and Referral Centre (*www.alzheimers.org*)
American Bar Association Commission on Law and Ageing (*www.abanet.org*)
American Geriatrics Society (*www.americangeriatrics.org/*)
American Medical Association (*www.ama-assn.org/*)
American Psychiatric Association (Alzheimer's disease) (*www.psych.org/public_
     info/alzheim.cfm*)
Behavioral and Social Research (*www.nia.nih.gov/ResearchInformation/
     ExtramuralPrograms/BehavioralAndSocialResearch/*)
Biology of Ageing (*www.nia.nih.gov/ResearchInformation/ExtramuralPrograms/
     BiologyOfAgeing/*)
Centers for Disease Control and Prevention (*www.cdc.gov*)
Centers for Medicare and Medicaid Services (*www.cms.hhs.gov*)
Department of Health and Human Services (*www.hhs.gov*)
Elderly Health Care (*www.ahrq.gov/research/elderix.htm*)
Food and Drug Administration (*www.fda.gov*)
General Accounting Office (GAO) (*www.gao.gov*)
Geriatric Education Centres (*http://bhpr.hrsa.gov/interdisciplinary/gec.html*)
Geriatrics and Clinical Gerontology (GCG) (*www.nia.nih.gov/Research
     Information/ExtramuralPrograms/GeriatricsAndClinicalGerontology/*)
Gerontological Society of America (*www.geron.org/*)
Health Resources and Services Administration (*www.hrsa.gov/*)
Indian Health Service Elder Care Initiative (*www.ihs.gov/MedicalPrograms/
     ElderCare/index.asp*)
National Advisory Council on Ageing (*www.nia.nih.gov/AboutNIA/NACA/*)
National Center for Health Statistics (*www.cdc.gov/nchs*)
National Institute on Ageing (*/www.nia.nih.gov/*)
Neuroscience and Neuropsychology (*/www.nia.nih.gov/ResearchInformation/
     ExtramuralPrograms/NeuroscienceOfAgeing/*)
Veterans Health Administration Alzheimer's/Dementia Program (*http://www1.va.
     gov/GeriatricsSHG/page.cfm?pg=21*)

CHAPTER 12

Future directions

JANE MAXIM AND KAREN BRYAN

Where are we now?

In the UK, the National Service Framework for Older People (DH 2001) set out the standards for promoting independence and well-being for older people and for supporting them wherever they live. Targets for service delivery have been set across both health and social care, encompassing prevention as well as intervention. This broad focus is an ambitious agenda which relies on the idea of service champions and service case studies (available on the Department of Health website, *www.dh.gov.uk*) for successful implementation. Although some areas of health care targeted by the National Service Framework have progressed well (stroke, for example), the range of need for people with a dementia and their carers is both great and complex and progress on implementing the National Service Framework has not been comprehensive. We now have extensive knowledge of what these needs are although our ideas for how to meet them are still developing.

The UK Priorities and Planning Framework for 2003–06 required that by April 2004 protocols would be in place across all health and social care systems for the care management of older people with mental health problems. The National Service Framework for Older People set a similar target for primary care trusts to ensure that every general practice would be using a protocol agreed with local specialist services, health and social services to diagnose, treat and care for patients with depression or a dementia. These initiatives have highlighted the need for change in the way services are developed and delivered for older people, with explicit targets for service delivery but, however excellent in intention, targets do need to be implemented in a consistent and timely manner in order to benefit older people with a dementia and their carers.

Speech and language therapy (SLT) services are perceived as a necessary part of such service delivery. The mental health standard (Standard 7)

319

of the National Service Framework explicitly states that commissioning arrangements (protocols for the service and for referrals) should be in place. Although new initiatives may require funding and certainly require commitment, innovation is also possible by flexible use of existing resources. This emphasis on target-driven approaches has the potential to reduce service variability but, for smaller services such as SLT and dietetics, there is a problem in becoming a visible part of key targets.

Although the UK government claims an improvement in services for common conditions in old age, findings from voluntary organizations still describe delivery of services as variable. Policy-driven agendas have promised much for older people but are always susceptible to newer initiatives which require immediate attention and which may actively undermine existing provision. Recent consultations by the National Institute for Clinical Excellence (NICE), for example, on the prescription of drugs for people with Alzheimer's disease may contribute to the uncertainty that older people, their carers and their GPs report on best treatment for people with the disease and how to access it.

Policies also now assume consumer involvement, but often the perceptions and choices of older people are largely ignored so that consumer involvement becomes a token issue. However, all the evidence is that older people do have a view and are able to evaluate the services that they are offered. This is illustrated, for example, by a recent study conducted by the Alzheimer's Society, the leading UK charity for people with dementia and their carers, which found that:

- half of all carers delay visiting their GP after first noticing something was wrong – the average length of delay was 3 years.
- less than a third of GPs and nurses feel confident about giving a diagnosis or talking to someone about their diagnosis of dementia.
- over a fifth of carers said no one had given them the diagnosis.

These findings suggest that major issues for older people's health care are in:

- the approachability of health and social care services
- the communication of the diagnostic process
- ensuring that older people get timely access to services.

In order to achieve good-quality care for people with a dementia, a number of key issues need to be addressed:

Access to services throughout the disease process

The UK Department of Health claims that older people can access up to 6 weeks' active convalescence and rehabilitation, that new housing schemes are providing flexible 24-hour support from social care and health teams, that provision of equipment is now faster and that there are increased home-care packages available. Access to services throughout the disease process is a vital part of any package of care and certainly, in Health Action Zones, set up where need is particularly great, progress towards service delivery has been made; but it is still variable, and not all areas of the UK have benefited from such initiatives. Even where there is good service provision, such services may not be widely publicized. Services such as assessment of memory problems are usually only available within a hospital-based service, which immediately limits access. Preventive interventions which promote independence and primary care services provided for older people with a dementia or depression are also central to the delivery of a service for older people (Wanless 2002), but their availability remains patchy.

Rehabilitation and intermediate care

Access to rehabilitation and intermediate care is still not automatic for older people with mental health problems, and there is particular difficulty in accessing these services for older people who are in residential and nursing homes. Services, now often geared towards response after a crisis, need to change and enable improved access to services such as psychology, occupational therapy, SLT and counselling. The Royal Commission on Long Term Care (1999) explicitly recommends that 'the opportunity for rehabilitation should be included as an initial part of any care assessment before any irreversible decisions on long term care are taken' (p. 4).

Training

The need for training is a key component of the National Service Framework for Older People, but greater joint working between social and health services is required. Training initiatives for care staff in the residential and nursing care sectors are now recognized, but there is still great variability and statutory requirements are limited and not incorporated into monitoring processes in terms of accessing the impact on care of older people, particularly those with dementia. In primary care, accredited training for nurses in the identification and initial management of mental health needs in older people (the dementias, depression and other conditions) is now vital. Better services, including training where necessary, should be available to both formal and family carers. SLT services should take any opportunity to engage with such initiatives, which should include the joint development of basic protocols to assist primary care staff in making appropriate referrals to SLT.

Consultancy and career frameworks

The potential for nurses in primary care to take on new roles is exemplified by that of the nurse practitioners, whose role may be as lead specialist providing training for other staff and enabling service developments such as assessment of older people and providing memory rehabilitation (Wanless 2002, RCGP 2004). Equally, the SLT profession needs to use the current opportunity to develop SLT consultant posts in the care of older people (RCSLT 2005).

Long-term care

The Royal Commission on Long Term Care (1999), set up to examine options for funding long-term care for older people, recommended that the costs of long-term care should be split between living, housing and personal care costs. It found that, for the UK, there was no demographic timebomb (as there is in Germany and Italy, for example), and recognized that the care needs of those with a dementia should be met 'just as much as those who suffer from cancer' (p. 2). While recognizing that the state cannot meet all long-term care costs, the Commission recommended that services could be underwritten by general taxation, with living and housing costs met from the individual's own income while personal care would be met by the state. The Commission acknowledged that any system set up required pooling of budgets across health and social services.

Social inclusion for older people

If access is to be equitable, then the motivation for all health and social care workers is to ensure that older people are treated as individuals whose care is devised to meet their individual needs across health and social services. Principles of social inclusion which need to be addressed are:

- partnerships with older people so that they can actively influence policy and practice at strategic and local levels within partner organizations
- involvement of black and other ethnic minority older people
- encouraging peer group (same age) health mentors who work with older people in the community
- setting up culture- and language-appropriate dementia services which have advisors and carers from minority ethnic groups
- development of culture- and language-specific information material for use by health workers.

A service agenda for speech and language therapists

New episodes of care for older people within hospital-based geriatric medicine make up about 10% of all SLT initial contacts in the UK, and 24% of all SLT initial contacts were with people of 75 years of age and older

(DH 2003). If SLT services are to be accessible, there needs to be more engagement with primary care in the community, more cross-sector working and use of innovative funding streams, with the following areas being of great importance:

- There needs to be a national-level agreement on access to SLT in private sector residential and nursing care, with equal access for older people to assessment and rehabilitation irrespective of whether they are in long-term care or in their own homes.
- The profession needs to press for a statutory requirement for the provision of rehabilitation in the private care sector.
- SLT services need to engage more with primary care initiatives to ensure that primary care nurses in particular are aware of what SLT can offer and make appropriate referrals.

In reviewing the current emphasis on hospital based services, the SLT profession should ensure that the recommendations of the RCSLT position paper (2005) on standards for SLT services for older people with dementia are disseminated and implemented. SLT services for older clients should be organized to facilitate continuity of care for clients which can respond flexibly to their changing needs such as entering day care and later full residential care. Some key issues are:

- the development of SLT consultant posts for care of older people
- linked to this development, greater emphasis in pre-registration SLT training and in continuing professional development on dementia awareness
- increasing SLT involvement in the multidisciplinary team
- ensuring that speech and language therapy clinical specialists and/or managers are included in local planning of all services for older people
- promotion of clinic-based research programmes to develop and evaluate working practices.

Towards evidence-based practice

The Alzheimer's Society has set out its research priorities under the headings of cause, cure and care, to make explicit that each of these areas requires a programme of research:

Alzheimer's Society research priorities

Cause
- cause of dementia and mechanism of disease progression (including basic brain physiology and biochemistry in diseases causing dementia)
- brain bank

- epidemiological research into environmental, health history and lifestyle factors predisposing for dementia
- genetics
- early onset of dementia

Cure
- stem cell therapy
- any cure/vaccine/complementary strategies
- evaluation of existing drugs for various stages of Alzheimer's; new drugs and availability of drugs
- early and better diagnosis
- prevention

Care
- increasing quality of life for the dementia patient
- better GP/primary care including effect of specific dementia training for staff
- alleviating distressing behavioural symptoms
- detection of pain and discomfort in non-verbal patients
- availability of medication, care and treatment
- hospitalization of the dementia patient
- the projected future needs for NHS and social support for dementia

Source: Alzheimer's Society
(*www.alzheimers.org.uk/Research/index.htm*)

This agenda highlights the vast amount of research still to be done in order for us to understand the disease processes in the dementias and to put into place services which will increase the quality of life for people with dementia and their carers. We can now differentiate between different forms of dementia, and between a dementia and depression. We know that different types of dementia require different approaches to support the person and their carers, but what we know is still very limited. In the area of SLT, some of the vital areas of research are:

- further evaluations of therapy practices, using more specific and sensitive indicators of change which will detect changes in language, cognition and functional communication
- joint research initiatives with practice nurses and GPs to develop structured interview 'conversational' formats for health screening for older people
- studies of the language breakdown in mild cognitive impairment (MCI), in Lewy body dementia and in vascular dementia.
- assessments which accurately define abilities and areas of deficit in language and cognition so that therapy input can be targeted
- given that only a minority of GPs and nurses in primary care are confident in providing and discussing a diagnosis (even when the diagnosis

has been made by a specialist team), shorter, more effective diagnostic screening tests for language and cognitive function which might include a carer questionnaire need to be developed

- efficacy guidelines for intervention and management of older people with a dementia
- evaluating different training packages on dementia and depression awareness and assessment for primary care
- evaluating care given by nurse practitioners against current models of care to consider best practice
- evaluating best practice in assessment and support for people with young onset dementia.

The Royal Commission on Long Term Care (1999) recommended a national strategy on rehabilitation which was government led and embedded in the performance frameworks of both health and social services, with longitudinal research to consider the efficacy of preventive interventions and their impact on quality of life. Wanless (2002) set out a vision of care provided in the community 'by nurses and other health and social care professionals in community based settings' (p. 58). Such an agenda would deliver better care to older people with a dementia and their carers.

References

DH (2001) National Service Framework for Older People. Department of Health, London.

DH (2003) NHS Speech and Language Therapy Services Summary Information for 2002–03. Department of Health, London.

RCGP (2004) Information sheet No. 19. Royal College of General Practitioners, London   (*www.rcgp.org.uk/rcgp/information/publications/information/ infosheets*).

RCSLT (2005) Speech and Language Therapy Service Provision for People with Dementia. Position Paper. Royal College of Speech and Language Therapists, London.

Royal Commission on Long Term Care (1999) With Respect to Old Age: long term care – rights and responsibilities. Royal Commission on Long Term Care, London.

Wanless D (2002) Securing Our Future Health: taking a long-term view. HM Treasury, London.

Index